Abdominal and Pelvic Pain

FROM DEFINITION TO BEST PRACTICE

Mission Statement of IASP Press®

IASP brings together scientists, clinicians, health care providers, and policy makers to stimulate and support the study of pain and to translate that knowledge into improved pain relief worldwide. IASP Press publishes timely, high-quality, and reasonably priced books relating to pain research and treatment.

Abdominal and Pelvic Pain

FROM DEFINITION TO BEST PRACTICE

Bert Messelink

Urologist-sexologist, University of Groningen, University Pelvic Care Center, Groningen, The Netherlands

Andrew Baranowski

Consultant and Honorary Senior Lecturer in Pain Medicine, NHNN, University College London Hospitals Foundation Trust, London, United Kingdom

John Hughes

Pain Medicine, The James Cook University Hospital, Middlesbrough, United Kingdom

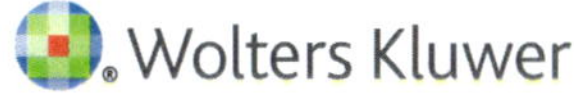

Philadelphia • Baltimore • New York • London
Buenos Aires • Hong Kong • Sydney • Tokyo

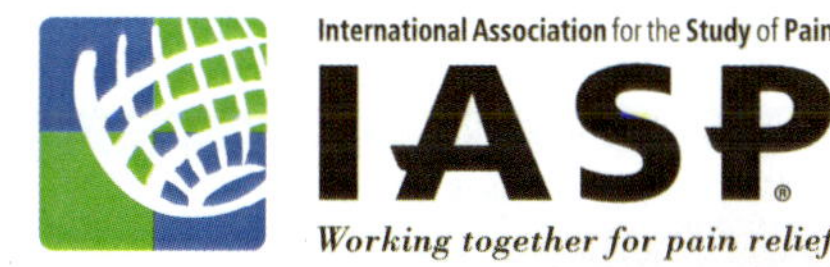

Acquisitions Editor: Keith Donnellan
Product Development Editor: Nicole Dernoski
Editorial Assistant: Kathryn Leyendecker
Production Project Manager: Alicia Jackson
Design Coordinator: Joan Wendt
Manufacturing Coordinator: Beth Welsh
Marketing Manager: Dan Dressler
Prepress Vendor: S4Carlisle Publishing Services

9 8 7 6 5 4 3

Printed in the United States of America

ISBN 13: 978-1-4963-0618-0
ISBN 10: 1-4963-0618-X

Library of Congress Cataloging-in-Publication Data

Available upon request

LWW.com

PREFACE

The subject of this book, "Abdominal and Pelvic Pain", could be characterised as an adolescent in the world of pain. It has a history of growing knowledge and changes in ideas. Now it is time to become an adult. This book shows us where we are in our evolution.

In the last decade of the 20th century, the International Association for the Study of Pain instituted a Special Interest Group named, Pain of UroGenital Origin, shortened to PUGO. Within this group many disciplines were represented. The name of the group clearly shows the leading ideas at that time. It denotes that the focus was on the bladder, the prostate, and the genitals. It also shows us that the origin of the pain was thought to be within these organs. From within PUGO, new insight in mechanisms and the pathophysiology of chronic pain in the urogenital region was developed. Apart from PUGO, the European Association of Urology became a partner in changing the leading thoughts in this area. The focus was re-oriented and became wider. The pelvis was recognised as a place where many different organs are situated. All these organs are working in close relation to each other. In the same time span, the pelvic floor muscles and their role in the function of the pelvic organs were clarified. Next, myofascial pain was found in many patients with urogenital pain. As a result, the pelvis became the central item in this area of chronic pain and, as a consequence, the focus became directed to the pelvis and the terminology was adapted likewise. Chronic pelvic pain became the updated term. This term fit well in the new ideas about the origin and nature of the pain. Pelvic pain was no longer seen as pain originating in pelvic organs but as pain perceived in these organs. The origin could be in the organs, in the muscles and in the nervous system.

In the world of pain, three organisations with a mission to spread the knowledge of pelvic pain and, thereby improve the care for patients with pelvic pain, started working together. Apart from PUGO, there are the International Pelvic Pain Society and Convergences Pelvi-Perineal. For an adolescent and, similarly for abdominal and pelvic pain, it is important to have good friends to discuss the sometimes difficult aspects of growing up. Bundling strength and ideas is a helpful trick in that period of life. The subsequent working together of these three organisations was the basis for the 1st World Congress on Abdominal and Pelvic Pain. It was organised in de Beurs van Berlage in Amsterdam from May 30 – June 2, 2013. The meeting was held during the IASP global year against visceral pain. In the talks with IASP about this relation, we found out that abdominal and pelvic pain are related in many ways. That was the first step to introduce another change in the world of pelvic pain: add the abdomen. As a consequence PUGO was renamed into IASP Special Interest Group on Abdominal and Pelvic Pain. The logo was adapted to this new name, as were the mission statements. During the 1st world congress, there was a plenary session with all the disciplines represented in the faculty and the audience, illustrating an optimal multifactorial and multidisciplinary approach. With 550 participants from more than 40 countries and more than 10 disciplines, the meeting is clearly marking the end of the adolescent period. The book that is in your hands is written by the faculty of this meeting, although it is not just a congress book. It is a textbook with the most up to date information on the subject of abdominal and pelvic pain. Reading this book will let you realise what has happened in the world of abdominal and pelvic pain. It will also show the work that has to be done in the next decade: from definition to best practice. We have ended puberty and stand at the doorstep of maturity. The editors want to express the wish that this book will be the guide for the first years in the grown up world.

Bert Messelink, Andrew Baranowski, and John Hughes

CONTENTS

PART I – **General Aspects**

1 **Societal Impact of Abdominal and Pelvic Pain** 3
Luke Mordecai and Andrew Baranowski

2 **Defining Abdominal and Pelvic Pain** 17
John Hughes

3 **From Animal Data to Human Practice** 25
Tony Buffington

4 **The Importance of Central Sensitization** 37
Timothy J. Ness, Meredith Robbins, and Alan Randich

5 **The Role of Gender in Abdominal and Pelvic Pain** 51
Natasha Curran

PART II – **Phenotyping Aspects**

Musculoskeletal

6 **Body, Mind, and Brain in Pelvic Pain** 59
Carolyn Vandyken and Sandra Hilton

7 **Referred Soft Tissue Phenomena** 71
Stephanie Prendergast

8 **Pelvic Floor Muscle Pain and Trigger Points** 79
Helena Frawley

Psychological/Sexological

9 **Understanding the Psychological Components of Pain** 89
Dean A. Tripp and J. Curtis Nickel

10 **Sexual Dysfunctions** 101
Ellen Laan, Lisa B.A. Bloemendaal, and Rik van Lunsen

11 **Addressing Psychosexual Components of Pelvic Pain** 113
Talli Rosenbaum

12 **Research, Assessment, and Treatment of Sex Related Pain** 123
Katy Vincent

Urological

13 **Bladder pain** 137
Ursula Wesselmann and Peter Czakanski

14 **Male genital pain** 149
Bert Messelink

Gynecological

15 **Gynaecological Aspects of Chronic Pelvic Pain** 159
Suzy Sohier Elneil

16 **Mechanisms and Treatment of Endometriosis Related Pain** 171
Rukset Attar and Erkut Attar

17 **Diagnosis and Treatment of Female Genital Pain** 187
Ahinoam Lev-Sagie

Gastro-Intestinal

18 **Functional Disorders of the Gastro-Intestinal Tract** 201
Lalit Kumar and Anton Emmanuel

19 **Anorectal Dysfunctions and Chronic Pain** 211
Marc Beer-Gabel

PART III –**Management Aspects**

Specific Treatment and Management

20 **Primary Care Management of Abdominal and Pelvic Pain** 221
Huibertien Oosterlee

21 **Physiotherapy in Assessment and Management of Pain** 229
Rebecca McLoughlin, Katrine Petersen, and Suzanne Brook

22 **Psychology in Assessment and Management of Pain** 239
Sarah Edwards, Katherine Herron, and Amanda C de C Williams

23 **Neuromodulation of Abdominal and Pelvic Pain** 249
Melissa Farmer

24 **Pharmacotherapy in Neuropathic Pain** 259
Gregory Gordon, Pei Ge, Jeffrey Segal, and Immaculada Silos-Santiago

Pain Patient Pathways

25 **European Association of Urology Algorithms** 269
Bert Messelink

26 **British Pain Society Patient Pathways** 277
Gareth Greenslade

27 **Developing a Structure for Delivery of Care** 283
Andrew Baranowski and Luke Mordecai

28 **Generating the Evidence Base for Chronic Pelvic Pain in the Future** 293
Seema Tirlapur and Khalid Khan

29 **The Future of Abdominal and Pelvic Pain Management** 299
Maria Adele Giamberardino, Claudio Tana, Giannapia Affaitati, Francesca Massimini, and Raffaele Costantini

30 **The Role of Patient Organizations** 311
Judy Birch, Françoise Watel, Jane Meijlink, Lisa Kruse, Sally Crowe, and Jennifer Birch

Index 321

CONTRIBUTORS

Giannapia Affaitati

Erkut Attar, MD, PhD
Department of Obstetrics and Gynecology, Division of Reproductive Endocrinology and Infertility, Istanbul University, School of Medicine, Istanbul, Turkey

Rukset Attar
Department of Obstetrics and Gynecology, Division of Reproductive Endocrinology and Infertility, Istanbul University School of Medicine, Istanbul, Turkey

Andrew Baranowski, BScHons, MBBS, FRCA, MD, FFPMRCA
Consultant and Honorary Senior Lecturer in Pain Medicine, NHNN, University College London Hospitals Foundation Trust, London, United Kingdom

Marc Beer-Gabel
Head Neurogastroenterology and Pelvic Floor Unit, Gastroenterology Department, Sheba Medical Center, Tel Aviv University, Sackler Faculty of Medicine, Ramat Aviv, Israel

Jennifer Birch, MSc, MA (Cantab)
Trustee, Pelvic Pain Support Network, Dorset, United Kingdom

Judy Birch, B Ed
Pelvic Pain Support Network, Dorset, United Kingdom

Lisa B.A. Bloemendaal

Suzanne Brook

Tony Buffington, BS, MS, PhD, DVM, DACVN
Department of Veterinary Clinical Sciences The vOhio State University, Columbus, Ohio

Amanda C de C Williams
Academic & Clinical Psychologist, Research Department of Clinical, Educational & Health Psychology, University College London, London, United Kingdom

Raffaele Costantini

Sally Crowe
Director, Crowe Associates Ltd, Member of International Pelvic Pain Partnership

Natasha Curran, MD, ChB(Hons), FRCA, FFPMRCA
University College Hospital, Pain Management Centre, National Hospital for Neurology and Neurosurgery, Queen Square, London, United Kingdom

Sarah Edwards
National Hospital of Neurology & Neurosurgery, University of College London Hospitals

Suzy Sohier Elneil
Consultant in Urogynaecology and Uro-neurology, National Hospital for Neurology and Neurosurgery, London, United Kingdom

Anton Emmanuel, MD, FRCP
GI Physiology Unit, University College Hospital, Department of Internal Medicine, London, United Kingdom

Melissa Farmer
Research Associate, Northwestern University, Feinberg School of Medicine, Chicago, Illinois, USA

Helena Frawley, PhD, FACP
Physiotherapist
Associate Professor Allied Health, La Trobe University
Senior Research Consultant Allied Health, Cabrini Health, Melbourne Australia,
Health Professional Research Fellow, National Health and Medical Research Council, Australia

Pei Ge

Maria Adele Giamberardino

Gregory Gordon

Gareth Greenslade
Pain Consultant, University College Hospital London, Dept. of Histopathology, London, United Kingdom

Katherine Herron, BSc, MSc, PhD, DClinPsy
Pain Management Centre, National Hospital for Neurology and Neurosurgery, UCLH Hospitals Queen Square, London, United Kingdom

Sandra Hilton

John Hughes
Pain Medicine, The James Cook University Hospital, Middlesbrough, United Kingdom

Khalid Khan, BSc, MBCHB
Women's Health and Clinical Epidemiology, London, United Kingdom

Lisa Kruse, BSN, RN

Lalit Kumar, MRCS, AFHEA
Research Fellow

Ellen Laan, Ph.D
Department of Sexology and Psychosomatic Gynaecology, Academic Medical Center, Amsterdam

Ahinoam Lev-Sagie
Clinical Senior Lecturer,
Hadassah University Hospital, Clinic for Vulvovaginal Disorders, Jerusalem, Israel

Francesca Massimini

Rebecca McLoughlin, MSc, BSc(Hons)
Clinical Specialist Physiotherapist, University College London Hospitals NHS Foundation Trust (UCLH), London, United Kingdom

Jan Meijink, BA Hons, MITI, MCIJ
Chairman, International Painful Bladder Foundation (IPBF)

Bert Messelink
Urologist-sexologist, University Pelvic Care Center, Groningen, The Netherlands

Luke Mordecai
Specialty Registrar in Anaesthetics, London, United Kingdom

Timothy J. Ness, MD, PhD
University of Alabama at Birmingham, Department of Anesthesiology, Birmingham, Alabama, USA

J. Curtis Nickel

Huibertien Oosterlee
General Practitioner, Dedemsvaart, The Netherlands

Katrine Petersen, BSc(Hons), MSc
Physiotherapist in Pain Management, Pain Management Department, Queen Square

Stephanie Prendergast
Physiotherapist, Partner at the Pelvic Health and Rehab Center, San Francisco/Berkeley/Los Gatos/Los Angeles, USA

Meredith Robbins

Alan Randich

Talli Rosenbaum, MSc
Individual and Couples Therapist,
Certified Sex Therapist,
Pelvic Floor Physiotherapist,
Inner Stability, Ltd, Jerusalem and Tel Aviv, Israel

Jeffrey Segal

Inmaculada Silos-Santiago
Sr. Director Pharmacology, Ironwood Pharmaceuticals, Inc, Cambridge, Massachusetts, USA

Claudio Tana

Seema Tirlapur

Dean A. Tripp, PhD
Queen's University, Departments of Psychology, Anesthesiology & Urology, Kingston, Ontario, Canada

Carolyn Vandyken
The Centre for Pelvic Health, Cambridge, Ontario, Canada

Rik van Lunsen

Katy Vincent, MRCOG, Dphil
Academic Clinical Lecturer, John Radcliffe Hospital NHS Trust, Nuffield Department of Obstetrics and Gynaecology, Oxford, United Kingdom

Francois Watel
Chairwoman of Patients Groups AFCI and RDCP

Ursula Wesselmann
Professor of Anesthesiology and Neurology
University of Alabama at Birmingham School of Medicine,
Department of Anesthesiology/Division of Pain Management,
Birmingham, Alabama, USA

Introduction

Bert Messelink, Andrew Baranowski and John Hughes.

The subject of this book: "Abdominal and pelvic pain" could be characterised as an adolescent in the world of pain. It has a history of growing knowledge and changes in ideas. Now it is time to become an adult. This book shows us where we are in our evolution.

In the last decade of the 20th century the International Association for the Study of Pain instituted a Special Interest Group named: Pain of UroGenital Origin, shortened to PUGO. Within this group many disciplines were represented. The name of the group clearly shows the leading ideas at that time. It denotes that the focus was on the bladder, the prostate and the genitals. It also shows us that the origin of the pain was thought to be within these organs. From within PUGO new insight in mechanisms and the pathophysiology of chronic pain in the urogenital region was developed. Apart from PUGO the European Association of Urology became a partner in changing the leading thoughts in this area. The focus was re-oriented and became wider. The pelvis was recognised as a place where many different organs are situated. All these organs are working in close relation to each other. In the same time span the pelvic floor muscles and their role in the function of the pelvic organs were clarified. Next to that myofascial pain was found in many patients with urogenital pain. As a result the pelvis became the central item in this area of chronic pain and as a consequence the focus became directed to the pelvis and the terminology was adapted likewise. Chronic pelvic pain became the updated term. This term fitted well in the new ideas about the origin and nature of the pain. Pelvic pain was no longer seen as pain originating in pelvic organs but as pain perceived in these organs. The origin could be in the organs, in the muscles and in the nervous system.

In the world of pain three organisations with a mission to spread the knowledge of pelvic pain and thereby improve the care for patients with pelvic pain started working together. Apart from PUGO there are the International Pelvic Pain Society and Convergences Pelvi-Perineal. For an adolescent and similarly for abdominal and pelvic pain it is important to have good friends to discuss the sometimes difficult aspects of growing up. Bundling strength and ideas is a helpful trick in that period of life. The subsequent working together of these three organisations was the basis for the 1st World Congress on Abdominal and Pelvic Pain. It was organised in de Beurs van Berlage in Amsterdam from May 30 – June 2, 2013. The meeting was held during the IASP global year against visceral pain. In the talks with IASP about this relation we found out that abdominal and pelvic pain are related in many ways. That was the first step to introduce another change in the world of pelvic pain: add the abdomen. As a consequence PUGO was renamed into IASP Special Interest Group on Abdominal and Pelvic Pain. The logo was adapted to this new name as were the mission statements. During the 1st world congress there was a plenary session with all the disciplines represented in the faculty and the audience, illustrating an optimal multifactorial and multidisciplinary approach. With 550 participants from more than 40 countries and more than 10 disciplines, the meeting is clearly marking the end of the adolescent period. The book that is in your hands is written by the faculty of this meeting, although it is not just a congress book. It is a textbook with the most up to date information on the subject of abdominal and pelvic pain. Reading this book will let you realise what has happened in the world of abdominal and pelvic pain. It will also show the work that has to be done in the next decade: from definition to best practice. We have ended puberty and stand at the doorstep of maturity. The editors want to express the wish that this book will be the guide for the first years in the grown up world.

PART 1

General Aspects

Chapter 1 **Societal Impact of Abdominal and Pelvic Pain**

Chapter 2 **Defining Abdominal and Pelvic Pain**

Chapter 3 **From Animal Data to Human Practice**

Chapter 4 **The Importance of Central Sensitization**

Chapter 5 **The Role of Gender in Abdominal and Pelvic Pain**

CHAPTER 1

Societal Impact of Abdominal and Pelvic Pain

Luke Mordecai and Andrew Baranowski

INTRODUCTION

This chapter will review the societal impacts of abdominal and pelvic pain. The major aetiologies will be briefly discussed before looking at how they affect the people that suffer with them. Central to the chapter will be the frequent difficulty in diagnosis owing to a combination of absence of proven underlying circuitous routes of referral, and historically confusing classifications all contributing to a vicious circle worsening symptoms. The increasing prevalence of chronic pain syndromes and their impact on healthcare provision, or lack thereof, will also be discussed as well as the emerging concept of pain being considered as a diagnosis in its own right.

DESCRIBING THE SUBJECT

Defining the Problem

The World Health Organisation's (WHO) World Mental Health Survey estimated that across ten developed countries, 37% of adults suffer from chronic pain conditions, which extrapolates to at least 116 million people in the United States alone [62]. Recent figures from Europe report that almost one in five people describe moderate to severe chronic pain, with almost 90% of those having had symptoms for over two years and a third not receiving any treatment [7]. There have been several high profile and similar publications from the United Kingdom [UK], which reiterate these findings. The Chief Medical Officer's Report in 2008 identified chronic pain as one of England's top five health priorities and emphasised the impact it had across all ages, on social and physical function, and the economy [26]. The Health survey for England, 2011, published the prevalence of chronic pain in the UK at 31% and 37% for men and women respectively as well demonstrating a strong socioeconomic correlation [25]. Finally, the National Pain Audit carried out in 2011-12 described the very poor quality of life reported by chronic pain sufferers, the significant amount of healthcare utilisation, and the inequalities that existed within the healthcare system with only 40% of specialist pain services fulfilling truly multidisciplinary criteria [72].

There is a great deal published regarding the prevalence and impact of "chronic pelvic pain" (CPP) as an all-encompassing entity whilst there is far less corresponding work regarding the abdominal variety.

With regards to women, there was not a widely acknowledged definition for chronic pelvic pain until very recently. The most widely accepted duration of pain in definitions in women is recurrent or constant pain in the lower abdominal region that has lasted for at least six months [64]. This duration is at odds with the standard three months usually required to define chronic pain [71]. In the first and seminal population study regarding CPP Mathias uses women who have reported greater than six months of pain in her study group [37], although she also states that accurate recall regarding healthcare events and symptoms diminishes rapidly after 3 months.

The second difficulty regarding defining CPP relates to the nature and position of the pain. In Mathias' study, she questioned women regarding "pain below the belly button or in the female organs" [37]. In a study of New Zealand women, Grace questioned regarding "pain in the lower abdomen, of at least six months duration that is not associated with menstruation or sexual activity" [20] and three UK studies asked regarding "abdominal pain occurring more than six times in the past year" [23,31,60]. The results for the latter were significantly higher given the inclusion of upper abdominal pain.

The aetiology underlying CPP in women comprises a wide range of disorders with somatic (such as endometriosis [34]), nonsomatic and with no apparent cause [49] at polar ends of the spectrum. Additionally, there is a wide variety of poorly understood terminology used in the literature such as Bladder Pain Syndrome, Painful Bladder syndrome, Interstitial Cystitis, Hypersensitivity Bladder Syndrome [27], Pelvic Pain Syndrome [50], and Pervalgia [48].

The cumulative effect of the above was a great deal of confusion and disagreement and an almost absolute inability to perform meaningful epidemiological studies. This was rectified in 2003 when a special interest group named Pain of Urogenital Origin (PUGO), under the auspices of IASP, and in collaboration with the European Association of Urologists (EAU), drafted a definition, published in 2004. This definition was fine-tuned with several publications over the years and adapted by IASP in 2012 and is as follows:

> "Chronic pelvic pain is chronic or persistent pain perceived in structures related to the pelvis of either men or women. It is often associated with negative cognitive, behavioural, sexual and emotional consequences as well as with symptoms suggestive of lower urinary tract, sexual, bowel, pelvic floor or gynaecological dysfunction".

Furthermore, the Chronic Pelvic Pain Syndrome is formally defined as: "the occurrence of chronic pelvic pain where there is no proven infection or other obvious local pathology that may account for the pain. It is often associated with negative cognitive, behavioural, sexual or emotional consequences as well as with symptoms suggestive of lower urinary tract, sexual, bowel or gynaecological dysfunction."

As already mentioned CPP is not the exclusive preserve of women. One accepted classification of male urogenital pain has existed since 1995, when the all encompassing and nonspecific diagnosis of prostatodynia was disbanded [36]. This has allowed international elucidation of epidemiology.

Major Contributing Pathology: Incidence & Prevalence

Abdominal

Inflammatory bowel disease creates a massive burden of work for health systems. There are between 400,000 and 600,000 Crohn's sufferers in Northern America [12] and prevalence for Europe is estimated at 27-48 per 100,000 [4]. The similarly important ulcerative colitis (UC) has up to 20 new cases per 100,000 per year and a prevalence of between 8-246 per 100,000 individuals [1]. Whilst acute pain is a well described symptom, chronic pain is also a problem with 20% of sufferers with endoscopic remission still reporting symptoms and up to one sixth of all inflammatory bowel disease patients taking long term opiates [5].

Chronic pancreatitis has a marked spectrum of disease and a variety of causes, but chronic abdominal pain is a common theme. The incidence of chronic pancreatitis is between 1.6 to 23 cases per 100,000 per year worldwide and this is on the rise most likely due to unhealthy lifestyles. In the US alone, the disease results in more than 122,000 outpatient visits and 56,000 hospitalisations, with abdominal pain accounting for up to 80% of the latter [66].

Irritable bowel syndrome [IBS] remains a contentious diagnosis as pathophysiology is poorly described and the spectrum of symptoms is significant, especially in severity. There are many epidemiological studies with prevalence varying greatly by geography. The prevalence in the UK and US was reported as 8.2% [17] and 14.1% [28] respectively whilst in Mexico is has been reported as high as 46% [47]. What is certain is that chronic pain is a problem for sufferers to the extent when classifying the syndrome "Pain Pre-dominant" is one of the four specified presentations [24].

Functional Abdominal Pain Syndrome [FAPS] is a debilitating disorder characterised by constant or nearly constant abdominal pain persisting for greater than six months and associated with a loss of daily functioning [52]. Pain appears to be caused by amplified central perception of normal visceral input rather than enhanced peripheral stimulation and it is differentiated from IBS based on normal bowel habit and eating. Few epidemiological studies have focused on FAPS alone perhaps because IBS is currently under a much larger spotlight, however those that have, estimate a not insignificant prevalence of between 0.5% [14] and 1.7% [61].

Before laparoscopic cholecystectomy became the norm, open procedures were associated with post-operative symptoms in 5-40% [70] of cases, and more recently a small study into post nephrectomy donors found that 33% experienced prolonged pain and 26% described long-term chronic pain [43].

Female Pelvic

CPP may arise from any structure in or related to the pelvis, which includes the abdominal and pelvic walls. Three major general population studies have estimated the total population prevalence at 14.7% in the US [37], 24% in the UK [73], and 25.4% in New Zealand [20]. The figure for the US is lower than the other two as their study excluded mid-cycle pain.

Endometriosis is thought to be the most common cause of CPP and has an estimated prevalence worldwide of between 6-10% [8] and although pain is the most common presenting complaint, the association is not entirely straightforward. Whilst women with endometriosis are more likely to complain of pain [57], studies conflict regarding symptoms and severity of disease as seen on laparoscopy regarding position and number of implants [48]. Additionally, some women with documented disease do not complain of pain [2] and some experts even believe endometriosis may be a normal physiological state [32].

Pelvic Inflammatory Disease [PID] is thought to be another important cause of CPP affecting 750,000 women in America annually, and is said to cause infertility in 100,000 of those [58]. In a recent review of patients with pain thought to be secondary to adhesions, adhesiolysis resulted in pain relief in 60-90% cases [15] the evidence of cause and effect is not clear.

The leading urological causes of CPP are Bladder Pain Syndrome [BPS], historically known as Interstitial Cystitis [IC], and Urethral Syndrome [US], which are thought to be a spectrum of the same condition [68]. Less common aetiologies also exist such as urethral diverticulum, urinary calculi, neoplasias, and radiation cystitis. BPS/IC is characterised by pain and bladder symptoms. Whilst estimates of prevalence for BPS/IC vary from 10 to 500 per 100,000 [30], chronic pain is a very common feature effecting 60% of sufferers [33].

Myofascial trigger points on the abdominal wall are also implicated in up to 71% of patients with unexplained CPP [51]. Pelvic Girdle Pain during pregnancy can also meet the definition for CPP and effects up to half of all women, 30% suffering severe pain [44].

There are many psychological contributors and examples include negative coping strategies, catastrophising, a feeling of no control over the pain, and a belief that the pain represents ongoing tissue damage. Depression and sleep disorders are more prevalent in women with CPP although this is thought to be a consequence, rather than a cause of the pain [39]. An important social factor when considering the development of chronic pain syndromes is a history of physical and/or sexual abuse and studies have shown that the prevalence of abuse is higher amongst women with CPP than among pain-free women [63]. Additionally, other studies have demonstrated an increased prevalence of major sexual abuse in populations suffering from CPP compared to women with other pain syndromes [65]. Despite this, the evidence is not clear and extreme caution has to be undertaken when considering cause and effect. In clinical practice, previous negative sexual encounters have to be identified and acknowledged and exploration of the patient's beliefs around the relationship to the pain have to be undertaken in a sympathetic manner. However, in many cases the previous negative sexual encounter is not apparently directly relevant to the pain.

Male Pelvic

In the United States, a variety of "prostatitis" is diagnosed in 8% of all urological consults and 1% of all primary care presentations [11].

Chronic Pelvic Pain Syndrome (CPPS), defined by IASP as: Chronic pelvic pain syndrome (CPPS) is the occurrence of chronic pelvic pain where there is no proven infection or other obvious local pathology that may account for the pain. It is often associated with negative cognitive, behavioral, sexual, or emotional consequences as well as with symptoms suggestive of lower urinary tract, sexual, bowel, or gynecological dysfunction. CPPS is a subdivision of chronic pelvic pain (see above).

CPPS, formerly known as chronic nonbacterial prostatitis, accounts for 95% of all prostatitis diagnoses [21]. The official definition is perineal pain without evidence of urinary infection lasting greater than three months [10], which further demonstrates the lack of durational concordance that exists within chronic pain timeframes. The annual prevalence of CPPS is 0.5% [59] and yet when presented with a hypothetical scenario, 38% of primary care physicians say that they have not encountered such a patient [59]. This demonstrates the scale of the problem as well as raising the possibility of a great deal of misdiagnosis.

SOCIETAL IMPACT – A REVIEW OF THE LITERATURE

Patients who suffer with chronic pain more often than not suffer from one of more other chronic long term conditions therefore dissecting out the impact of pain alone amongst other symptoms may not be possible.

Societal impact may be considered in terms of three broad categories: direct costs to the healthcare system, indirect costs to the economy as a whole, and impact of the condition on sufferers' quality of life.

We have already mentioned the seminal paper on this topic written by Mathias [37]. This was the first attempt to quantify the impact of female chronic pelvic pain and was relevant because it was a telephone questionnaire from a random sample across the United States, hence not from a "by definition" biased healthcare seeking population. She specifically asked regarding healthcare utilisation and out-of-pocket payments, such as for prescription medication, directly related to CPP. From extrapolation, she estimated the annual national cost of physician visits to be $881.5 million with a further $1.9 billion spent by individuals on pain medication making a total input of $2.8 billion. This figure is from 1996 so today's extrapolated figure given inflation and the rising cost of US healthcare would be far higher.

Of those surveyed, 71% with CPP were employed and of those 15% indicated that they had taken time off work because of the pain in the last month. The mean amount of paid work missed was between 14.8 and 25.5 hours per month in comparison to between 2.2 and 11.2, the global monthly amount of hours missed for all employed women. Extrapolating from these figures, and taking employment and wage statistics into account from the population as a whole, the indirect costs of CPP from lost productivity was estimated at $555.3 million. Questions were also posed regarding the quality of life of sufferers of CPP. Disregarding the issue of causality, 47% reported feeling "downhearted and blue" some, most, or all of the time, 26% said that they had stayed in bed for at least half a day in the last month specifically because of the pain and 88% reported pain after intercourse, some, most of all of the time in the past month. Respondents with CPP also reported significantly poorer general health. Finally, this study states that 61% of women with CPP had no diagnosis. It could be suggested that this uncertainty, anxiety, and potential fear of serious undiagnosed yet underlying pathology, would do nothing to augment quality of life.

The effects on quality of life were re-iterated in a study performed in Southampton, England, where women attending their first gynaecology outpatients' appointment completed a Short-Form 36 Health Questionnaire [SF-36], to assess health status. The results from this were compared with women suffering from other chronic conditions and healthy controls. Data suggested that whilst the physical capabilities and roles of women with CPP were affected less than suffers of comparative conditions, namely diabetes, congestive cardiac failure and hypertension, the burden of disease demonstrated itself in the "emotional, social, pain, energy, and psychological" categories where only those with clinical depression scored consistently lower [56]. This same study also included interview data with women who suffered with CPP, which confirmed reports from other studies that whilst the condition causes substantial distress and disruption there are often few objective indications of functional limitation as women do not allow the pain to disturb physical function [45].

A more recent New Zealand study broke down SF-36 data into a Physical Component Summary [PCS] and a Mental Component Summary [MCS] and compared general health, comorbidity, and sleep problems between CPP sufferers and the general population [20]. Both the PCS and MCS were significantly lower in the CPP group. Additionally women with CPP were more likely to have had other longstanding chronic illness and disability, such as fibromyalgia and temporomandibular disorders, and indeed other pain syndromes; an association already postulated. This study also demonstrated the impact on activities and work with almost half of CPP sufferers unable to carry out normal living without taking analgesics or resting, and 10% reported being restricted by lethargy and fatigue, possibily related to the sleep disturbance already observed. Interestingly, and in disagreement with

Mathias, although women reported significant restriction because of pain, those with CPP did not appear to take more time off work when compared to a healthy parallel population. The study also commented on the psychological aspect of causality in CPP with concern over not understanding the origin of pain being overwhelmingly the more troubling aspect, greater even than the pain itself.

Hatchett published the first qualitative study of urological chronic pelvic pain syndromes, which included both men and women [22]. An unexpected result in this paper was fatigue, which was described as a consequence and symptom by patients and was said to merit further investigation. It was also observed that the desire of patients to return to their premorbid state signifies a lack of acceptance and understanding of the condition, and indeed chronic pain at large, with regard to management rather than cure.

In a study similar to the one described above, New Zealand male patients completed a Short-Form 12 [SF-12] and the disease specific NIH-CPSI QOL subscale, to measure Health Related Quality of Life [HRQOL], which also generated PCS and MCS scores. This study found that both mental and physical domains of HRQOL scores were significantly impaired in sufferers, and worse scores were correlated with worse symptoms [40]. Male patients with CPP fared worse in the mental scores than their counterparts with diabetes and congestive cardiac failure. The mental component is re-iterated in another study from Finland, the findings from which suggest that psychological stress is common in male sufferers of CPP and consultation with a psychiatrist should be considered [41].

Sexual dysfunction is another major component when considering the impact of CPP in the male population, and is self-reported in up to 75% of sufferers [35]. Men with sexual dysfunction describe substantially worse QOL and NIH-CPSI scores than those with pain alone and a multi-centre study found 88% were unhappy with their condition [42]. Adverse consequences on relationships are also reported with chronic "prostatitis" causing marriage difficulties in 17% of men and a further 4% attributing divorce to the syndrome [41].

There is less literature regarding the economic impact of male chronic pelvic pain. One study from the US states that prostatitis accounts for 2 million consultations per annum although this figure includes acute sub-types. The estimated cost is $84 million for 2007 and chronic prostatitis accounts the majority of this burden in terms of prevalence and also because the absence of effective treatment results in multiple and recurrent presentations. Indirect economic costs are mentioned although not quantified [16].

Another American study looked at the direct and indirect costs using questionnaires to assess healthcare utilisation over a three-month period in chronic prostatitis clinic attendees. Total medical costs were $126,915 and 26% of the men reported time off work valued at an average of $551. The average total cost over the study per participant was $1099, which extrapolated to annual costs of $4397 [9].

Where evidence exists in the literature, the societal impact of chronic abdominal pain is equally as pronounced. A systemic review investigating HRQOL in sufferers of IBS was published in 2002 looking at all relevant papers since 1980 [18]. This revealed, as with CPP, both PCS and MCS domains of HRQOL were significantly reduced.

Another systematic review focused on the prevalence of suicidal behavior in sufferers of chronic abdominal pain and IBS [55]. The link with functional pain syndromes and psychiatric illness, especially depression and anxiety disorders [67] is well described and although the direction of causality is still hotly debated the societal impact is self-evident. One half of community based IBS patients meet criteria for the diagnosis of psychiatric disorders and this increases to 90% in those referred to tertiary care [67]. The literature confirms an association between chronic abdominal pain and both suicidal ideation and suicide, the rates in this cohort of patients being higher than the general population and those suffering with other chronic pain syndromes. Significantly, the increase in suicidal behaviour is stated to be at least partially independent from the otherwise most common risk factor – depression.

Evaluating the economic cost related to chronic abdominal pain is also difficult because it is well known that a significant proportion goes unknown to the medical system [3]. However, due to the chronicity and often young age of onset of symptoms along with the detrimental impact of productivity, IBS is thought to be one of the top ten most expensive gastrointestinal diseases in the US [29]. Calculated on the basis of 18 studies from the US, published between 1991 and 2003, the average direct medical costs per IBS patient were between $341 and $8750 [38]. An American study showed that in the employed population, sufferers of IBS have three times as many sick days as healthy colleagues [6], whilst a Canadian publication stated this demographic missed an average of 13.4 days per annum specifically because of IBS symptoms which equated to an annual cost to the employer of CAD $2,200 per IBS patient [14].

PRACTICAL IMPLICATIONS

Abdominal pelvic pain is still considered a niche condition that is not well understood or treated. There are several possible reasons for this.

The lack of robust classifications means that past data and studies have relied on ambiguous and un-agreed criteria subsequently leading to inaccurate epidemiology. Additionally, the subjective nature of the syndromes in question result in widespread inter-clinician variation. This can be demonstrated in the case of IBS with regard to the Rome criteria. One paper demonstrated a 1.5 fold difference in prevalence of IBS in the same cohort of patients depending on varying interpretations of Rome II [54] whilst another demonstrated an intra-cohort four-fold difference in prevalence [53].

Another problem associated with this general absence of understanding relates to the patient journey. With the symptoms discussed in this chapter patients can be referred to a number of specialties including urology, gynaecology, gastroenterology, pain medicine, genitourinary medicine, sexual health, and rheumatology each with their own specific and perhaps non-holistic way of investigating the symptoms of CPP. This non-linear and certainly not integrated pathway may explain why 61% of US women, 50% of UK women and 47.7% of New Zealand women in the general population described symptoms of CPP but had no formal diagnosis [20]. There are other downstream effects of this protracted referral process such as a loss in faith and disengagement from the medical system before appropriate treatment has been initiated or worse initiation of the wrong treatment. Evidence coming from the US states that opiate prescriptions for non-malignant pain has doubled over the last ten years [13].

Finally, use of a generic questionnaire, such as the SF-36, whilst validated, is limited in scope. Questions refer to a limited time frame and there is no ability for patients to express how the condition has evolved over a continuum. Additionally, it does not address relevant issues to the chronic pain population such as depression and specific pain avoidance behaviours.

LOOKING AT THE FUTURE

There is no doubt that the medical fraternity is finally waking up to the enormous burden that pain has been quietly amassing on health systems and society. Additionally, pain is beginning to be recognised as a condition in its own right and cannot always be explained as the unwanted consequence of other underlying pathology, however counterintuitive this might seem. Furthermore the optimum treatment of chronic pain is not with increasing doses of stronger pain medications. Therefore, with this in mind, one can see large-scale changes that are essential and hopefully on the horizon such as the proliferation of truly multidisciplinary pain clinics, the gold standard in pain management, but also currently a scarce resource.

Hopefully with the recent development of IASP classifications, CPP patients will be able to be triaged more appropriately to the correct specialty and with more universal agreement over classification, epidemiological data will improve shedding more accurate light on the conditions and allowing better resource allocation as well as further work into areas such as risk factor analysis. Furthermore, with a standardised referral system, multidisciplinary conversations could occur regarding more appropriate treatment pathways than for example the often negative, yet highly invasive diagnostic laparoscopy that many women presenting for the first time undergo under the assumption that they have endometriosis. Initial work has shown that medical treatment with a GnRH analogue could be employed instead of laparoscopy, which is not only less invasive but would also have a significant cost implication [69].

Finally, pain specialists, and indeed sub-specialists, need to fully engage with primary care doctors and patients to raise awareness of the problem and what should and can be done about it. Pelvic pain, in particular, should not be normalized within society and early presentation should be encouraged to avoid a potential downward spiral of sensitization and worsening of symptoms. Similarly, clear treatment algorithms, such as the British Pain Society's Map of Medicine, Chronic pelvic pain [in men and women], England view 2012, should be published by specialist organisations and made widely available to enhance awareness and guide early management. This should help achieve the ultimate goal and perhaps Holy Grail of medicine which is ensuring that the right patient sees the right professional at the right time.

TAKE HOME MESSAGES

- Chronic abdominal and pelvic pain affects many people and accounts for a significant financial burden and reduction in HRQOL.
- Classification of chronic abdominal and pelvic pain syndromes is fraught with difficulty leading to confusion, mis-diagnosis, and inappropriate referrals.
- Whilst the societal burden is known to be significant, accurate estimates are difficult because of the high proportion of pathology that goes undiagnosed both from failure to present and failures of awareness within the medical profession.
- Pain needs to be considered as a diagnosis in its own right and does not by definition require an underlying cause.
- People presenting with chronic abdominal and pelvic pain need to be identified quickly and referred to an appropriate multi-disciplinary service experienced in dealing with the problem.

REFERENCES

1. Anese S, Fiocci C. Ulcerative colitis. N Engl J Med. 2011; 365:1713–25.
2. Balasch J, Creus M, Fábregues F, et al. Visible and non-visible endometriosis at laparoscopy in fertile and infertile women and patients with chronic pelvic pain: a prospective study. Hum Repod 1996; 11: 387–91.

3. Bentkover JD, Field C, Greene EM, et al. The economic burden of irritable bowel syndrome in Canada. Can J Gastroenterol. 1999;13: 89A–96A.
4. Bernstein CN, Wajda A, Svenson LW, et al. The Epidemiology of Inflammatory Bowel Disease in Canada: A Population-Based Study. Am J Gastroenterol. 2006: 101; 1559–68.
5. Bielefeldt K, Davis B, Binion DG. Pain and inflammatory bowel disease. Inflamm Bowel Dis. 2009;15: 778–88.
6. Boivin M. Socioeconomic impact of irritable bowel syndrome in Canada. Can J Gastroenterol 2001;15: 8B–11B.
7. Breivik H, Eisenberg E, O'Brien T. The individual and societal burden of chronic pain in Europe: the case for strategic prioritisation and action to improve knowledge and availability of appropriate care. BMC Public Health 2013 ;13:1229.
8. Bulletti C, Coccia ME, Battistoni S, Borini A. Endometriosis and infertility. J. Assist. Reprod. Genet. 2010; 27: 441–7.
9. Calhoun EA, McNaughton Collins M, et al; Chronic Prostatitis Collaborative Research Network. The economic impact of chronic prostatitis. Arch Intern Med. 2004; 164:1231–6.
10. Clemens JQ, Meenan RT, O'Keeffe Rosetti MC, et al. Incidence and clinical characteristics of National Institutes of Health type III prostatitis in the community. J Urol 2005; 174: 2319–22
11. Collins MM, Stafford RS, O'Leary MP, Barry MJ. How common is prostatitis? A national survey of physician visits. J Urol. 1998; 159: 1224–8.
12. Cosnes J. Tobacco and IBD: Relevance in the understanding of disease mechanisms and clinical practice. Best Pract Res Clin Gastroenterol. 2004; 18: 481–96.
13. Daubresse M, Chang HY, Yu Y, et al. Ambulatory Diagnosis and Treatment of Nonmalignant Pain in the United States, 2000–2010. Med Care, 2013; 51: 870–8.
14. Drossman DA, Li Z, Andruzzi E, et al. U.S. householder survey of functional gastrointestinal disorders. Prevalence, sociodemography, and health impact. Dig Dis Sci. 1993; 38: 1569–80.
15. Duffy DM, DiZarega GA. Adhesion controversies. Pelvic pain as a cause of adhesions, crystalloids in preventing them. J Reprod Med. 1996; 41:19–26.
16. Duloy AM, Calhoun EA, Clemens JQ. Economic impact of chronic prostatitis. Curr Urol Rep. 2007;8: 336–9.
17. Ehlin AG, Montgomery SM, Ekbom A, et al. Prevalence of gastrointestinal diseases in two British national birth cohorts. Gut. 2003; 52: 1117–21.
18. El-Serag HB, Olden K, Bjorkman D. Health related quality of life among persons with irritable bowel syndrome: a systematic review. Aliment Pharmocol Ther. 2002; 16: 1171–1185.
19. Grace V, Zondervan KT. Chronic Pelvic Pain in New Zealand: Comparative Well-Being, Co-morbidity, and Impact on Work and Other Activities. Health Care Women Int. 2006; 27: 585–99.
20. Grace VM, Zondervan KT. Chronic pelvic pain in New Zealand prevalence, pain, severity, diagnoses and use of health services. Aust N Z J Public Health. 2004; 28: 369–75.
21. Habermacher GM, Chason JT, Schaeffer AJ. Prostatitis/chronic pelvic pain syndrome. Annu. Rev. Med. 2006 ; 57: 195–206.
22. Hatchett L, Fitzgerald MP, Potts J, et al. Life Impact of Urological Pain Syndromes. J Heath Psychol 2009; 14: 741.
23. Heaton KW, O'Donnell LJD, Braddon FEM. Symptoms of Irritable Bowel Syndrome in British Urban Community. Consulters and Non-Consulters. Gastroenterology 1992: 102; 1962–1967.
24. Holten KB, Wetherington A, Bankston L. Diagnosing the patient with abdominal pain and altered bowel habits: is it irritable bowel syndrome? Am Fam Physician 2003; 67: 2157–62.
25. Health survey for England - 2011, health, social care, and lifestyles [NS]. Volume 1, Chapter 9. https://catalogue.ic.nhs.uk/publications/public-health/surveys/heal-surv-eng-2011/HSE2011-Ch9-Chronic-Pain.pdf. Last Accessed September 10, 2014.
26. Donaldson L. 150 years of the Annual Report of the Chief Medical Officer: On the state of public health 2008. Crown copyright, 2009. http://www.dh.gov.uk/prod_consum_dh/groups/dh_digitalassets/documents/digitalasset/dh_096233.pdf. Last accessed September 20, 2014.
27. Hughes J. Defining Abdomino-pelvic pain to include overlapping pain conditions. May 30, 2013. Last accessed July 16, 2014. *http://www.pelvicpain-meeting.com/fileadmin/docs/J_Hughes__Defining_AbdominoPelvic_Pain_130530_publish.pdf*
28. Hungin AP, Chang L, Locke GR, et al. Irritable bowel syndrome in the United States: prevalence, symptom patterns and impact. Aliment Pharmacol Ther. 2005; 21:1365–75.
29. Inadomi JM, Fennerty MB, Bjorkman D. Systematic review: The economic impact of irritable bowel syndrome. Aliment Pharmacol Ther. 2003; 18 :671–82.
30. Jones CA, Nyberg L. Epidemiology of interstitial cystitis. Urology 1997: 49; 2–9.
31. Jones R, Lydeard S. Irritable Bowel syndrome in the general population. BMJ. 1992; 304: 87–90.

32. Koninckx PR. Is mild endometriosis a disease? Hum Reprod 1994; 9: 2202–2211.
33. Koziol JA, Carlk DC, Gittes RF, Tan EM. The natural history of interstitial cystitis, a survey of 374 patients. J Urol 1993; 149: 465–469.
34. Kresch AJ, Seifer DB, Sachs LB, Barrese I. Laparoscopy in 100 women with chronic pelvic pain. Obstet Gynecol 1984; 64: 672–4
35. Lee SWH, Liong ML, Yuen KH, et al. Adverse Impact of sexual dysfunction in chronic prostatitis/chronic pelvic pain syndrome. Urology. 2008; 71; 79–84.
36. Litwin MS, Mc-Naughton-Collins M, Fowler FR Jr, et al. The National Institutes of Health Chronic Prostatitis Index: development and validation of a new outcome measure. Chronic Prostatitis Collaborative Research Network. J Urol 1999; 162: 369–75.
37. Mathias SD, Kuppermann M, Liberman RF, et al. Chronic pelvic pain: prevalence, health-related quality of life, and economic correlates. Obstet Gynecol. 1996; 87: 321–7.
38. Maxion-Bergemann S, Thielecke F, Abel F, Bergemann R. Costs of irritable bowel syndrome in the UK and US. Pharmacoeconomics. 2006; 24: 21–37.
39. McGowan LPA, Clark-Carter DD, Pitts MK. Chronic Pelvic Pain; a meta-analytic review. Psychology and Health 1998; 13: 937–951.
40. McNaughton Collins M, Pontari MA, et al; Chronic Prostatitis Collaborative Research Network. Quality of Life Is Impaired in Men with Chronic Prostatitis: The Chronic Prostatitis Collaborative Research Network. J Gen Intern Med. 2001; 16: 656–662.
41. Mehik A, Hellström P, Sarpola A, et al. Fears, sexual disturbances and personality features in men with prostatitis: a population-based cross-sectional study in Finland. BJU Int. 2001; 88: 35–8.
42. Nied R, Penson DF, Dhanani N. Effects of erectile dysfunction on quality of life. J Urol 1997; 157: 427A.
43. Owen M, Lorgelly P, Serpell M. Chronic pain following donor nephrectomy--a study of the incidence, nature and impact of chronic post-nephrectomy pain. Eur J Pain. 2010; 14: 732–4.
44. Persson M, Winkvist A, Dahlgren L, Mogren I. "Struggling with daily life and enduring pain": a qualitative study of the experiences of pregnant women living with pelvic girdle pain. BMC Pregnancy Childbirth. 2013; 13: 111.
45. Pearce S. The Concept of Psychogenic Pain: a psychological investigation of women with chronic pelvic pain. Curr Psychol Res Rev 1987; 6: 219–228.
46. Pepper MM, Nezhat F, Goldstein H. Dysmenorrhoea is related to the number of implants in endometriosis patients. Fertil Steril. 1995: 63; 500–503.
47. Quigley EM, Locke GR, Mueller-Lissner S, et al. Prevalence and management of abdominal cramping and pain: a multinational survey. Aliment. Pharmacol. Ther. 2006; 24: 411–9.
48. Reiter RC. A profile of women with chronic pelvic pain. Clin Obstet Gynecol. 1990; 33: 130–136.
49. Reiter RC, Gambone JC. Non gynaecological somatic pathology in women with chronic pelvic pain and negative laparoscopy. J Reprod Med 1991; 36: 253–9.
50. Robinson JC. Chronic Pelvic Pain. Current opinion in obstretics and gynecology. 1993: 5; 740–743.
51. Slocumb JC. Neurogenic factors in chronic pelvic pain: trigger points. Am J Obstet Gynecol. 1984; 149: 536–543.
52. Sperber AD, Drossman DA. Review article: the functional abdominal pain syndrome. Aliment Pharmacol Ther. 2011; 33: 514–24.
53. Sperber AD, Shvartzman P, Friger M, Fich A. A comparative reappraisal of the Rome II and Rome III diagnostic criteria: Are we getting closer to the 'true' prevalence of irritable bowel syndrome? Eur J Gastroenterol Hepatol. 2007; 19: 441–7.
54. Sperber AD, Shvartzman P, Friger M, Fich A. Unexpectedly low prevalence rates of IBS among adult Israeli Jews. Neurogastroenterol Motil. 2005; 17: 207–11.
55. Spiegel B, Schoenfeld P, Naliboff B. Systematic review: the prevalence of suicidal behaviour in patients with chronic abdominal pain and irritable bowel syndrome. Aliment Pharmcol Ther. 2007; 26: 183–193.
56. Stones RW, Selfe SA, Fransman S, Horn SA. Psychosocial and economic impact of chronic pelvic pain. Baillieres Best Pract Res Clin Obstet Gynaecol. 2000; 14: 415–31.
57. Stout AL, Steege JF, Dodson WC, Hughes CL. Relationship of laparoscopic findings to self report of pelvic pain. Am J Obstet Gynecol 1991; 164:73–79.
58. Sutton MY, Sternberg M, Zaidi A, et al. Trends in pelvic inflammatory disease hospital discharges and ambulatory visits, United States, 1985–2001. Sex Transm Dis 2005; 32: 778–84.
59. Taylor BC, Noorbaloochi S, McNaughton-Collins M, et al; Urologic Diseases in America Project. Excessive antibiotic use in men with prostatitis. Am. J. Med. 2008; 121: 444–9.
60. Thompson WG, Heaton KW. Functional bowel disorders in apparently healthy people. Gastroenterology 1980; 79: 283–288.

61. Thompson WG, Irvine EJ, Pare P, et al. Functional gastrointestinal disorders in Canada, First population based survey using Rome II criteria with suggestions for improving the questionnaire. Dig Dis Sci 2002; 47: 225–35.
62. Tsang A, Von Korff M, Lee S, et al. Common chronic pain conditions in developed and developing countries: gender and age differences and comorbidity with depression-anxiety disorders. J Pain. 2008; 13: 883–891.
63. Walker E, Katon W, Harrop-Griffiths J. Relationship of chronic pelvic pain to psychiatric diagnoses and childhood sexual abuse. Am J Psychiatry 1988; 145: 75–80.
64. Waller KG, Shaw RW. Endometriosis, pelvic pain and psychological functioning. Fertil Steril 1995; 63: 796–800.
65. Walling MK, Reiter RC, O'Hara MW, et al. Abuse history and chronic pain in women: Prevalences of sexual abuse and physical abuse. Obstet Gynecol 1994;84:193–199.
66. Warshaw AL, Banks PA, Fernández-Del Castillo C. AGA technical review: Treatment of pain in chronic pancreatitis. Gastroenterology. 1998: 115; 765–776.
67. Whitehead WE, Palsson O, Jones KR. Systematic review of the comorbidity of irritiable bowel syndrome with order disorders: what are the causes and implications? Gastroenterology 2002; 122: 1140–56.
68. Wilkins EGL, Payne SR, Pead PJ, et al. Interstitial Cystitis and the urethral syndrome. A possible answer. Br J Urol 1989; 64: 39–44.
69. Winkel CA. Modelling of medical and surgical treatment costs of chronic pelvic pain: new paradigms for making clinical decisions. Am J Manag Care 1999; 5: S276-S290.
70. Womack NA, Crider RL. The Persistence of Symptoms Following Cholecystectomy. Ann. Surg. 1947; 126: 31–55.
71. The British Pain Society. *www.britishpainsociety.org/media_faq.htm* Last accessed July 16, 2014.
72. The British Pain Society. National Pain Audit Final Report 2010–2012. www.britishpainsociety.org/members_articles_npa_2012.pdf Last accessed July 16, 2014.
73. Zondervan KT, Yudkin PL, Vessey MP, et al. The community prevalence of chronic pelvic pain in women and associated illness behaviour. Br J Gen Pract. 2001; 51: 541–7.

CHAPTER 2

Defining Abdominal and Pelvic Pain

John Hughes

INTRODUCTION

Abdominal and pelvic pain is not new, with documented descriptions going back to 1886[13] and beyond. As an area of specific study and understanding there has been a growing interest, particularly in pelvic pain, over the last 15 to 20 years. One of the principal difficulties has been that patients may be referred to one or more separate specialties that have traditionally worked independently of each other.

Running in parallel to this a number of special interest groups developed, often with focused remits (e.g. International Society for the study of Bladder Pain Syndrome (ESSIC), The British Society for the Study of Vulval Disease (BSSVD)) involving clinicians, other health care workers, and often, patient groups. These organisations have provided support and recourses to patients and developed management and research strategies. These, however, tended to be diagnosis or specialist orientated providing benefit for some patient groups, but not always encompassing a truly integrated package. They developed individual sets of terminology resulting in multiple terms for the same or very similar condition. As a result despite best intentions there was a degree of confusion.

Over the last decade, there has been a discussion between these groups to develop a consensus that allows the individual groups to flourish but also share and integrate their ideas and understanding with the ultimate aim of improving patient care. This has led to a set of broadly agreed definitions for abdominal and pelvic pain that have been accepted and ratified by the International Association for the Study of Pain (IASP)[7] and used by the European Association of Urology (EAU)[4].

This chapter aims to discuss the confusion that existed in the terminology and how it developed to the current position. It will provide a definition of chronic pelvic pain and chronic pelvic pain syndrome (there being no current equivalent for abdominal pain) and fit it to a standardised classification as well as a proposed alternative. Then briefly suggest opportunities for the future.

BASIC ASPECTS

Pain is defined as "An unpleasant sensory and emotional experience associated with actual or potential tissue damage, or described in terms of such damage"[7]. This underpins the notion that pain has both sensory and emotional components and both need to be considered together. There is no requirement for there to be actual tissue damage in order to experience pain or that pain is necessarily protective. Often pain has a protective role, but there are occasions when it does not (e.g. Trigeminal neuralgia, phantom pain). Under these circumstances the pain becomes the condition in its own right. There is always a requirement at presentation to assess for a known treatable condition and manage it accordingly. If no such condition can be found or it is managed optimally but the pain persists then it is reasonable to manage the pain as a condition and not persist with interventions that are unlikely to provide any benefit. The focus of management moves away from the organ that is assumed to be involved and encompasses a broader biopsychosocial model.

Development of the Terminology

There has been a development of multiple terms for the same condition or several definitions for the same term. This has resulted in confusion for both patients and clinicians. It makes it difficult to compare studies, perform meaningful metanalysis or develop focused research strategies. One example is highlighted by Berry et al.[2] who noted that there was no standard case definition in existence for interstitial cystitis/painful bladder syndrome. This study was looking at the epidemiology of the condition and concluded that in order to assess the prevalence two definitions should be used. This group felt that an international consensus was required. Further to this, other terms that have been used for this condition include Hypersensitivity Bladder Syndrome and Bladder Pain Syndrome. Some terms suggested an underlying pathology (e.g. infection in Interstitial Cystitis) or that the end organ (the bladder in painful bladder syndrome) is the cause of the problem and the research has tended to be focused in this direction. Similar situations can be argued for pain in the region of the prostate and vulva.

Part of the difficulty is that patients with pain perceived in the pelvis may be seen by clinicians from primary care as well as several specialities including: gynaecology, urology, urogynaecology, dermatology, general or specialist surgery, gastroenterology, physiotherapy, pain medicine, genitourinary medicine, sexual health and rheumatology. Frequently patients would be transferred or referred in and out of these services over a period of years. There may be little or no co-ordination of care with patients often undergoing repeat procedures and interventions that proved no benefit and on occasion's significant harm. They are given a variety of explanations and management strategies resulting in at best confusion and worst exacerbation of their overall quality of life. This often goes on over years, consuming a significant amount of time and health care resource.

The revolving door of referral and intervention results in patients receiving several diagnoses or labels depending on whom they see. These include: Painful Bladder Syndrome, Endometriosis, Irritable Bowel Syndrome, Chronic Pelvic Pain Syndrome or even Fibromyalgia. It suggests poor understanding of the aetiology of the conditions, the terms not being very specific along with a degree of confusion amongst the professionals seeing these patients. This is not to denigrate the conscientiousness of the clinicians or patients but acts to emphasise the complexity of the variety of presentations and systems involved.

In approximately 1998, a special interest group of the International Association for the Study of Pain (IASP) developed with the aim of bringing together individuals with an interest and expertise in managing this patient group. The group was called Pain of Urological Origin (PUGO) which changed its name in 2012 to the Special Interest Group on Abdominal and Pelvic Pain to better represent the science, clinical work and patients that are actually being considered. The group includes a mix of basic scientists, researchers, psychologists, physicians, nursing, sexologists, physiotherapy and patient groups. From this and the involvement of other groups there were a variety of international conferences and meetings some being outlined in Table 1. There was a degree of common ground and

TABLE 1 Some of the Organisations and Meetings Involved in Developing the Current Consensus

The European Association for Urology (EAU) - working party for Chronic Pelvic Pain guidelines - 2004, 2008, 2010, 2012, 2013

International Society for the study of Bladder Pain Syndrome (ESSIC) – 2008

Pain of Urogenital Origin (PUGO) - Update on Urogenital Pain, Current Issues and Controversies – 2008, 2010, 2012

National Institute of Health (NIH): workshop on Interstitial Cystitis, Bethesda. November 2006; and Defining the urologic chronic pelvic pain syndromes, Bethesda. June 2008

International Consultation on IC - Forging an International Consensus: progress in painful bladder syndrome/interstitial cystitis 2004. Interstitial cystitis/painful bladder syndrome/bladder pain syndrome: the evolution of a new paradigm 2008

a desire to reduce some of the confusion and develop a terminology that had the potential to provide ease for clinicians but also be helpful at a research level. Following a PUGO meeting in Glasgow in 2008 a working group developed (Table 2). This group has a broad membership covering several countries, disciplines, and interests. Some members were also members of some of the special interest groups in the field. Therefore, a broad range of interested parties were involved whilst maintaining a manageable number in the group. There followed a series of frank discussions, debates, and meetings from which a set of definitions was agreed and presented to the IASP Taxonomy Taskforce for ratification. This occurred in December 2012[7] and the same set of definitions has been used by the European Association of Urology (EAU) in their Chronic Pelvic Pain Guidelines[4] and by the British Pain Society Map of Medicine pathway[11]. This is the culmination of over 10 years of work.

The IASP Taxonomy[7] of definitions referred to in this chapter are titled, 'Visceral and other Syndromes of the Trunk apart form Spinal and Radicular Pain'. This covers a variety of well known and clearly described conditions (e.g. Chronic Gastric Ulcer, Carcinoma of the Stomach and Familial Mediterranean Fever) and some of the Chronic Pelvic Pain Syndromes (e.g. Bladder Pain Syndrome, Prostate Pain Syndrome, Vulvar Pain Syndrome and Endometriosis-Associated Pain Syndrome). The concept is to divide the various abdominal and pelvic pains into those that are well described and have clear management pathways associated with them (e.g. Bladder Infection) and those where there is poorer understanding of the underlying mechanisms (e.g. Bladder Pain Syndrome).

TABLE 2 Members of the Taxonomy Working Group

Andrew Baranowski, Chairman of PUGO's Classification Committee (UK Pain)	Fred Howard (USA Gynaecology)
Paul Abrams (UK Urology)	John Hughes (UK Pain)
Richard Berger (US Urology)	Curtis Nickel (Canady Urology)
Tony Buffington (US Veterinary Science)	Jorgen Nordling (Denmark Urology)
Beverly Collett (UK Pain)	Dean Tripp (Canada Psychology)
Anton Emmanuel (UK Gastroenterology)	Katy Vincent (UK Gynaecology)
Magnus Fall (Sweden Urology)	Ursula Wesselmann (US Neurology)
Phil Hanno (US Urology)	Amanda C de C Williams (UK Psychology)

Definitions and Taxonomy[7]

The definitions are starting to be used at both a clinical and research level. Below are those for pelvic pain as they have been ratified and accepted. Currently there is no direct equivalent for abdominal pain and is an area for further discussion. With regard to pelvic pain the definitions relate to both men and women with pain perceived in the region of the anatomical pelvis and includes the external genitalia.

Chronic pelvic pain (CPP) is "chronic or persistent pain perceived in structures related to the pelvis of either men or women. It is often associated with negative cognitive, behavioural, sexual and emotional consequences as well as with symptoms suggestive of lower urinary tract, sexual, bowel, pelvic floor or gynaecological dysfunction".

The term perceived is used in the definition to indicate that the patient and clinician, to the best of their ability from the history, examination, and investigations (where appropriate) has localised the pain as being perceived in the specified anatomical pelvic area.

Cyclical or recurrent pain "In the case of documented nociceptive pain that becomes chronic or persistent through time, the pain must have been continuous or recurrent for at least 6 months. That is, it can be cyclical over a six month period, such as the cyclical pain of dysmenorrhea. If non-acute and central sensitization pain mechanisms are well documented, then the pain may be regarded as chronic, irrespective of the time period". This part of the definition stipulates a six month period before the pain can be considered as chronic. This is arbitrary but chosen as it was considered that three months was not long enough when including cyclical pain. With cyclical pain being included, dysmennorhea should be considered as a CPP if it is persistent and associated with negative cognitive, behavioural, sexual, or emotional consequences.

These general definitions of pelvic pain can be broadly subdivided into two principal groups:

Specific disease related chronic pelvic pain – e.g. infection, cancer.

Chronic Pelvic Pain Syndromes – those where no obvious pathology is identified, e.g. bladder pain syndrome, generalised vulvar pain syndrome.

Chronic pelvic pain syndrome (CPPS) is defined as "the occurrence of chronic pelvic pain where there is no proven infection or other obvious local pathology that may account for the pain. It is often associated with negative cognitive, behavioural, sexual, or emotional consequences as well as with symptoms suggestive of lower urinary tract, sexual, bowel, or gynaecological dysfunction."

These patients have symptoms suggestive of structures related to the pelvis (the anatomical pelvis including the external genitalia in men and women). The term Syndrome is being used to indicate that although there may be peripheral mechanisms involved that central nervous system neuromodulation may be more important, or at a clinical level, we do not fully understand the mechanisms.

Pain perceived in the pelvis in CPPS may be focused in the region of a single organ, when clinicians may feel like including the end organ (e.g. Bladder Pain Syndrome), more than one pelvic organ (e.g. bladder and rectal components) where keeping the term CPPS will be more appropriate. CPPS may also be associated with systemic symptoms such as chronic fatigue syndrome or fibromyalgia.

These definitions can then be applied to the IASP taxonomy grid (Table 3). This has a use as a taxonomy structure but is less helpful in understanding the potential interactions between the axis when moving across the table. At a clinical level, it is often difficult to move beyond axis I. It is common for patients to have several elements in axis II and III

TABLE 3 **IASP Taxonomy for Pelvic Pain (From EAU Guidelines [4])**

Axis I Region		Axis II System	Axis III End organ as pain syndrome as identified from Hx, Ex and Ix	Axis IV Referral characteristics	Axis V Temporal characteristics	Axis VI Character	Axis VII Associated symptoms	Axis VIII Psychological symptoms
Chronic pelvic pain	Specific disease associated pelvic pain OR Pelvic pain syndrome	Urological	Prostate Bladder Scrotal Testicular Epididymal Penile Urethral Post-vasectomy	Suprapubic Inguinal Urethral Penile/clitoral Perineal Rectal Back Buttocks Thighs	ONSET Acute Chronic ONGOING Sporadic Cyclical Continuous TIME Filling Emptying Immediate post Late post TRIGGER Provoked Spontaneous	Aching Burning Stabbing Electric	UROLOGICAL Frequency Nocturia Hesitance Dysfunctional flow Urge Incontinence GYNAECOLOGICAL Menstrual Menopause GASTROINTESTINAL Constipation Diarrhoea Bloatedness Urge Incontinence NEUROLOGICAL Dysaesthesia Hyperaesthesia Allodynia Hyperalgesia SEXOLOGICAL Satisfaction Female dyspareunia Sexual avoidance Erectile dysfunction Medication MUSCLE Function impairment Fasciculation CUTANEOUS Trophic changes Sensory changes	ANXIETY About pain or putative cause of pain Catastrophic thinking about pain DEPRESSION Attributed to pain or impact of pain Attributed to other causes Unattributed PTSD SYMPTOMS Re-experiencing Avoidance
		Gynaecological	Vulvar Vestibular Clitoral Endometriosis associated CPPS with cyclical exacerbations Dysmenorrhea					
		Gastrointestinal	Irritable bowel Chronic anal Intermittent chronic anal					
		Peripheral nerves	Pudendal pain syndrome					
		Sexological	Dyspareunia Pelvic pain with sexual dysfunction					
		Psychological	Any pelvic organ					
		Musculo-skeletal	Pelvic floor muscle Abdominal muscle Spinal Coccyx					

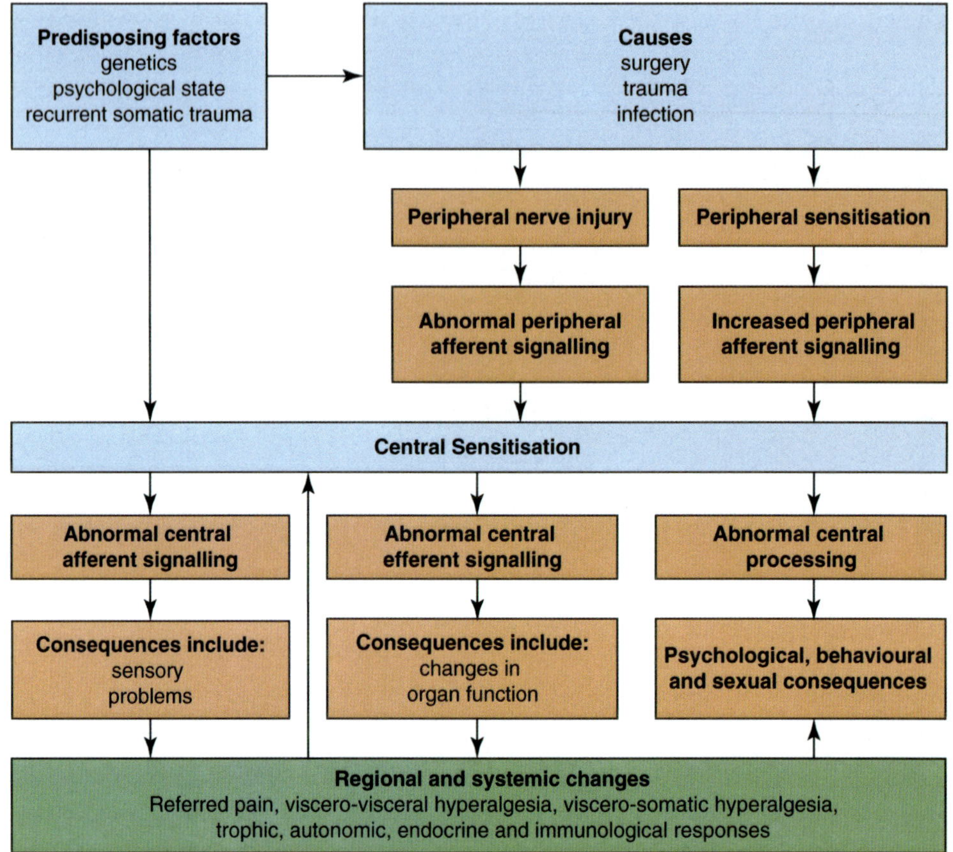

FIGURE 1 Predisposing factors, cause, central and peripheral mechanisms[4] (from EAU guidelines).

(e.g. bladder, vaginal and pudendal). Psychological disturbance is common and may occur with many conditions but are not considered until axis VII.

A newer and different representation of the classification has been developed by the EAU in order to aid both an academic and clinical understanding of this patient group (Fig. 1)[4]. This covers the predisposing factors, causes, central and peripheral mechanisms. Some detail can be added to each of the boxes but it is also understood that there remains a significant amount to be elucidated.

It is not prescriptive about a cause but does suggest predisposing factors. The basic science elements have a significant amount of understanding but gaps remain. This model allows alterations in organ function that may have a central component, altered sensory perception, changes in psychological, behavioural, and sexual function. This is true for all the pelvic pain syndromes and the balance and complexion of presentation will vary from patient to patient which again this model allows.

FUTURE DEVELOPMENTS

Along with this strand of work there has been a significant amount of parallel developments and potential avenues for further exploration.

Guidelines and pathways have become very popular over recent years in many countries. The European Association of Urology[4] has taken this to heart and the chronic pelvic pain guidelines have been well received and frequently downloaded by a wide range of specialities. They are updated very regularly and have open access for download. There are other published guidance documents from organisations such as: American Urological Association[6], American committee of obstetrics and gynaecology[1], Royal College of Obstetrics and Gynaecology[8,9], British Society for the Study of Vulval Disease (BSSVD) [10], International Consultation on Incontinence[5], this is not an exhaustive list. Often the guidance is aimed at relatively specific groups such as endometriosis, vulvodynia, bladder pain syndrome but some are broader in direction. More recently the British Pain Society[11] in conjunction with the map of medicine have developed a patient pathway which is evidence based, reference graded and externally reviewed with the aim of supporting primary care physicians manage this patient population and a second part for secondary care. The committee that developed the pathway included patients and was truly multiprofessional.

Education in pain management is poorly taught across many disciplines in a general sense [3,12,14]. There has been debate as to what and how to train health care workers with regard to pelvic and abdominal pain. This includes what and at what depth but also who to develop and how to make the teams managing these patients most effective. The clarification of terminology and growing understanding of management strategies should help develop this strand of work.

Research opportunities are now becoming more apparent with greater consistence in terminology. It should be easier to evaluate published papers and potentially compare them. With the increasing involvement of patient organizations and growing understanding of the underlying factors influencing pelvic and abdominal pain the research agenda is broadening its focus.

Joint working, traditionally there have been growing numbers of groups (patient and professional) looking at elements of pelvic pain, all having their own meetings and published guidance. The development of unifying the terminology has allowed connections to be made between these groups and realization of mutual understanding. It has become possible to have meetings supported and organized by groups working together such as the 19th International Pelvic Pain Society annual scientific meeting in 2011 (Turkey) and this, the 1st World Congress on Abdominal and Pelvic Pain 2013 (Amsterdam). None of the member groups looses its autonomy or focus but a much greater integration of our understanding can occur between the institutions, patients groups, and professionals working in the field.

In summery there was a great deal of confusion with regard to the terminology used for patients with pelvic and abdominal pain. This hindered our understanding of the problem and how best to manage it. The research data was difficult to compare and understand whilst being largely focused on end organ disease. There were a growing number of organisations developing with an interest in often localised elements of these problems and little cross communications between them. The development of broader interest groups, the involvement of the EAU and pelvic pain guidelines (in Europe) and some individuals being members of more than one interested organisation allowed a task force to form looking specifically at the terminology and attempt to unify it. This came to fruition with the IASP ratifying the taxonomy on 2012. Although there continues to be debate and discussion, a much greater degree of mutual understanding has occurred with potential benefits for clinicians, researchers, and above all patients. This is only the beginning and highlights more questions and opportunities than it solves but with greater mutual understanding a way forward can continue to be developed.

TAKE HOME MESSAGES

- Using the agreed terminology eases communication for clinicians, researchers, and patients.
- Pain is multidimensional in nature having biological, psychological, and social components. Using the suggested schema provides an outline of potential areas involved, how they interact and can be developed as our understanding continues
- Bringing together the organisations and individuals involved in pelvic and abdominal pain is allowing a better understanding of the bigger picture, reducing the risk of duplication of work and further confusion for professionals and patients alike.
- There is growing awareness of this population, increasing research activity, guidance on management, and a desire to increase professional education on management strategies for both the generalist who occasionally sees this population, as well as, the specialist in abdominal and pelvic pain.

REFERENCES

1. ACOG Practice Bulletin No. 51. Chronic pelvic pain. Obstet Gynecol 2004;103(3):589–605.
2. Berry SH, Bogart LM, Pham C, et al. Development, validation and testing of an epidemiological case definition of interstitial cystitis/painful bladder syndrome. J Urol 2010;183(5):1848–1852.
3. Briggs EV, Carr EC, Whittaker MS. Survey of undergraduate pain curricula for healthcare professionals in the United Kingdom. Eur J Pain 2011;15(8):789–795.
4. Engeler D, Baranowski AP, Elneil S, et al. EAU guidelines on chronic pelvic pain: European Association of Urology, 2012.
5. Hanno P, Lin A, Nordling J, et al. Bladder Pain Syndrome Committee of the International Consultation on Incontinence. Neurourol Urodyn 2010;29(1):191–198.
6. Hanno PM, Burks DA, Clemens JQ, et al. AUA guideline for the diagnosis and treatment of interstitial cystitis/bladder pain syndrome. J Urol 2011;185(6):2162–2170.
7. IASP Taxonomy Working Group. Classification of Chronic Pain. Descriptions of Chronic Pain Syndromes and Definitions of Pain Terms. Second Edition (revised). In: JD Loeser editor: IASP Press, 2012.
8. Kennedy SH, Moore J. Guideline No. 41. The Initial Management of Chronic Pelvic Pain, Vol. Guideline No. 41: Royal College of Obstetricians and Gynaecologists, 2005.
9. Kennedy SH, Moore J. Guideline No. 24. The Investigation and Management of Endometriosis., Vol. Guideline No. 24: Royal College of Obstetricians and Gynaecologists, 2006.
10. Mandal D, Nunns D, Byrne M, et al. Guidelines for the management of vulvodynia. Br J Dermatol 2010;162(6):1180–1185.
11. Map of Medicine, The British Pain Society. Chronic pelvic pain (in men and women). England View. . London: Map of Medicine, 2012.
12. Mezei L, Murinson BB. Pain education in North American medical schools. J Pain 2011;12(12):1199–1208.
13. Thomas TG. Practical Treatise on the Diseases of Women. Philadelphia: Henry C Lea, 1868.
14. Watt-Watson J, McGillion M, Hunter J, et al. A survey of prelicensure pain curricula in health science faculties in Canadian universities. Pain Res Manage 2009;14(6):439–444.

CHAPTER 3

From Animal Data to Human Practice

Tony Buffington

INTRODUCTION

The study of chronic abdominal and pelvic pain syndromes is in a healthy stage of ferment. From my perspective as a veterinary clinical scientist studying one of these syndromes, interstitial cystitis (IC), also known by the International Association for the Study of Pain (IASP) as Bladder Pain Syndrome (BPS), in domestic cats and human beings, answers to basic questions about the causes of these syndromes that has hindered progress for centuries finally seem clearer. This clarity is particularly significant from the perspective of development of useful animal models of these syndromes, because some agreement on the causes of these syndromes will improve the relevance of contributions from animal models to our understanding of the etiopathogenesis and treatment of these syndromes.

For animal data to inform treatment of human beings with naturally occurring disease, the data obtained from the animals must be relevant to the disease modeled. The utility of animal models of chronic abdominal and pelvic pain syndromes thus depends on how closely the model resembles the condition to which it is compared. Helpful criteria [93] for considering the usefulness of animal models include:

Face validity—the degree of phenomenological similarity between the model and the disease modeled. Although necessary, this criterion is not sufficient due to the limited repertoire of responses to noxious stimuli available to most organ systems.

Construct validity—the extent to which the model has a sound theoretical rationale. This criterion first requires a good theoretical understanding of the etiopathogenesis of the condition modeled, then evidence of congruency of the model with this understanding.

Predictive validity—the similarity in response of the model and naturally occurring disease to disease-modulating interventions.

DESCRIBING THE SUBJECT

Face Validity

The two most common types of animal models of human disease are those of induced disease (or signs of disease) in otherwise healthy animals and investigation of spontaneously occurring disease in animals that bear some resemblance to the human disease of interest. A variety of injuries have been inflicted on healthy animals of various species to study the responses of the abdominal and pelvic organs to different types of noxious stimuli of acute or persistent duration. These studies have revealed important differences in nociceptive responses based on the location, type and duration of the nociceptive stimulus, as well as on the species, strain, age, sex, context, and environmental history of the animal to which it is applied.

Data from both nociceptive and neuropathic injuries of healthy animals and from animals with naturally occurring chronic pain states have contributed importantly to our current understanding of chronic abdominal and pelvic pain syndromes in animals and humans. My introduction to these syndromes occurred during the course of investigations of the etiopathogenesis of lower urinary tract signs (LUTS) in domestic cats (signs as cats can't talk!),[9] a syndrome that shares many features in common with Bladder Pain Syndrome/ Interstitial Cystitis (BPS/IC), a chronic pain syndrome of human beings. We termed the syndrome in cats feline IC (FIC)[13] since the cats seemed to share a comparable disease history and course, and to meet all the applicable inclusion and exclusion criteria for the research diagnosis of IC promulgated by the National Institutes of Diabetes, Digestive and Kidney Diseases[37] that could reasonably be applied to animals.

Induced Models of Etiopathogenesis

Noxious Local Stimuli

Many models of acute abdominal and pelvic injury in healthy animals have been investigated for their potential relevance to human disease. For example, a variety of toxins, including acetone, a variety of acids, turpentine, mustard oil, and croton oil have been instilled into the abdominal and pelvic organs of animals[7,40,42,51,88]. Immune sensitization also has been used to characterize features of the acute response to noxious luminal stimuli. Unfortunately, although many studies have investigated the effects of intraluminally administered agents, and may be of value to further understanding basic mechanisms of the responses of these organs to noxious stimuli, the absence of a demonstrated toxin or other noxious luminal agent involved in these syndromes in human beings, the acute time course, and the histological and functional alterations induced by toxins make these studies difficult to relate to patients with chronic abdominal and pelvic pain syndromes.

Noxious Systemic Stimuli

In addition to local instillation of irritants, the abdominal and pelvic organs also are known to respond to systemic challenges. For example, intravenous injection of Substance P or lipopolysaccharide induced cystitis and increased plasma extravasation in normal, but not in mast cell-deficient mice, indicating that mast cells participate in the inflammatory response of the bladder in these mice[6]. Infection with animals with viruses at remote sites also can inflame abdominal and pelvic organs. In one model, injection of pseudorabies virus into the tail base of healthy rats resulted in inflammation of the bladder, (and colon and prostate gland of some animals) by activation of central nervous system circuits[43].

Irritation of other pelvic organs also affects abdominal and pelvic function by a phenomenon called viscero-visceral hyperalgesia, wherein injury to one visceral organ sometimes can affect function of the others. Examples include ureteral[36] and bladder[29] injury affecting uterine function, and bidirectional cross-sensitization of the colon and lower urinary tract following either acute bladder irritation or colorectal distension[64].

Although the pathways mediating this phenomenon remain to be identified, these models may help explain the commonly observed presence of co-morbid pelvic organ disorders in patients with some forms of abdominal and pelvic pain.

Noxious Environmental Stimuli

Stressful circumstances seem to aggravate symptoms of some patients with chronic abdominal and pelvic pain syndromes, and the effects of some noxious external stimuli have been studied in animal models by exposing them to stressors like prolonged restraint[72] or illumination[44], water avoidance or cold temperature[32,33], and maternal separation[65]. Evaluation of the urothelium of animals exposed to some of these conditions revealed disruption of tight junctions between superficial urothelial cells and desquamation of superficial cells, which exposed the underlying intermediate cells to the bladder lumen and its contents. Desquamation appears to be a non-specific bladder defense mechanism, also occurring after E. coli adherence[22; 59], administration of lipopolysaccharide [44], ischemia[50], systemic administration of hydrocortisone or norepinephrine, or removal of calcium[83], and also occurs in the colon [69], intestine [94], lung [38], and skin [25] in response to a variety of noxious stimuli. Desquamation may increase epithelial permeability, permitting increased access of external stimuli to neurons and inflammatory cells, which may mediate part of the organism's response to noxious environmental stimuli.

These studies of the role of external stimuli on epithelial integrity suggest that complex mechanisms mediate central nervous system activation of local inflammation during stressful circumstances. The inflammatory response to acute external stressors may partially explain the observation of submucosal petechial hemorrhages (glomerulations) in healthy women undergoing tubal ligation; one might imagine that they may have perceived this procedure as stressful[86].

Corticotrophin releasing factor (CRF) appears to be one mediator of the range of stress responses to internal and external stimuli[78]. CRF over expressing (CRF-OE) mice show a number of physiologic and behavioral features that parallel those seen in chronically stressed animals and humans[21]. For example, 60 minutes of restraint stress, exposure to a novel environment (individually placed into a novel cage for 60 min) or 2 minutes of handling of adult female wild type and CRF-OE mice did not affect frequency of either defecation or micturition, which increased from baseline in both groups. However, exposure to novel environment and brief handling significantly increased frequency of defecation and urination, as well as time spent grooming and rearing, in CRF-OE mice only. These data provide evidence that chronically increased stress reactivity can increase abdominal and pelvic organ responsiveness to additional mild stressors, whereas the response to more severe stimuli (restraint) is similar to that of control mice[58].

Studies of healthy animals have thus provided an essential description of the complexity of responses of the abdominal and pelvic organs to a variety of insults, and have demonstrated that both local and distant factors can result in pathology. The relevance of these models to the cause(s) of chronic abdominal and pelvic pain syndromes, however, is less clear. The identified responses usually are not specific to a particular organ, and when the stimulus is removed, healthy animals appear to return to normal rather quickly[32].

Naturally Occurring Models of Etiopathogenesis

Naturally occurring models of abdominal and pelvic distress also have been reported, including colitis in cotton-topped tamarins,[96] endometriosis in primates,[40] and FIC in domestic cats[9]. Because I am most familiar with FIC, and because it is the most developed of these models, I will focus on it.

Depending on one's perspective, FIC appears to have the greatest face validity for IC of any animal model currently available. The syndrome of BPS/IC in cats and humans is remarkably similar[11]. FIC primarily resembles non-ulcer IC in humans [13] (Bladder Pain Syndrome Type 2 according to the ESSIC Criteria [82]), although ulceration and inflammatory infiltrates occasionally have been reported in cats [12]. Patients of both species have abnormalities of local bladder factors, as well as involvement of the afferent, central, and efferent limbs of the nervous system [11] and a common serum infrared spectral pattern[68]. Variable combinations of comorbid disorders also have been identified in patients of both species [11,14,77]. Moreover, the occurrence of comorbid disorders often precedes the occurrence of LUT signs and symptoms in these patients [Buffington, CAT Unpublished observations [84,97]. These comorbid disorders also appear to occur more commonly in close relatives of human patients [18,27,87] and evidence of adverse early experiences has been reported in patients with FIC [91] and BPS/IC [8].

Like the induced models of bladder injury, FIC also has limitations as a model of BPS/IC. One is the seemingly different gender distribution between affected males and females of the two species. In cats, both genders are affected roughly equally, whereas in humans, early studies suggested that 90% of patients were women[45]. Recent reports, however, suggest that the gender difference in humans may not be as large as originally thought [20,45], if it exists at all[57,76].

Another limitation to using cats with FIC to investigate etiologic mechanisms of BPS/IC is that affected animals are not easy to acquire without veterinarian and owner cooperation. Additionally, cats are more expensive to maintain in laboratory animal facilities than are rodents, are outbred, and many molecular probes have not been validated for use in this species. Despite these limitations, studies of cats with FIC have duplicated many results obtained in humans with BPS/IC, and even predicted some abnormalities that were subsequently found in humans with BPS/IC[26,80]. Moreover, a wealth of bladder and stress neuroscience research conducted in cats is available to compare anatomic and functional alterations in the CNS caused by BPS/IC in ways not currently possible in humans or induced models.

Construct Validity

Animal models of chronic abdominal and pelvic pain syndromes struggle to demonstrate construct validity, because no good theoretical understanding of the etiopathogenesis of these conditions has yet been agreed to. For example, BPS/IC has been thought to be an inflammatory disorder of the bladder for centuries[63]. A syndrome of chronic frequency, urgency, dysuria and pelvic pain in the absence of demonstrable etiology was described in a textbook published in 1836, and BPS/IC still is described like this by some to the present day[28].

Unfortunately this situation has left many basic scientists interested in contributing to a better understanding of these disorders in a position reminiscent of the blind men and an elephant[92]. In these stories, some blind men touch an elephant to learn what elephants are like. Each one feels a different part and describes their findings to each other, only to find out that they are in complete disagreement about what elephants are like. With regard to abdominal and pelvic organs, for example, in the absence of an accepted etiopathogenesis cell physiologists have generally focused on epithelial surfaces, immunologists on immune cells and function, endocrinologists on hormones, and neurophysiologists on peripheral nerves to produce face valid models of isolated features of these syndromes.

Part of the problem is embedded in the very nosology of terms such as "chronic abdominal and pelvic pain syndromes". Nosology refers to the naming of diseases, which may be designated according to etiology, pathogenesis, affected organ system(s) and by presenting signs and symptoms. Feinstein[34] recently concluded that, "An important principle in naming apparently new ailments is to avoid etiologic titles until the etiologic agent has been suitably demonstrated. A premature causal name can impair a patient's recovery from the syndrome and impede research that might find the true cause."

A significant challenge to accurate nosology exists because diseases often are named based on prominent signs and symptoms long before research identifies their etiology and pathogenesis. For example, traditional terminology like "abdominal and pelvic pain", "IC (and its many recent variant names)", "irritable bowel syndrome", "vulvodynia", and "endometriosis" seem to suggest to many patients, clinicians, and researchers that the organ included in the name represents the source of the problem. Whereas prominent presenting symptoms may result in naming a disease for the organ associated with them, the disease may not originate in the affected organ, and many diseases affect more than one organ.

Although terms such as "abdominal and pelvic pain", "IC", "irritable bowel syndrome", "vulvodynia", and "endometriosis" fairly accurately describe the currently recognized diagnostic criteria for the organ-specific aspects of these disorders, recent clinical research has revealed that they no longer seem to capture the extent of the problems occurring in many patients to whom these labels are applied[56,85]. These labels all focus on a peripheral organ, reflecting the prominent presenting signs and organ-focused diagnostic testing specific to the particular medical or surgical (sub)specialist evaluating the patient, rather than reflecting the results of a thorough evaluation of the entire patient[47].

More recent, comprehensive investigations of these patients has resulted in the suggestion of a variety of rather vague descriptive terms such as "medically unexplained syndrome"[71], "functional somatic syndrome"[1], or "central sensitivity syndrome"[98] to describe the multiple abnormalities often observed in these patients, whereas the IASP has chosen to use the term "chronic pelvic pain". The list of chronic disorders proposed to be covered by these names is long, and includes problems addressed by most of the medical subspecialties[8]. These names also seem to violate Feinstein's admonition, however, so it seems that some generic umbrella term comparable to "cancer" or "infection" might be preferable for the present. I have suggested adoption of "Pandora Syndrome" as an interim name for FIC until the most biologically appropriate nosological term is identified in cats[9].

One fairly consistent recent finding has been a role for early life experiences in creating vulnerability for development of chronic disease syndromes later in life,[3] including a variety of chronic pain and other "medically unexplained" syndromes[17,39,46,52,61,66,95]. Some animal models of these events also have been investigated, including maternal separation, provision of limited nesting material, and neonatal irritation of the colon[2] or bladder[24]. Animals subjected to the maternal separation or limited nesting material interventions develop changes in hypothalamic-pituitary-adrenal activity, and have been used extensively in mental health-related research[4]. It also has been found that these treatments also can result in visceral hypersensitivity in adulthood[62]. Additionally, neonatal colonic irritation by infusion of mustard oil or repeated distension [2] and exposure of the neonatal bladder to zymosan [24] have also been shown to cause visceral hypersensitivity.

These models might even be more useful if investigators with interest in different organs or processes could collaborate to more comprehensively investigate the effects of these manipulations on the animals subjected to them. An example of the value of such integration is a presented in a recent review [62] which describes the components of the brain–gut axis individually and how they are altered by maternal separation in rodents. Animals that had been exposed to maternal separation had alterations of intestinal barrier function and balance of enteric microflora, as well as exaggerated stress responses and visceral hypersensitivity as adults, all of which occur in humans with the modeled disease - irritable bowel syndrome. It is easy to imagine that thorough scrutiny of other organs might yield additional discoveries[49,55].

There possibly also are different kinds of "BPS/IC"[85], although the extent to which these represent distinct diseases or variability in the clinical manifestations of a common underlying etiology currently is unknown. Baranowski, et al.[5], have suggested that there may be three groups; patients with bladder symptoms only, patients with more generalized pelvic pain, and patients with multiple systemic symptoms. As shown in Table 1, two studies subsequently evaluated the distribution of patients in each of these groups:

Warren, et al. [84], used eleven syndromes to categorize patients, whereas Nickel, et al. [60], used three in their 2010 study. If these classifications apply to cats, those with Pandora Syndrome may have acceptable construct validity as a model of patients with multiple systemic symptoms[9].

Predictive Validity

Induced Models of Treatment

Pharmacological treatment of animals with induced models of chronic abdominal and pelvic pain syndromes has been reported, but to my knowledge none of the agents tested has been translated into effective clinical therapy to date. In contrast, effects of social and environmental manipulations of mice three months after induction of chronic neuropathic pain recently were reported[81]. In this study, seven to eight week-old male CD-1 mice underwent surgery to induce the spared nerve injury model of neuropathic pain or sham condition, after which they were assigned to one of four groups: nerve injury with enriched environment, nerve injury with impoverished environment, sham surgery with enriched environment, or sham surgery with impoverished environment (n = 8-9 per group). The effects of environmental manipulations on cutaneous mechanical heat and cold sensitivities, motor impairment, spontaneous exploratory behavior, anxiety-like behavior, and depression-like phenotype were assessed one and two months after the environmental changes.

Environmental enrichment attenuated nerve injury-induced hypersensitivity to mechanical and cold stimuli, while the impoverished environment exacerbated mechanical hypersensitivity; no antidepressant effects of enrichment were observed in this study. The authors concluded that environmental enrichment was a safe, inexpensive, and easily implemented non-pharmacological intervention that might play an important role in

TABLE 1 **Evaluation of Different Kinds of BPS/IC**

	Patient Group		
Study	Bladder only	Other Pelvic Symptoms	Systemic symptoms
Warren, et al.[82]	7%	2%	91%
Nickel, et al.[60]	56%	27%	16%
Nickel, et al.[59]	13%		87%

the rehabilitation of chronic pain patients well after the establishment of chronic pain. Although this study investigated chronic somatic rather than abdominal and pelvic pain, similar effectiveness has been found in cats with FIC, as described below.

Naturally Occurring Model of Treatment

In cats with FIC, laboratory studies have revealed that environmental enrichment was associated not only with reduction in LUT signs, but with normalization of circulating catecholamine concentrations, bladder permeability, cardiac function [89,90], and reduced responses to acoustic startle[41]. We also conducted a ten-month prospective observational study of client-owned cats with moderate to severe FIC[10]. In addition to their usual care, clients were offered individualized recommendations for multimodal environmental modification based on a detailed environmental history obtained from the owner. In addition to significant reductions in LUT signs, decreased fearfulness, nervousness, signs referable to the respiratory tract, and a trend toward reduced fear-like behaviors were identified.

We have also observed sickness behaviors after environmental enrichment, both in healthy cats and in cats with FIC, in response to unusual external events[73]. Sickness behaviors refer to a group of nonspecific clinical and behavioral signs and symptoms that include variable combinations of vomiting, diarrhea, anorexia or decreased food and water intake, fever, lethargy, somnolence, enhanced pain-like behaviors, decreased general activity, body-care activities, and social interactions[23]. These behaviors are well-documented physiologic and behavioral responses to infection found in all species studied, and also occur in response to aversive environmental events[54]. Psychological stressors recently have been linked to immune activation and pro-inflammatory cytokine release[67] as well as to changes in mood and pathological pain[75]. Thus, sickness behaviors can result both from activation of either peripheral (e.g., infection) or central (e.g., psychological) pathways, or both.

Increasing age and weeks when unusual external events occurred, but not disease status, resulted in a significant increase in total sickness behaviors observed in the cats when controlled for other factors. Unusual external events were associated with significantly increased risks for decreases in food intake and elimination, increases in defecation and urination outside the litter box. These results suggest that some of the abnormalities observed in cats with FIC may represent amplifications of responses observed in healthy animals, possibly due to differences in genetics, early life experience, or disease chronicity, as appears to be the case in humans with BPS/IC and other chronic abdominal and pelvic pain syndromes[18].

Warren et al. [85], recently suggested three hypotheses about the causes of BPS/IC that accommodate the presence of multiple systemic symptoms in these patients: (1) that BPS/IC initiates a pathophysiology that results in other disorders, (2) that these disorders initiate a pathophysiology that results in other disorders and in BPS/IC, and (3) that a preceding pathophysiology results in both. One way to exclude one or more of these hypotheses would be a to conduct a prospective longitudinal study of healthy individuals. Another would be to treat patients with BPS/IC to determine the effect on their systemic symptoms. If other symptoms remained in recovered patients, hypothesis 1 would be excluded, if other symptoms were treated and BPS/IC remained, hypothesis 2 would be excluded, and if a hypothesized underlying pathology was treated and BPS/IC remained, hypothesis 3 would be excluded.

Effective environmental enrichment might be conceptualized as one treatment approach to test these hypotheses. What we have found in both in cage-confined and client-owned cats with FIC is that enrichment results in statistically and clinically significant improvements in all disease signs, arguing against exclusion of hypothesis 3. The fact that these improvements occurred in the absence of any treatment directed at the bladder or any other peripheral organ provides evidence for exclusion of hypotheses 1 and 2. I await comparable studies in human beings with BPS/IC to determine the extent to which these results are predictive of responses in them.

PRACTICAL IMPLICATIONS

Animal models appear to have made relatively few documentable contributions to drugs that can be used in practical situations by clinicians treating patients with chronic abdominal and pelvic pain syndromes, or for any other chronic pain condition for that matter[30]. In contrast, environmental enrichment has resulted in statistically and clinically significant improvements in both a chronic induced model and a naturally occurring model of neuropathic pain, one of which serves as a model for BPS/IC.

But what does environmental enrichment mean for clinicians? One significant difference between human and non-human animals is their level of consciousness. While animals may be said to have primary consciousness to varying degrees, only humans appear to have secondary consciousness – understanding the potential meaning of symptoms for their personal, social and financial futures. This knowledge can be a double-edged sword. On the one hand, as natural and understandable as it is, ruminating and catastrophizing about one's pain can exacerbate it[31,35]. On the other hand, effective doctor-patient communications [16,19], empathy[53] and cognitive behavioral therapy[48] may reduce pain and other symptoms in patients with chronic medically unexplained syndromes, and might be conceptualized as "environmental enrichment". While cognitive and emotional control are disrupted in chronic pain patients,[15] recent studies of cognitive behavioral therapy have shown that multiple functional somatic symptoms improve with effective therapy [70], as has been found for environmental enrichment for cats.

LOOKING AT THE FUTURE

To return to the blind men and the elephant, stories differ in how violent the conflict between the differing perspectives becomes, and how (or if) the conflicts are resolved. In some versions, they stop talking, reminding one of Max Plank's observation that "*...a new scientific truth does not triumph by convincing its opponents and making them see the light, but rather because its opponents eventually die, and a new generation grows up that is familiar with it.*" In other versions, they start listening and collaborating with each other so that all can eventually "see" the full elephant – the choice is ours.

TAKE HOME MESSAGES

The most important things I have learned from the study of BPS/IC in both cats and people that may be pertinent to other chronic abdominal and pelvic pain syndromes are:

- These are complex syndromes; current evidence suggests to me that BPS/IC is more likely to be a syndrome affecting the bladder than a bladder disease in most cases. If this is the case, urologists, as acute care-focused subspecialty surgeons, are more suited to the diagnosis of BPS/IC than the ongoing care of patients with a chronic medical syndrome. Perseverative efforts to force the disease back into the bladder seem unlikely to succeed.

- Although animal models have provided a wealth of basic scientific information about abdominal and pelvic organ responses to a range of noxious stimuli, these models were based on the presumption that the diseases modeled arose in the organ for which they were named; this no longer seems to be the case for many patients with BPS/IC. One hopes that collaboration among investigators with interest in different organs or processes will permit more thorough evaluation of ecologically relevant models of stress and disease. Such investigations could simultaneously accelerate acquisition of knowledge and reduce the number of animals subjected to these noxious procedures.
- Novel therapies may become more available based on classification of these disorders as central sensitivity syndromes as appropriate. These may include pharmacological agents that modulate gene expression [74,79], as well as online and coaching-based self-management – if evidence for their effectiveness can be demonstrated.

FURTHER READING

Books

Pain in women; A Clinical Guide. New York: Springer; 2013.

Bladder Pain Syndrome A Guide for Clinicians. New York: Springer; 2013.

Smith's Patient-Centered Interviewing – an evidence-based method.

Review articles

Franklin TB, Saab BJ, Mansuy IM. Neural mechanisms of stress resilience and vulnerability. *Neuron.* Sep 6 2012;75(5):747–761.

Larauche M, Mulak A, Tache Y. Stress and visceral pain: From animal models to clinical therapies. *Experimental Neurology.* Jan 2012;233(1):49–67.

Mayer EA, Tillisch K. The brain-gut axis in abdominal pain syndromes. *Annual review of medicine.* 2011;62:381–396.

REFERENCES

1. Ablin K, Clauw DJ. From Fibrositis to Functional Somatic Syndromes to a Bell-Shaped Curve of Pain and Sensory Sensitivity: Evolution of a Clinical Construct. Rheum Dis Clin N Am 2009;35(2):233–251.
2. Al-Chaer ED, Kawasaki M, Pasricha PJ. A new model of chronic visceral hypersensitivity in adult rats induced by colon irritation during postnatal development. Gastroenterology 2000;119(5):1276–1285.
3. Anda RF, Felitti VJ, Bremner JD, et al. The enduring effects of abuse and related adverse experiences in childhood - A convergence of evidence from neurobiology and epidemiology. Eur Arch Psyc Clin Neurosci 2006;256(3):174–186.
4. Bale TL, Baram TZ, Brown AS, et al. Early Life Programming and Neurodevelopmental Disorders. Biolog Psych 2010;68(4):314–319.
5. Baranowski AP, Abrams P, Berger RE, et al. Urogenital pain--time to accept a new approach to phenotyping and, as a consequence, management. Eur Urol 2008;53(1):33–36.
6. Bjorling DE, Jerde TJ, Zine MJ, et al. Mast cells mediate the severity of experimental cystitis in mice. J Urol 1999;162(1):231–236.
7. Bjorling DE, Wang ZY, Bushman W. Models of inflammation of the lower urinary tract. Neurourol Urodyn 2011;30(5):673–682.
8. Buffington CA. Developmental influences on medically unexplained symptoms. Psychother Psychosom 2009;78(3):139–144.
9. Buffington CA. Idiopathic cystitis in domestic cats-beyond the lower urinary tract. J Vet Intern Med 2011;25(4):784–796.
10. Buffington CA, Westropp JL, Chew DJ, Bolus RR. Clinical evaluation of multimodal environmental modification (MEMO) in the management of cats with idiopathic cystitis. J Feline Med Surg 2006;8(4):261–268.
11. Buffington CAT. Comorbidity of Interstitial Cystitis with other Unexplained Clinical Conditions. J Urol 2004;172:1242–1248.

12. Buffington CAT, Chew DJ, Woodworth BE. Animal model of human disease - feline interstitial cystitis. Comp Pathol Bull 1997;29(1):3,6.
13. Buffington CAT, Chew DJ, Woodworth BE. Feline Interstitial Cystitis. J Am Vet Med Assoc 1999;215(5):682–687.
14. Buffington CAT, Westropp JL, Chew DJ, Bolus RR. A case-control study of indoor-housed cats with lower urinary tract signs. J Am Vet Med Assoc 2006;228(5):722–725.
15. Bushnell MC, Ceko M, Low LA. Cognitive and emotional control of pain and its disruption in chronic pain. Nature Reviews Neuroscience 2013;14(7):502–511.
16. Butow P, Sharpe L. The impact of communication on adherence in pain management. Pain 2013;154 (Suppl 1):S101–107.
17. Chaloner A, Greenwood-Van Meerveld B. Early life adversity as a risk factor for visceral pain in later life: importance of sex differences. Frontiers Neurosci 2013;7:13.
18. Chelimsky G, Heller E, Buffington CA, et al T. Co-morbidities of interstitial cystitis. Frontiers Neurosci 2012;6(114):1–6.
19. Chelimsky TC, Fischer RL, Levin JB, et al. The primary practice physician program for chronic pain ((c) 4PCP): outcomes of a primary physician-pain specialist collaboration for community-based training and support. Clin J Pain 2013;29(12):1036–1043.
20. Clemens JQ, Meenan RT, Rosetti MC, et al. Prevalence and incidence of interstitial cystitis in a managed care population. J Urol 2005;173(1):98–102; discussion 102.
21. Coste SC, Murray SE, Stenzel-Poore MP. Animal models of CRH excess and CRH receptor deficiency display altered adaptations to stress. Peptides 2001;22(5):733–741.
22. Dalal E, Medalia O, Harari O, Aronson M. Moderate stress protects female mice against bacterial infection of the bladder by eliciting uroepithelial shedding. Infect Immun 1994;62(12):5505–5510.
23. Dantzer R, O'Connor JC, Freund GG, et al. From inflammation to sickness and depression: when the immune system subjugates the brain. Nat Rev Neurosci 2008;9(1):46–56.
24. DeBerry J, Ness TJ, Robbins MT, Randich A. Inflammation-induced enhancement of the visceromotor reflex to urinary bladder distention: modulation by endogenous opioids and the effects of early-in-life experience with bladder inflammation. J Pain 2007;8(12):914–923.
25. Denda M, Tsuchiya T, Elias PM, Feingold KR. Stress alters cutaneous permeability barrier homeostasis. Am J Physiol-Regul Integr Comp Physiol 2000;278(2):R367-R372.
26. Dimitrakov J, Joffe HV, Soldin SJ, et al. Adrenocortical hormone abnormalities in men with chronic prostatitis/chronic pelvic pain syndrome. Urology 2008;71(2):261–266.
27. Dimitrakov JD. A case of familial clustering of interstitial cystitis and chronic pelvic pain syndrome. Urology 2001;58(2):281.
28. Diniz S, Dinis P, Cruz F, Pinto R. Bladder pain syndrome/interstitial cystitis: present and future treatment perspectives. Minerva Urol Nefrol 2013;65(4):263–276.
29. Dmitrieva N, Berkley KJ. Contrasting effects of WIN 55212–2 on motility of the rat bladder and uterus. J Neurosci 2002;22(16):7147–7153.
30. Dworkin RH, Turk DC, Peirce-Sandner S, et al. Considerations for improving assay sensitivity in chronic pain clinical trials: IMMPACT recommendations. Pain 2012;153(6):1148–1158.
31. Eccleston C, Crombez G. Worry and chronic pain: a misdirected problem solving model. Pain 2007;132(3):233–236.
32. Ercan F, San T, Cavdar S. The effects of cold-restraint stress on urinary bladder wall compared with interstitial cystitis morphology. Urol Res 1999;27(6):454–461.
33. Erin N, Ercan F, Yegen BC, et al. Role of capsaicin-sensitive nerves in gastric and hepatic injury induced by cold-restraint stress. Digest Dis Sci 2000;45(9):1889–1899.
34. Feinstein AR. The Blame-X syndrome: Problems and lessons in nosology, spectrum, and etiology. J Clin Epidemiol 2001;54(5):433–439.
35. Flink IL, Boersma K, Linton SJ. Pain Catastrophizing as Repetitive Negative Thinking: A Development of the Conceptualization. Cogn Behav Ther 2013;42(3):215–223.
36. Giamberardino MA, Berkley KJ, Affaitati G, et al. Influence of endometriosis on pain behaviors and muscle hyperalgesia induced by a ureteral calculosis in female rats. Pain 2002;95(3):247–257.
37. Gillenwater JY, Wein AJ. Summary of the National Institute of Arthritis, Diabetes, Digestive and Kidney Diseases workshop on interstitial cystitis. J Urol 1988;140:203–206.
38. Godfrey RWA. Human airway epithelial tight junctions. Microsc Res Techn 1997;38(5):488–499.
39. Gonzalez A, Boyle MH, Kyu HH, et al. Childhood and family influences on depression, chronic physical conditions, and their comorbidity: findings from the Ontario Child Health Study. J Psych Res 2012;46(11):1475–1482.
40. Grummer R. Animal models in endometriosis research. Human Reprod Update 2006;12(5):641–649.

41. Hague DW, Stella JL, Buffington CA. Effects of interstitial cystitis on the acoustic startle reflex in cats. Am J Vet Res 2013;74(1):144–147.
42. Jabr RI, Fry CH. Animal Models of Lower Urinary Tract Dysfunction. Animal Models for the Study of Human Disease 2013:461–481.
43. Jasmin L, Janni G, Manz HJ, Rabkin SD. Activation of CNS circuits proceeding a neurogenic cystitis: Evidence for centrally induced peripheral inflammation. J Neurosci 1998;18(23):10016–10029.
44. Jezernik K, Medalia O, Aronson M. A comparative study of the desquamation of urothelial cells during gestation and in adult mice following moderate stress or endotoxin treatment. Cell Biology International 1995;19(11):887–893.
45. Jones CA, Nyberg L. Epidemiology of interstitial cystitis. Urology 1997;49(5A):2–9.
46. Jones GT, Power C, Macfarlane GJ. Adverse events in childhood and chronic widespread pain in adult life: Results from the 1958 British Birth Cohort Study. Pain 2009;143(1–2):92–96.
47. Kartha GK, Kerr H, Shoskes DA. Clinical phenotyping of urologic pain patients. Curr Opin Urol 2013;23(6):560–564.
48. Kerns RD, Sellinger J, Goodin BR. Psychological treatment of chronic pain. Ann Rev Clin Psych 2011;7:411–434.
49. Kinkead R, Gulemetova R. Neonatal maternal separation and neuroendocrine programming of the respiratory control system in rats. Biol Psychol 2010;84(1):26–38.
50. Korosec P, Jezernik K. Early cellular and ultrastructural response of the mouse urinary bladder urothelium to ischemia. Virchows Arch 2000;436(4):377–383.
51. Larauche M, Mulak A, Tache Y. Stress and visceral pain: from animal models to clinical therapies. Exp Neurol 2012;233(1):49–67.
52. Li Q, Winston JH, Sarna SK. Developmental origins of colon smooth muscle dysfunction in IBS-like rats. Am J Physiol Gastrointest Liver Physiol 2013;305(7):G503–512.
53. Lumley MA, Cohen JL, Borszcz GS, et al. Pain and emotion: a biopsychosocial review of recent research. J Clin Psychol 2011;67(9):942–968.
54. Marques-Deak A, Cizza G, Sternberg E. Brain-immune interactions and disease susceptibility. Molec Psych 2005;10(3):239–250.
55. Martisova E, Aisa B, Guerenu G, Ramirez MJ. Effects of early maternal separation on biobehavioral and neuropathological markers of Alzheimer's disease in adult male rats. Curr Alzheimer Res 2013;10(4):420–432.
56. Mayer EA, Tillisch K. The brain-gut axis in abdominal pain syndromes. Ann Revi Med 2011;62:381–396.
57. Miller JL, Rothman I, Bavendam TG, Berger RE. Prostatodynia and interstitial cystitis: one and the same? Urology 1994;45:587–590.
58. Million M, Wang L, Stenzel-Poore MP, et al. Enhanced pelvic responses to stressors in female CRF-overexpressing mice. Am J Physiol 2007;292(4):R1429-R1438.
59. Mulvey MA, Schilling JD, Martinez JJ, Hultgren SJ. Bad bugs and beleaguered bladders: Interplay between uropathogenic Escherichia coli and innate host defenses. Proc Natl Acad Sci USA 2000;97(16):8829–8835.
60. Nickel JC, Tripp DA, Pontari M, et al. Interstitial cystitis/painful bladder syndrome and associated medical conditions with an emphasis on irritable bowel syndrome, fibromyalgia and chronic fatigue syndrome. J Urol 2010;184(4):1358–1363.
61. Nickel JC, Tripp DA, Pontari M, et al. Childhood sexual trauma in women with interstitial cystitis/bladder pain syndrome: a case control study. Can Urol Assoc J 2011;5(6):410–415.
62. O'Mahony SM, Hyland NP, Dinan TG, Cryan JF. Maternal separation as a model of brain-gut axis dysfunction. Psychopharmacology 2011;214(1):71–88.
63. Parsons JK, Parsons CL. The historical origins of interstitial cystitis. J Urol 2004;171(1):20–22.
64. Pezzone MA, Liang R, Fraser MO. A model of neural cross-talk and irritation in the pelvis: implications for the overlap of chronic pelvic pain disorders. Gastroenterology 2005;128(7):1953–1964.
65. Pierce AN, Ryals JM, Wang R, Christianson JA. Vaginal hypersensitivity and hypothalamic-pituitary-adrenal axis dysfunction as a result of neonatal maternal separation in female mice. Neuroscience 2014;263:216–230.
66. Plante AF, Kamm MA. Life events in patients with vulvodynia. BJOG 2008;115(4):509–514.
67. Raison CL, Miller AH. When not enough is too much: the role of insufficient glucocorticoid signaling in the pathophysiology of stress-related disorders. Am J Psych 2003;160(9):1554–1565.
68. Rubio-Diaz DE, Pozza ME, Dimitrakov J, et al. A candidate serum biomarker for bladder pain syndrome/ interstitial cystitis. Analyst 2009;134(6):1133–1137.
69. Santos J, Saunders PR, Hanssen NPM, et al. Corticotropin-releasing hormone mimics stress-induced colonic epithelial pathophysiology in the rat. Am J Physiol-Gastrointest Liver Physiol 1999;40(2):G391-G399.
70. Schroder A, Rehfeld E, Ornbol E, et al. Cognitive-behavioural group treatment for a range of functional somatic syndromes: randomised trial. Br J Psych 2012;200(6):499–507.

71. Schur EA, Afari N, Furberg H, et al. Feeling bad in more ways than one: comorbidity patterns of medically unexplained and psychiatric conditions. J Gen Intern Med 2007;22(6):818–821.
72. Spanos C, Pang XZ, Ligris K, et al. Stress-induced bladder mast cell activation: implications for interstitial cystitis. J Urol 1997;157(2):669–672.
73. Stella JL, Lord LK, Buffington CAT. Sickness behaviors in response to unusual external events in healthy cats and cats with feline interstitial cystitis. J Am Vet Med Assoc 2011;238(1):67–73.
74. Stone LS, Szyf M. The emerging field of pain epigenetics. Pain 2013;154(1):1–2.
75. Strouse TB. The relationship between cytokines and pain/depression: a review and current status. Curr Pain Headache Rep 2007;11(2):98–103.
76. Suskind AM, Berry SH, Ewing BA, et al. The Prevalence and Overlap of Interstitial Cystitis/Bladder Pain Syndrome and Chronic Prostatitis/Chronic Pelvic Pain Syndrome in Men: Results of the RAND Interstitial Cystitis Epidemiology Male Study. J Urol 2013;189(1):141–145.
77. Suskind AM, Berry SH, Suttorp MJ, et al. Health-related quality of life in patients with interstitial cystitis/bladder pain syndrome and frequently associated comorbidities. Qual Life Res 2013;22(7):1537–1541.
78. Tache Y, Martinez V, Wang L, Million M. CRF1 receptor signaling pathways are involved in stress-related alterations of colonic function and viscerosensitivity: implications for irritable bowel syndrome. Br J Pharmacol 2004;141(8):1321–1330.
79. Tran L, Chaloner A, Sawalha AH, et al. Importance of epigenetic mechanisms in visceral pain induced by chronic water avoidance stress. Psychoneuroendocrinology 2013;38(6):898–906.
80. Twiss C, Kilpatrick L, Craske M, et al. Increased startle responses in interstitial cystitis: evidence for central hyperresponsiveness to visceral related threat. J Urol 2009;181(5):2127–2133.
81. Vachon P, Millecamps M, Low L, et al. Alleviation of chronic neuropathic pain by environmental enrichment in mice well after the establishment of chronic pain. Behav Brain Funct 2013;9:22.
82. van de Merwe JP, Nordling J, Bouchelouche P, et al. Diagnostic criteria, classification, and nomenclature for painful bladder syndrome/interstitial cystitis: an ESSIC proposal. Eur Urol 2008;53(1):60–67.
83. Veranic P, Jezernik K. The response of junctional complexes to induced desquamation in mouse bladder urothelium. Biol Cell 2000;92(2):105–113.
84. Warren JW, Howard FM, Cross RK, et al. Antecedent nonbladder syndromes in case-control study of interstitial cystitis/painful bladder syndrome. Urology 2009;73(1):52–57.
85. Warren JW, van de Merwe JP, Nickel JC. Syndromes Associated with Bladder Pain Syndrome as Clues to its Pathogenesis. In: Nordling J, van de Merwe JP, Cervigni M, Fall M (eds). Bladder Pain Syndrome A Guide for Clinicians. New York: Springer, 2013: 103–114.
86. Waxman JA, Sulak PJ, Kuehl TJ. Cystoscopic findings consistent with interstitial cystitis in normal women undergoing tubal ligation. J Urol 1998;160(5):1663–1667.
87. Weissman MM, Gross R, Fyer A, et al. Interstitial Cystitis and Panic Disorder: A Potential Genetic Syndrome. Arch Gen Psych 2004;I61(3):273–279.
88. Westropp JL, Buffington CAT. In Vivo Models of Interstitial Cystitis. J Urol 2002;167(2):694–702.
89. Westropp JL, Kass PH, Buffington CA. Evaluation of the effects of stress in cats with idiopathic cystitis. Am J Vet Res 2006;67(4):731–736.
90. Westropp JL, Kass PH, Buffington CA. In vivo evaluation of alpha(2)-adrenoceptors in cats with idiopathic cystitis. Am J Vet Res 2007;68(2):203–207.
91. Westropp JL, Welk KA, Buffington CAT. Small adrenal glands in cats with feline interstitial cystitis. J Urol 2003;170(6 (Pt 1)):2494–2497.
92. Wikipedia. Blind men and an elephant; http://en.wikipedia.org/wiki/Blind_men_and_an_elephant. Accessed 05/19/2014.
93. Willner P. Stress and depression: Insights from animal models. Stress Med 1997;13(4):229–233.
94. Wilson LM, Baldwin AL. Environmental stress causes mast cell degranulation, endothelial and epithelial changes, and edema in the rat intestinal mucosa. Microcirculation 1999;6(3):189–198.
95. Winston JH, Sarna SK. Developmental origins of functional dyspepsia-like gastric hypersensitivity in rats. Gastroenterology 2013;144(3):570–579 e573.
96. Wood JD, Peck OC, Tefend KS, et al. Evidence that colitis is initiated by environmental stress and sustained by fecal factors in the cotton-top tamarin (Saguinus oedipus). Digest Dis Sci 2000;45(2):385–393.
97. Wu EQ, Birnbaum H, Kang YJ, et al. A retrospective claims database analysis to assess patterns of interstitial cystitis diagnosis. Curr Med Res Opin 2006;22(3):495–500.
98. Yunus MB. Central sensitivity syndromes: a new paradigm and group nosology for fibromyalgia and overlapping conditions, and the related issue of disease versus illness. Semin Arthr Rheum 2008;37(6):339–352.

CHAPTER 4

The Importance of Central Sensitization

Timothy J. Ness, Meredith Robbins, and Alan Randich

INTRODUCTION

The experience of visceral pain requires a sensitization process to occur. When healthy, our viscera are minimally sensate, save for pressure, gurgles, a sense of fullness or occasional skipped beats. At a conscious level, we are not particularly aware of our internal organs; they perform their visceral functions and our brain is allowed to concentrate on our external world. However, when disease occurs, sensations associated with these same organs come to dominate all sensory processes.

Pain can exist without the activation of a primary afferent neuron due to the pathological activity of central nervous system (CNS) substrates of pain-related sensation. These substrates, intertwined throughout the CNS, form what Melzack termed, the "neuromatrix" which has components at cortical, thalamic, brainstem, cerebellar, and craniospinal levels [14] and it is possible to have pain due to pathology of those structures. More commonly, visceral pain occurs when normal visceroceptive inputs to our CNS, which in their normal physiological state minimally activate the "neuromatrix," become profoundly activating through the mechanisms of sensitization. These mechanisms can occur at the level of the primary afferent or can be due to processes occurring at CNS sites (Table 1) (Fig. 1). Research from the last 25 years performed by ourselves and with colleagues such as Gerald Gebhart, suggests that the key to understanding this sensitization process lies with discerning the dynamic alterations that occur at the level of the second-order neuron where this "central" sensitization process includes both facilitatory and inhibitory mechanisms. We present a summary of that research here.

BASIC ASPECTS

Dorsal Horn Components of Sensation

The spinal cord and brainstem nuclei are home to second-order neurons, the first site of sensory integration and processing. Second-order neurons are more than a simple relay for nociceptive information and any plan for the treatment of pain must understand the critical role these neurons play in the formation of painful sensation. The second-order neuron converts afferent input from multiple sites, and often multiple modalities, into an encoded message that is sent to other parts of the CNS. Those other parts of the CNS, in turn, modify the second-order neuron through both excitatory and inhibitory mechanisms. To define

TABLE 1 Mechanisms of Dorsal Horn Neuronal Sensitization

- I. Increased input from Primary Afferent Neurons
  - A. Peripheral release of neuroactive substances
  - B. Increased transduction/transmission
    1. Decreased thresholds for activation
    2. Increased action potential generation
    3. Due to ion channel/receptor induction, expression, modification
  - C. Increased number of afferents as part of development
  - D. Release of intraspinal transmission block (Lissauer's tract)
  - E. Peripheral expansion of receptive field distribution (branching)
  - F. Expansion of spinal branching to more segments, more laminae
  - G. Ganglionic interaction (paravertebral, prevertebral)
  - H. Increased central neurotransmitter release
    1. Greater synthesis
    2. More efficient release
    3. Less reuptake/local metabolism
- II. Increased Responsiveness of Second Order Neuron
  - A. C-fiber Wind-Up
  - B. Sustained noxious input - NMDA-linked sensitization
  - C. Reduced Inhibition
    1. Tonic segmental
    2. Evoked segmental
    3. Tonic heterosegmental intraspinal (propriospinal)
    4. Evoked heterosegmental intraspinal (propriospinal)
    5. Tonic heterosegmental supraspinal (descending)
    6. Evoked heterosegmental supraspinal (descending)
  - D. Increased Facilitation
    1. Tonic segmental
    2. Evoked segmental
    3. Tonic heterosegmental intraspinal (propriospinal)
    4. Evoked heterosegmental intraspinal (propriospinal)
    5. Tonic heterosegmental supraspinal (descending)
    6. Evoked heterosegmental supraspinal (descending)
  - E. Release of post-synaptic transmission block

a neuron as "visceroceptive", one must identify the type or modality of afferent information they receive from a given viscera (e.g., mechanical, chemical). Calling a visceroceptive neuron "nociceptive" is a more difficult proposition and there have been great debates related to this topic, which have recapitulated monumental arguments related to specificity theory, intensity theory and pattern theory [25]. Due to the observation that most, if not all, visceroceptive neurons are viscerosomatic neurons due to the presence of convergent cutaneous excitatory receptive fields, we have chosen to define a visceral nociceptive neuron as one which demonstrates an encoding of sensory information for stimuli that are in excess of normal function. We also relied on the presence or absence of convergent excitatory input from somatic structures where clear definitions of "noxious" and "non-noxious" intensities of cutaneous stimulation exist. Subsequent characterization methods have been able to identify where these neurons are located, how they are modulated and further have helped to identify where these neurons send their information via direct axonal projections.

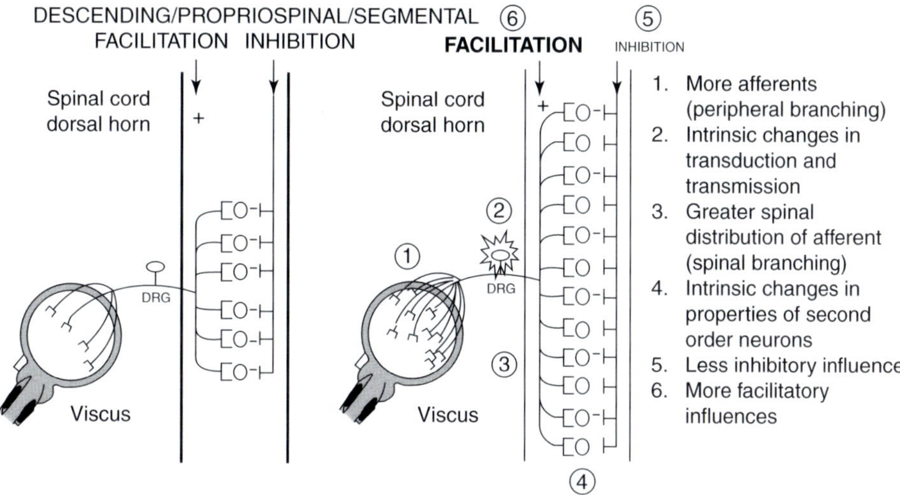

FIGURE 1 Potential sites of sensitization mechanisms associated with visceral pain. On left is a schematic diagram of the normal physiological state of an organism. On the right are indicated potential sites for sensitization mechanisms which are listed to the far right. Table 1 indicates more precise mechanisms located at these sites.

To properly describe spinal cord sensory processing, one must also consider the third-, fourth-, and higher-order neurons located within the spinal cord itself which form what we refer to as a Multisynaptic Nociceptive Network (MNN). Notably, many second-order neurons receive multisynaptic excitatory input from multiple distant (non-adjacent) spinal segments (e.g. heterosegmental sites) in addition to primary afferent input and so are, by definition, MNN neurons.

The overriding hypothesis that has driven studies in our laboratories for the last three decades is that the conscious perception of visceral pain is associated with the activation of at least two separate subsets of visceroceptive, nociceptive, second-order neurons. These neurons can broadly be categorized as (1) second-order neurons which are associated with focal activation within the spinal cord and (2) second order neurons which are associated with widespread activation within the spinal cord – MNN neurons. Widespread activation is relatively easy to mechanistically accomplish and can consist of either short or long axonal excitatory connections that are associated with a degree of reciprocity. Neuronal lattices with these features have been commonly identified to exist within craniospinal structures and have been described as propriospinal excitatory connections and intersegmental connections. Early neurophysiological studies of spinal visceroceptive neuronal interconnectivity immediately identified such interconnections [12,13]. In contrast, focal activation of spinal neuronal structures requires either a precise set of excitatory connections from the viscera and/or the presence of feedback inhibitory systems that focus the excitatory effects of transmission signals to a specific spinal location. Painful stimuli can activate such feedback inhibitory systems, a general phenomenon which we have previously referred to as nocigenic inhibition (NI) [26,27]; with specific cases described as conditioned pain modulation [43], diffuse noxious inhibitory controls [8–10,43], propriospinal inhibitory circuits and segmental inhibitory phenomena [16,17]. Based on our interpretation of neuroanatomic and functional studies and building on

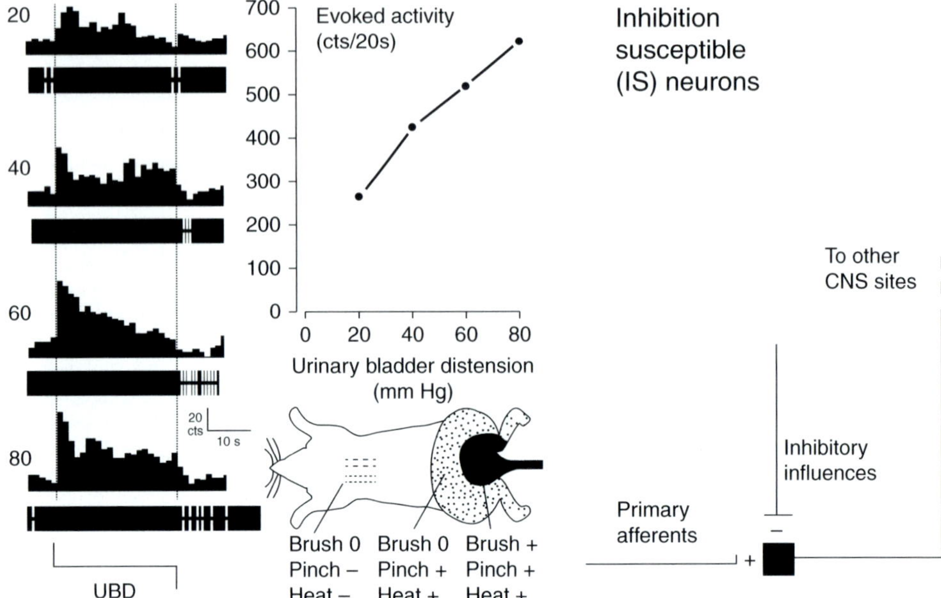

FIGURE 2 Typical example and schematic description of an Inhibition Susceptible (IS) neuron. At far left are peristimulus-time histograms and oscillographic tracings associated with an L6/S1 spinal dorsal horn neuron excited by graded intensities of urinary bladder distension (UBD; pressure of distension in mm Hg indicated at left). Dotted lines indicate onset and cessation of distending stimulus. The center upper graph indicates graphically the excitatory response of the same neuron – number of action potentials were counted (cts) for the 20 period of UBD and spontaneous activity subtracted out to give a measure of evoked activity. The center bottom graph is a cartoon indicating convergent cutaneous receptive field of neuron – notably pinch of the midscapular skin at a noxious intensity produced inhibition (indicated by "-") whereas light touch brush and noxious pinch and heat produced excitation (indicated by "+'; no response "0") of the neuron when presented in lumbosacral fields. At far right is schematic diagram indicating essential features of IS second order neurons. (Adapted from Ness TJ, Castroman P. Evidence for two populations of rat spinal nociceptive neurons excited by urinary bladder distension. Brain Res 2001; 923:147–156).

concepts championed by Lebars and colleagues [8–10], we have chosen to focus on NI influences as predictors of sensory function and so have utilized neuronal susceptibility to pain-activated inhibitory control systems as a defining functional characteristic. Our overriding hypothesis has therefore simplified to the assertion that visceral pain is due to the activity of two spinal dorsal horn neuronal subgroups: Inhibition Susceptible neurons (IS, Fig. 2) and MNN neurons (Fig. 3).

Quantitative characterization studies that have assessed for NI effects in viscero-ceptive neurons suggest that an important neurofunctional difference between visceral pain and cutaneous pain is that somatic-only (not viscerosomatic) nociceptive neurons are almost exclusively IS neurons [8–10,32] whereas a majority of viscerosomatic no-ciceptive neurons are non-IS neurons with a ratio slightly greater than 50:50 compared to IS neurons in quantitative studies of dorsal horn neurons excited by either colorectal distension or bladder distension [20,26]. Evidence that non-IS neurons are MNN neurons is that they are typically excited by noxious stimuli applied to distant (heteroseg-mental) parts of the body often including the entire body surface. It is the differential susceptibility of IS and MNN neurons to other inhibitory and facilitatory influences that may explain the necessity of central sensitization processes for the experience of visceral pain.

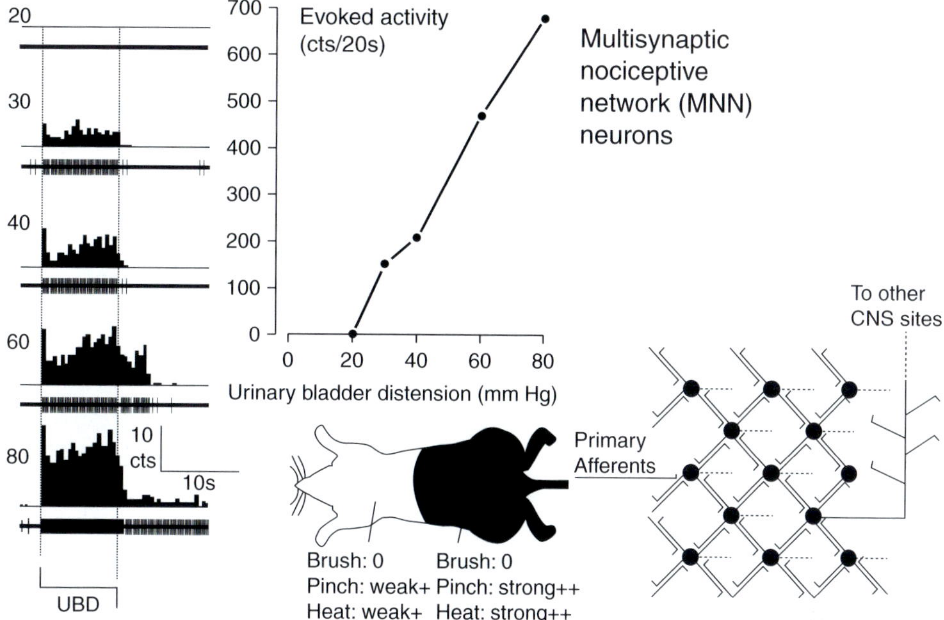

FIGURE 3 Typical example and schematic description of Multisynaptic Nociceptive Network (MNN) neuron. At far left are peristimulus-time histograms and oscillographic tracings associated with an L6/S1 spinal dorsal horn neuron excited by graded intensities of urinary bladder distension (UBD; pressure of distension in mm Hg indicated at left). Dotted lines indicate onset and cessation of distending stimulus. In center upper graph indicates graphically the excitatory response of the same neuron – number of action potentials were counted (cts) for the 20 period of UBD and spontaneous activity subtracted out to give a measure of evoked activity. In center bottom is a cartoon indicating convergent cutaneous receptive field of neuron – this neuron had strong excitatory responses to noxious pinch and heat (indicated by "++') when these stimuli were presented in lumbosacral fields; presentation in distant heterosegmental sites produced weak excitatory responses. In this neuron, non-noxious brush produced no response (indicated as "0") of the neuron. At far right is schematic diagram indicating essential features of MNN second order neurons which have reciprocal excitatory connections with multiple other spinal neurons. (Adapted from Ness TJ, Castroman P. Evidence for two populations of rat spinal nociceptive neurons excited by urinary bladder distension. Brain Res 2001; 923:147–156).

DESCRIBING THE SUBJECT

Studies of Visceroceptive Neurons Using Nocigenic Inhibition-Related Criteria

In our initial studies of visceral nociceptive neurons, which used the visceral stimulus of colorectal distension, there were neuronal subgroups that could be differentiated based on "temporal" characteristics of their responses. One subgroup abruptly terminated their excitatory discharges following cessation of the distending stimulus and hence were called ABRUPT neurons [22,23]. This was in contrast to a separate subgroup of neurons excited by colorectal distension that had a sustained after discharge following cessation of the distending stimulus and hence were called SUSTAINED neurons [22,23]. Only after introduction of neuronal characterization methods that included NI assessments did it become clear that all ABRUPT neurons were IS neurons [26]. The simplest explanation for their "abrupt" temporal characteristics was that a negative-feedback NI system was being activated by the visceral stimulus. The end result of this feedback inhibition would be an adapting response with a sharp reduction in neuronal activity as soon as the primary afferent excitatory signaling ceased. The same inhibitory phenomenon was not generally observed in SUSTAINED neurons, most of which were non-IS neurons. In many cases these lumbosacral neurons were excited by neurologically distant noxious stimuli (nose or front paw pinch in rats)[26]. This activation by heterosegmental stimuli gives strong evidence that these neurons received multisynaptic input making them at least third- or fourth-order spinal neurons, in addition to being second-order neurons. By our definition that made them MNN neurons. Identification of these neurons in spinally-transected rats indicated that the "network connections" did not require a brainstem circuit. When later utilizing urinary bladder distension as a noxious visceral stimulus, use of susceptibility to NI to determine neuronal subclasses became our routine as it resulted in empirically precise differentiation of neurons, in that individual neurons either met criteria or did not meet criteria in an unambiguous fashion [20].

IS neurons have been demonstrated to have many different characteristics than MNN neurons apart from their susceptibility to NI. In comparison with MNN neurons, IS neurons require lower pressures of visceral distension to be activated. They also have smaller convergent cutaneous receptive fields with distinct "inhibitory-surround" characteristics. That is, noxious stimuli applied outside the areas of excitation produce inhibition [20,22,23,26]. IS neurons are less inhibited than MNN neurons by systemic administration of traditional analgesics, such as opioids and lidocaine [18–20,24], but more inhibited by NMDA receptor antagonists [1]. Further, inflammation of visceral structures (e.g. colon, bladder) results in quantitatively less vigorous excitatory responses in samples of IS neurons [21,28,29] (Fig. 4 upper) as does the presentation of an experimental stressor [39] (Fig. 5 - upper). Stated in a converse fashion, this means that the MNN neurons, which represent a majority of visceroceptive neurons, when compared with IS neurons have larger convergent cutaneous receptive fields (often total body), are more inhibited by traditional analgesics and demonstrate more robust responses following manipulations known to increase clinical pain such as inflammation and stress/anxiety. Notably, differential modulation of the IS and MNN neurons occurred whether the "trigger" for sensitization was either a clearly primary afferent-related mechanism (inflammation) or due to supraspinal mechanisms (stress/anxiety). These modulators also increase visceral nociceptive reflexes in a similar fashion [36,38,40]. What is particularly notable when contrasting these two modulations is that IS neurons demonstrated susceptibility to stress-induced inhibitory influences in addition to the NI manipulations used to define that neuronal group. In contrast, MNN neurons demonstrated robust responsiveness to stress-induced facilitatory mechanisms. It is likely that inflammation also resulted in central facilitatory mechanisms that impacted on MNN function, but the effect of central facilitation is difficult to dissociate from the increased primary afferent inputs produced by inflammatory processes.

Features of Visceral Pain

So how might a difference in the populations of neurons excited by nociceptive stimuli help us understand other features of visceral pain? This type of pain has as its hallmark feature a diffuse localization. Much of the diffuse localization can be explained by the diffuse point of entry of primary afferents into the CNS from any particular visceral site. Cell bodies in the dorsal root ganglia spanning from midthoracic to lower sacral sites are labeled when pelvic organs are injected with neuronal tracers (e.g. [23]). Further, Sugiura et al [42] demonstrated that once a single visceral afferent C-fiber enters the spinal cord it often branches and may form weak synaptic contact with more than 10 spinal segments with branches

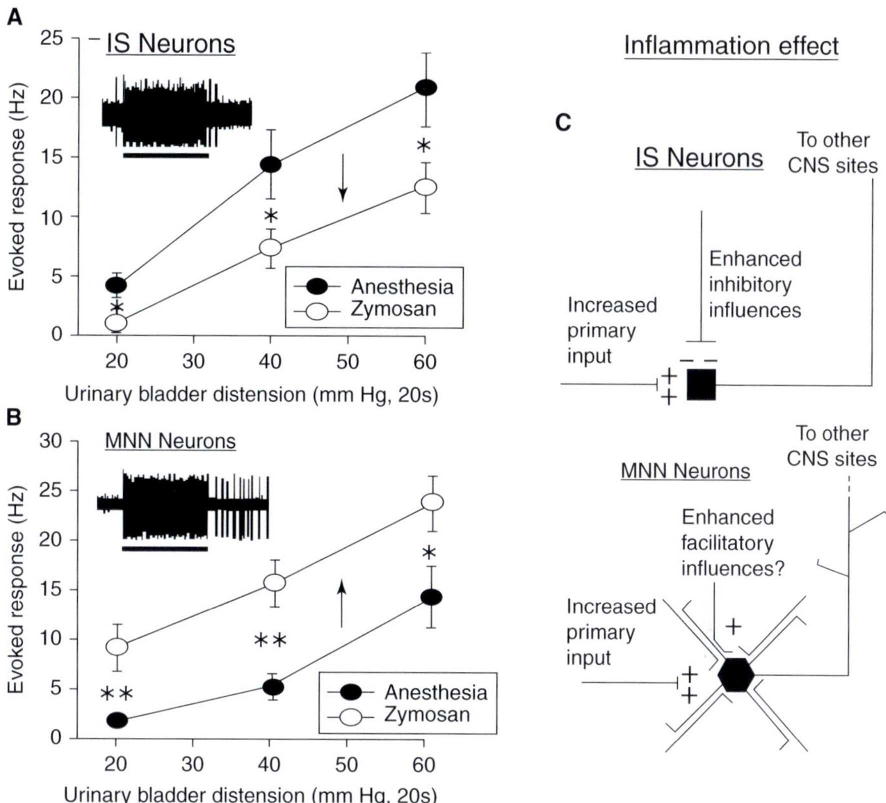

FIGURE 4 Effects of acute inflammation produced by intravesical zymosan administered 24 hours prior to study or control treatments (anesthesia only) on mean activities of IS and MNN neurons in rats. At left are graphical representations of the mean responses of neuron as mean discharge rate of action potentials for the 20 period of UBD minus spontaneous activity. Oscillographic tracings embedded in graphs at left are typical examples of responses to urinary bladder distension (60 mm Hg, 20s). IS neuronal responses in rats pretreated with zymosan were less robust that those measured in control rats. In contrast, MNN neuronal responses became more robust. At right is schematic diagram indicating proposed mechanisms affecting IS and MNN second order neurons following acute inflammation. (Data and figure adapted from Ness TJ, Castroman PJ, Randich A. Acute bladder inflammation differentially affects spinal visceral nociceptive neurons. Neurosci Lett, 2009; 467:150–4).

extending into multiple ipsilateral and contralateral spinal laminae. In contrast, single C-fiber afferents from cutaneous structures often form tight baskets of input to a limited number of second-order neurons within limited ipsilateral laminae of single spinal segments [42]. If one couples this neuroanatomic information, that suggests a diffuse distribution of visceral primary afferents synapsing onto neurons located in many laminae of many spinal segments, with the neurofunctional assessment that a majority of visceroceptive neurons have diffuse multisynaptic inputs from other craniospinal sites in addition to their visceral inputs, it is a small wonder that the visceral sensation which is processed would be interpreted by the brain such that the perception is "diffuse." A diffuse distribution of visceral afferents to second-order neurons would be expected to result in relatively weak excitatory inputs from any individual afferent to an individual second-order neuron. We assert that this would make sensations related to these afferents particularly sensitive to modulatory influences. Weak inputs would not be difficult to mask by even weak inhibitory influences and facilitation would be mandated if any robust excitatory responses were to be evoked.

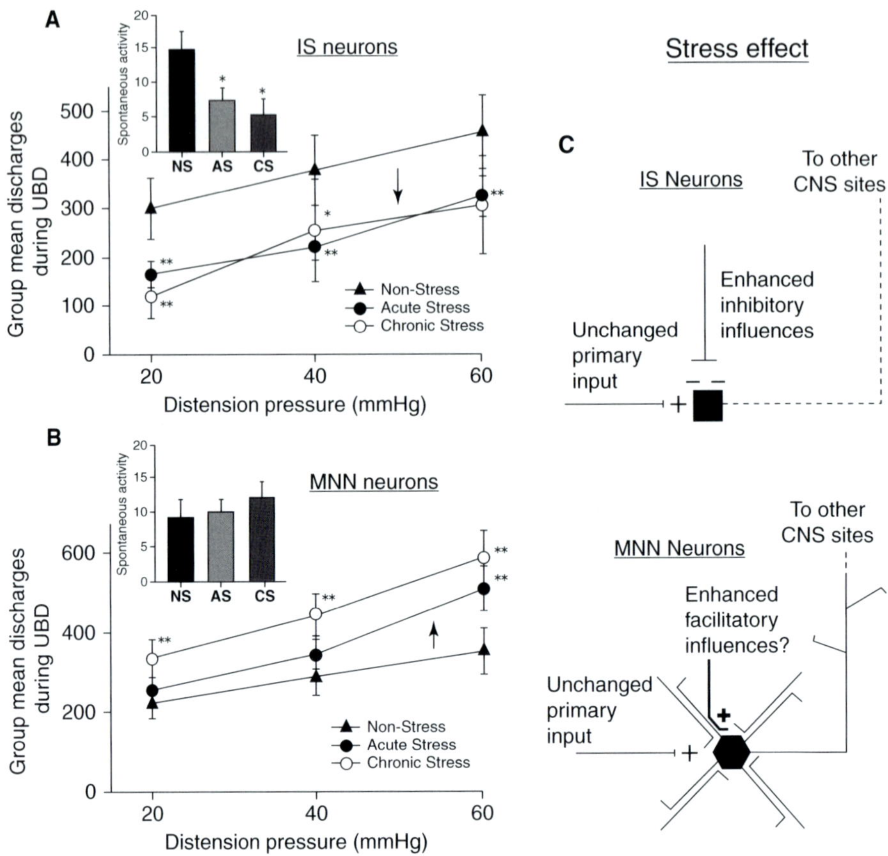

FIGURE 5 Effects of acute or chronic stress produced by 15 minute intermittent footshock sessions administered immediately prior to study (Acute Stress) or for six days prior to and on the day of study (Chronic Stress) or control treatments (Non-Stress) on mean activities of IS and MNN neurons in rats. At left are graphical representations of the total number of action potentials of neurons during the 20 period of graded urinary bladder distension. Inset graphs indicate mean spontaneous activities of these same neurons. IS neuronal responses in rats experiencing stress were less robust that those measured in control rats. In contrast, MNN neuronal responses became more robust following stress. At right is schematic diagram indicating proposed mechanisms affecting IS and MNN second order neurons following stress. (Data and figure adapted from Robbins MT, Deberry J, Randich, Ness TJ. Footshock stress differentially affects responses of two subpopulations of spinal dorsal horn neurons to urinary bladder distension in rats. Brain Res 2011; 1386: 118–26).

Models of Disease

Our discussion so far has centered around models of visceral pain in otherwise "healthy" animals which were then subjected to modulatory influences by the introduction of inflammatory or stress-related manipulations. In these models, there was some balance between increased neuronal activation of one group (MNN neurons) and decreased neuronal activation of a different group (IS neurons) – the two groups being differentiated by the presence of a susceptibility to NI. In healthy human subjects, painful stimuli such as immersion of the hand in ice water results in a raising of thermal pain thresholds and thermal pain tolerance temperatures when presented in heterosegmental sites. This effect is termed Conditioned Pain Modulation (CPM) by convention [43]. We have observed deficits/reductions in CPM correlated with episodic clinical pain in relatively healthy populations [3,4] and in chronic pain populations, CPM effects have often been demonstrated to be profoundly altered. For example, studies of subjects with temporomandibular disorder, irritable bowel syndrome, fibromyalgia and/or chronic fatigue syndrome have all been demonstrated to have CPM-related inhibitory mechanisms that are deficient (e.g. [6,7,15]). In our own studies, subjects with Bladder Pain Syndrome/ Interstitial Cystitis, who are hypersensitive to bladder-related stimuli [31] demonstrate not only a deficiency of CPM-related inhibition but also demonstrate an augmentation of their painful sensations [30]. In these subjects, thermal pain thresholds and thermal pain tolerances measured in dermatomes adjacent to spinal segments receiving bladder inputs were decreased rather than increased while the subject's hand was immersed in ice water [30]. These human clinical studies suggest that creating a nonhuman animal model that is focally or globally deficient in inhibitory pain control systems would be desirable and more relevant than acute pain model systems to the understanding of pathological pain. Although not our original intent, we have determined that the introduction of neonatal injuries can produce such deficiencies and hypersensitivity to visceral stimuli [37].

Studies of the neonatal development of the nervous system suggest that at birth sensory systems have very little modulation by inhibitory influences. This changes during development until inhibitory connections become the predominant form of CNS neurotransmission. In humans, the precise timing of both excitatory and inhibitory system maturation in nociceptive systems is not fully known, but based on experiments in non-human animals these systems appear highly plastic, with cell death-processes being as important as cell growth-processes in relation to the final developed nervous system [35]. Specific transcriptional factor expression has been used to track neuronal subgroup development and has demonstrated a profound role for pathological modification of nociceptive circuitry [44]. The general phenomenon of use-dependent growth (or preservation) appears to hold in multiple sensory systems ranging from taste to vision, with the nociceptive systems not withstanding. Ruda and colleagues [41] have demonstrated that injury during critical periods of development such as the neonatal period, has profound effects on the subsequent development of nociceptive systems. In rats, Fitzgerald and Koltzenburg [5] identified that inhibitory connections descending from the brainstem reach lumbosacral regions between 10 and 20 days of life. We therefore performed experiments in which bladder inflammation was induced in rat pups on days 14–16 of life. We postulated that increased primary afferent input at that critical period of development could disrupt normal maturation processes. This indeed proved to be the case. As adults, these rats have a definably changed CNS in that they lack an inducible opioid-dependent inhibitory system related to the bladder [2]. Notably, when we re-challenge these animal subjects by re-inflaming their bladders as adult, there is a profound change in the effect of the inflammatory stimulus on the activity of visceroceptive IS neurons [33]. Whereas "healthy" control rats demonstrate an attenuation of IS neuronal responses (left panels Fig. 6 – same phenomenon as in Fig. 4), rats which received neonatal bladder inflammatory treatments show an augmentation of the IS neuronal responses following re-inflammation (right panels Fig. 6). Further, the MNN neurons are augmented by inflammation in both control rats and in rats who's CNS was changed by a neonatal inflammatory event. We attribute this change in modulatory effect to a focal deficit in NI-related inhibitory mechanisms. Let us explain… Whereas the inflammation-increased nociceptive inputs from the bladder would normally activate a negative feedback modulatory NI effect on IS neurons, the absence of such negative feedback resulted in increased CNS activation due to a net increase in overall activity of neurons projecting to the brain: IS neuronal inputs were increased due to less inhibition and MNN neuronal inputs were increased due to a net increase in both primary afferent activity and convergent

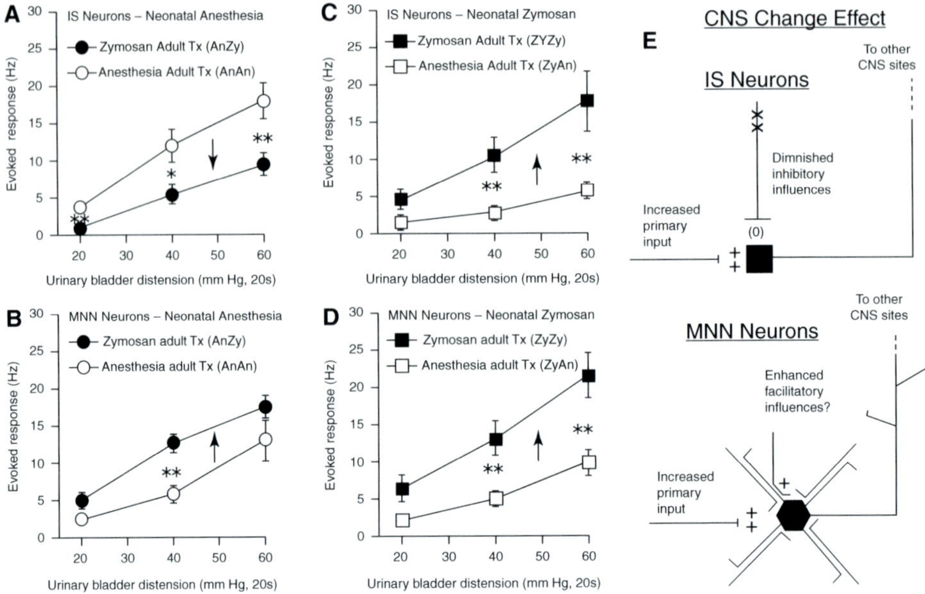

FIGURE 6 Graphic description of effects of acute inflammation produced by intravesical zymosan administered 24 hours prior to study (Zymosan Adult Tx) or control treatments (Anesthesia Adult Tx) on mean activities of IS and MNN neurons in rats which received control treatments as neonates (Neonatal Anesthesia: panels A,B) or had experienced neonatal bladder inflammation on P14–16 (Neonatal Zymosan; panels C, D). At left are graphical representations of the mean responses of neuron as mean discharge rate of action potentials for the 20 period of UBD minus spontaneous activity. IS and MNN neuronal responses in rats without a CNS change due to neonatal treatments (A,B) had responses similar to those noted in "normal" rats presented in Figure 4. However, rats pretreated with intravesical zymosan as neonates demonstrate a loss of the inhibition previously noted in IS neurons and instead, *both* IS and MNN neuronal responses were more robust following acute adult zymosan treatment. At right is schematic diagram indicating proposed mechanisms affecting IS and MNN second order neurons following acute inflammation when in a neonatal bladder inflammation-induced CNS changed state. (Data and figure adapted from Ness TJ, Randich A. Neonatal bladder inflammation alters activity of adult rat spinal visceral nociceptive neurons. Neurosci Lett 2010; 472, 210–214).

facilitatory input from other MNN neurons and potentially from other sites producing central facilitation. Ongoing dorsal horn neuronal studies using the manipulation of footshock-induced stress as a modulator of adult rat dorsal horn neuronal activity suggests similar "reversals" of the modulatory effects of stress on the activity of visceroceptive IS neurons. Instead of observing stress-induced inhibition of IS neurons, stress-induced augmentation is the observed phenomenon in rats with a CNS changed by neonatal bladder inflammation (unpublished data). Additional studies are needed to further support the conjectures derived from these observations, but this is what we believe constitutes the neural substrates of central sensitization in most subjects with chronic bladder pain syndromes.

PRACTICAL IMPLICATIONS

The clinician must synthesize these diverse pieces of information into a general model of visceral nociceptive processing and must accept that at this point in time the model is incomplete. The concept of central sensitization has been described clinically for almost a century by clinician-scientists such as Livingston and Noordenbos who proposed descriptions of networks of ascending nociceptive neurons and reverbatory circuits creating "internuncial pools" of CNS neurons that are *irritated* (facilitated) by pathological processes resulting in patients who are hypersensitive in focal or global ways[11,34]. Although useful when conceptualizing the clinical features observed in visceral pain patients, the general term central sensitization has not generally proven predictive of therapeutic interventions. Electrophysiological studies can now give some validity to the substrates of sensitization processes.

As stated before, visceral pain requires a sensitization process, but in the most vexing clinical pain conditions (to the clinician), no peripheral sensitization process which we understand (like inflammation) is apparent. This leaves us with the need for understanding the central processes that can cause changes that appear similar to mechanisms we do understand. As we have described in the preceding pages, an important take-home message for the clinician is that from the perspective of a visceroceptive second-order neuron (whether it be an IS or MNN neuron), the modulations produced by altered primary afferent activities (as with inflammation) are indiscernible from modulations due to purely central phenomena like acute stress/anxiety. Sensitization may occur due to multiple reasons: inflammation, stress, convergent deep tissue inputs, developmental alterations, neuronal injury and more. Once initiated, the mechanisms associated with these different manipulations appear to follow convergent pathways, and to date, one can explain most phenomena by specific patterns in the activity of second-, third-, fourth- and higher-order neurons. This is clinically relevant because patients often cannot tell what has made their pain worse. For example, Bladder Pain Syndrome / interstitial cystitis patients often cannot tell the difference between their typical pain (often made worse by stress) and the pain which they experience due to a urinary tract infection (an inflammatory process). If the pattern of alteration of the activity of elements of sensation does not appear to differ, one would not expect the evoked sensations to differ.

LOOKING AT THE FUTURE

The effectiveness of therapeutic interventions intended to treat pain is dependent upon the modulation of these substrates of nociception and so identification of the precise pharmacology which leads to changes in patterns of activity should lead us to potential therapeutics. Unfortunately, clinical data suggests that "normal" modulatory changes observed in healthy animals may not be reflective of the changes that will be observed when the CNS is altered by a pathological process (such as with neonatal injury) and so our animal model systems need to continue to mature and become more translatable. This is a back-and-forth process moving from animal to human and back again, but the prize of improved pain control for our patients is worth the effort.

TAKE HOME MESSAGES

- Sensitization phenomena associated with second order neurons in the spinal cord are representative of clinical phenomena: these include changes due to inflammation and stress.
- Sensitization phenomena are more than simple neuronal activation but represent a mixture of facilitatory and inhibitory influences.

FURTHER READING

Woolf C.J. Central sensitization: implications for the diagnosis and treatment of pain. Pain 2011 152 (supplement): S2-S15.

Farrell KE, Keely S, Graham BA, et al. A systematic review of the evidence for central nervous system plasticity in animal models of inflammatory-mediated gastrointestinal pain. Inflamm Bowel Dis 2014 20: 176–195.

Bardoni R, Takazawa T, Tong CK, et al. Pre- and postsynaptic inhibitory control in the spinal cord dorsal hor. Ann NY Acad Sci 2013 1279: 90–96.

ACKNOWLEDGEMENTS

The described studies have been performed thanks to the support of the United States National Institute of Diabetes, Digestive and Kidney Disease. TJN, MTR and AR are supported by DK51419.

REFERENCES

1. Castroman P, Ness TJ. Ketamine, an N-methyl-D-aspartate antagonist, inhibits the spinal neuronal responses to distension of the rat urinary bladder. Anesthesiology 2002; 96:1410–1419.
2. DeBerry J, Ness TJ, Robbins MT, Randich A. Inflammation-induced enhancement of the visceromotor reflex to urinary bladder distention: Modulation by endogenous opioids and the effects of early-in-life experience with bladder inflammation. J. Pain 2007; 8:914–23.
3. Edwards R, Fillingim R, Ness T. Age-related differences in endogenous pain modulation: a comparison of diffuse noxious inhibitory controls in healthy older and younger adults. Pain 2003; 101:155–165.
4. Edwards, R.R., Ness TJ, Weigent, DA, Fillingim RB. Individual differences in diffuse noxious inhibitory controls (DNIC): association with clinical variables. Pain 2003; 106: 427–37.
5. Fitzgerald M, Koltzenberg M. The functional development of descending inhibitory pathways in the dorsolateral funiculus of the newborn rat spinal cord. Brain Res. 1986; 389: 261–270.
6. King CD, Wong F, Currie T, et al. Deficiency in endogenous modulation of prolonged heat pain in patients with irritable bowel syndromone and temporomandibular disorder. Pain 2009;143: 172–178.
7. Lautenbacher S, Rollman G. Possible deficiencies of pain modulation in fibromyalgia. Clin. J. Pain 1997; 13: 189–196.
8. LeBars D. The whole body receptive field of dorsal horn multireceptive neurons. Brain Res Revs. 2002; 40: 29–44.
9. LeBars D, Dickenson AH, Besson JM. Diffuse noxious Inhibitory Controls (DNIC): I Effects on dorsal horn convergent neurones in the rat. Pain 1979; 6: 283–304.
10. LeBars D, Dickenson AH, Besson JM. Diffuse noxious Inhibitory Controls (DNIC): II Lack of effect on non-convergent neurons, supraspinal involvement and theoretical implications. Pain 1979; 6: 305–327.
11. Livingston WK. Pain and Suffering (Ed: H.L.Fields) Seattle: IASP Press, 1998
12. McMahon SB, Morrison JFB. Two group of spinal interneurones that respond to stimulation of the abdominal viscera of the cat. J Physiol. 1982;322:21–34.
13. McMahon SB, Morrison JFB. Spinal neurones with long projections activated from the abdominal viscera of the cat. J Physiol. 1982;322:1–20
14. Melzack R. Evolution of the neuromatrix theory of pain. Pain Pract. 2005;5:85–94.
15. Meeus M, Nijs J, Van de Wauwer N, et al. Diffuse noxious inhibitory control is delayed in chronic fatigue syndrome: an experimental study. Pain 2009; 139: 439–448.
16. Millan MJ. The induction of pain. Prog Neurobio. 1999; 57: 1–164.
17. Millan MJ. Descending control of pain. Prog Neurobio. 2002; 66:355–474.
18. Ness TJ. Kappa opioid receptor agonists differentially inhibit two classes of rat spinal neurons excited by colorectal distension. Gastroenterology 1999; 117:388–394.
19. Ness TJ. Intravenous lidocaine inhibits visceral nociceptive reflexes and spinal neurons in the rat. Anesthesiology 2000; 92:1685–1691.
20. Ness TJ, Castroman P. Evidence for two populations of rat spinal nociceptive neurons excited by urinary bladder distension. Brain Res 2001; 923:147–156.

21. Ness TJ, Castroman PJ, Randich A. Acute bladder inflammation differentially affects spinal visceral nociceptive neurons. Neurosci Lett, 2009; 467:150–4.
22. Ness TJ, Gebhart GF. Characterization of neuronal responses to noxious visceral and somatic stimuli in the medial lumbosacral spinal cord of the rat. J Neurophysiol 1987; 57:1867–92.
23. Ness TJ, Gebhart GF. Characterization of neurons responsive to noxious colorectal distension in the T13-L2 spinal cord of the rat. J Neurophysiol 1988; 60:1419–1438.
24. Ness TJ, Gebhart GF. Differential effects of morphine and clonidine on visceral and cutaneous spinal nociceptive transmission in the rat. J Neurophysiol 1989; 62:220–230.
25. Ness TJ, Gebhart GF. Visceral pain: a review of experimental studies. Pain 1990; 41:167–234.
26. Ness TJ, Gebhart GF. Interactions between visceral and cutaneous nociception. I. Noxious cutaneous stimuli inhibit visceral nociceptive neurons and reflexes. J Neurophysiol 1991; 66:20–28.
27. Ness TJ, Gebhart GF. Interactions between visceral and cutaneous nociception in the rat. II. Noxious visceral stimuli inhibit cutaneous nociceptive neurons and reflexes. J Neurophysiol 1991; 66:29–39.
28. Ness TJ, Gebhart GF. Acute inflammation differentially alters the activity of two classes of rat spinal visceral nociceptive neurons. Neurosci Lett 2000; 281:131–134.
29. Ness TJ, Gebhart GF. Inflammation enhances reflex and spinal neuron responses to noxious visceral stimulation in rats. Am J Physiol Gastrointest Liver Physiol 2001. 280:G649-G657.
30. Ness TJ, Lloyd LK, Fillingim RB. An endogenous pain control system is altered in subjects with interstitial cystitis. J Urol. 2014;191(2):364–70.
31. Ness TJ, Powell-Boone T, Cannon R et al. Psychophysical evidence of hypersensitivity in subjects with interstitial cystitis. J Urol 2005;173: 1983–1987.
32. Ness TJ, Randich A. Which spinal cutaneous nociceptive neurons are inhibited by intravenous lidocaine. Reg Anesth Pain Med. 2006; 31: 248–253.
33. Ness TJ, Randich A. Neonatal bladder inflammation alters activity of adult rat spinal visceral nociceptive neurons. Neurosci Lett 2010; 472, 210–214.
34. Noordenbos W. Pain. Amsterdam: Elsevier, 1959.
35. Pattinson D and Fitzgerald M. The neurobiology of infant pain: development of excitatory and inhibitory neurotransmission in the spinal dorsal horn. Reg. Anesth Pain Med. 2004; 29: 36–44.
36. Randich A, Uzzell TW, Cannon RS, Ness TJ. Inflammation and enhanced nociceptive responses to bladder distension produced by intravesical zymosan in the rat. BMC Urol. 2006; 6:2.
37. Randich A, Uzzell TW, DeBerry JJ, Ness TJ. Neonatal urinary bladder inflammation produces adult bladder hypersensitivity. J. Pain 2006; 7: 469–79.
38. Robbins MT, DeBerry J, Ness TJ. Chronic psychological stress enhances nociceptive processing in the urinary bladder in high-anxiety rats. Physiol Behav. 2007; 91:544–50.
39. Robbins MT, Deberry J, Randich, Ness TJ. Footshock stress differentially affects responses of two subpopulations of spinal dorsal horn neurons to urinary bladder distension in rats. Brain Res 2011; 1386: 118–26.
40. Robbins MT, Ness TJ. Footshock-induced urinary bladder hypersensitivity: role of spinal corticotrophin-releasing factor receptors. J. Pain. 2008; 9: 991–998.
41. Ruda MA, Ling QD, Hohmann AG, et al. Altered nociceptive neuronal circuits after neonatal peripheral inflammation. Science. 2000; 289:628–31.
42. Sugiura Y, Terui N, Hosoya Y. Difference in distribution of central terminals between visceral and somatic unmyelinated primary afferent fibers. J. Neurophysiol. 1989; 62: 834–840.
43. Yarnitsky D, Arendt-Nielsen L, Bouhassira D, et al. Recommendations on terminology and practice of psychophysical DNIC testing. Eur J Pain. 2010;14:339.
44. Zhang X, Bao L. The development and modulation of nociceptive circuitry. Curr Opin Neurobiol. 2006; 16: 460–466.

CHAPTER 5

The Role of Gender in Abdominal and Pelvic Pain

Natasha Curran

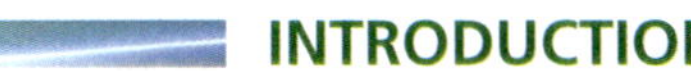

INTRODUCTION

The role of gender in abdominal and pelvic pain (APP) has been an area of increasing interest over the last twenty years as clinicians and researchers have begun to postulate and wonder if investigating differences between the sexes and or genders can expand our understanding of pain and offer potential treatments. At this point it becomes necessary to define and discuss the difference between sex and gender. According to the Oxford English Dictionary sex refers to 'either of the two main categories (male and female) into which humans and most other living things are divided on the basis of their reproductive functions' [25]. This, of course, is subject to some limitation if one considers intersex, discussion of which has become more prevalent in the media. The prevalence of intersex "restricted to those conditions in which chromosomal sex is inconsistent with phenotypic sex, or in which the phenotype is not classifiable as either male or female" is however only about 0.018%. [27]. Gender is 'the state of being male or female (typically used with reference to social and cultural differences rather than biological ones)' [25]. This chapter will thus use male and female to denote the biological sex type, and masculine and feminine in reference to behavioral gender type. One must accept however sex and gender influence each other and change at different stages of an individual's life. The 'complication' of sexuality that may influence further and may depend on how socially accepted certain sexualities are in different cultures, is not a topic that this chapter will address.

BASIC ASPECTS

History

It was Karen Berkley's 1992 paper, which revealed that only half of 100 articles in neuroscience journals reported the sex of their subjects which really brought sex and gender differences to the fore. She suggested that the differences between sexes can and should be exploited in scientific research [3]. In the later 1990s, several works interested in gender related differences in pain and analgesic response followed. In 1999, IASP's Special Interested Group (SIG) 'Sex, Gender and Pain' was born and its mission statement remains:

- Encourage basic and clinical research on how sex and gender affect pain mechanisms and all realms of its management
- Provide a central information resource on these issues
- Develop multidisciplinary discussion groups on subtopics of these issues

Epidemiology

Most (but not all) population-based studies have found a higher prevalence of pain in women in all societies and in all painful conditions. When looking at APP, there is less data available and this is hampered further by the different categorisations for pain experienced in the abdomen and pelvis [23]. Gerdel et al's large postal questionnaire (n = 7637) with a participation rate of 76.7%, found the prevalence (%) of pain in the previous week of all pains including the abdomen and pelvis to be higher in women (see Table 1) [13].

Irritable bowel syndrome, or IBS, has a female predominance with a female-to-male ratio of 2–2.5:1 in those who seek health care [1].

It is clear that women experience more 'normal' APP because of their physiology, having monthly menses, pain from intercourse, during pregnancy and a higher incidence of cystitis and so on. A systematic review from the United Kingdom revealed that in women, dysmenorrhoea has a prevalence as high as 45–97%, abdominal pain 23–29% and dyspareunia 8% [34]. Even when abdominal pain is separated from dysmenorrhoea, women still report more abdominal pain than men. It may be that dysmenorrhoea sensitises females for future abdominal and pelvic pain, as dysmenorrhoea is associated with long lasting central changes [32].

Vincent's study and others show that women with dysmenorrhoea have increased sensitivity to local and distant noxious somatic stimuli and also visceral stimuli. This raises the possibility that the menstrual and other pains women experience are responsible for viscero-viscero and viscero-somatic hyperalgesia; perhaps the reason that all other chronic pain states are more common in females. The most common cause for men to experience pain in their early years is secondary to trauma, which is not as prevalent in most societies.

The prevalence of bladder pain syndrome (BPS) is not clear, probably as a result of different definitions having been used over the years. A recent European Association of Urology review suggests between 0.06% - 30% of the population have BPS with women ten times more likely to have BPS than men, but this may partly be due to men being given different labels such as prostate pain syndrome as opposed to BPS [33].

Pain of the sex-specific organs and genitalia, for instance vulval pain or testicular pain, are experienced by one or the other sex so no direct comparison can be made, but it is worth noting that the prevalence of chronic male abdominal and pelvic pain is large and male patients with APP probably represent a huge unmet need. The prevalence of prostate pain for example is estimated to be between 2–10% of men worldwide [21], scrotal pain is present in 4.75% of all men presenting to urology clinics [7]. The only known incidence

TABLE 1 **Prevalence (%) of pain in previous week (n = 7637). (Adapted from Gerdel B, Jonas B, Coster L, et al. Prevalence of widespread pain and associations with work status: a population study. BMC Musculoskelet Disord 2008; 9:102)**

Region	Men	Women	All
Head	10.1	21.8	16.2
Upper back	33.2	44.8	39.2
Chest	5.6	6.8	6.2
Abdomen	3.8	6.1	5.0
Pelvis	5.4	10.3	8.0
Low back	29.1	36.6	3.0

of testicular pain is post vasectomy (15–19%) and the authors of this paper state that 'this condition represents a gender gap and a disparity in the knowledge for a subpopulation of men with chronic pain' [26].

Sex Differences in Pain and Analgesia

Most of the following data are not specific to abdominal and pelvic pain but demonstrate the role of gender in pain in general. Fillingim and colleagues excellent review article should be read by those wanting a more in depth understanding [10].

Overall females have lower pain thresholds, experience higher pain intensities and less pain tolerance when assessed in the laboratory [11]. It is difficult to pinpoint mechanisms as sex differences appear relatively consistent across multiple stimulus modalities. It is suggested that recent studies using deep tonic stimuli that mimic clinical musculoskeletal pain may be particularly sensitive to sex differences [10].

Sex differences also occur in endogenous pain modulation but the effects are quite variable and the authors conclude that the mechanisms and practical importance of these differences merit further investigation.

There is no consistent evidence of sex differences in experimental analgesic responses to opioid or non-opioid medication. Clinically, women use more analgesic drugs (and have more side effects) than men [18]. Women consume less morphine post-operatively via patient controlled analgesia (PCA) than men and men show lower morphine requirement when administered by a provider [24]. This would seem contradictory; one could speculate that men report pain less and/or are less willing to request analgesics, or that women use PCA less because of other factors, for instance, side effects or no contact with the provider. It has previously been demonstrated that psychological factors such as trait anxiety and locus of control affect PCA use [4] and expectations of gender such as 'strong men don't need painkillers' could be significant in any study assessing analgesic use. Variations in body composition between men and women, and hormonal effects on protein binding, gastrointestinal transit time, thermoregulation, and creatinine clearance can also influence drug pharmacokinetics and pharmacodynamics [28].

Sex Differences With Non-Pharmacological Treatments

Fillingim's review [10] demonstrates that different distractions prove more effective for one sex than the other with different types of experimental pain. For example, exercising is better for distracting women from cold pressor pain, whereas video games are a more effective distraction for men in this situation. The clinical relevance of this is yet to be elucidated but if different predictors for success of certain treatments exist for men and women, this might be helpful to target treatments. With interdisciplinary pain treatment for example, pretreatment pain tolerance predicts the reduction in pain severity and pain-related interference more strongly in women than men [9]. For physical therapy, duration of symptoms and baseline pain-related disability significantly predicted change in pain intensity for women whereas type of treatment and fear avoidance beliefs predicted the response in males [12]. Baseline pain intensity was predictive for both sexes.

The Role of Sex Hormones

A refresher: the testes produce mainly androgens, i.e. testosterone and the ovaries produce mainly oestrogens and progestins, as does the placenta. Testosterone is aromatized to oestradiol and the adrenal cortex also produces androgens in response to adrenocorticotrophic hormone (ACTH). Thus, both the testes and ovaries produce both sex hormones. In women, testosterone is produced by the adrenal cortex (25%), ovaries (25%), and biotransformation (50%). Although oestrogen levels are higher in females than males, testosterone is higher than oestrogen in females, but below the levels in males. After menopause ovarian production of oestrogens dramatically decreases and the adrenal cortex is responsible via aromatization of androgens to oestradiol in the peripheral tissue (fat). Men are subject to less hormonal variation than women, the most significant change for men being the reduction of testosterone with aging. In the menstrual cycle, oestrogen levels rise in the follicular phase with a peak near ovulation.

Hormonal Influences on Pain

The exact influences of gonadal steroid hormones in pain are not well understood but several clinical conditions lead us to the conclusion that hormones must be important in pain. The severity of symptoms varies across the menstrual cycle for several pain conditions. The menstrual cycle and hormonal influences on pain sensitivity have been reported, but the direction and magnitude of these influences are highly variable.

Prepubertal girls and boys have equal prevalence of migraine, but the lifetime prevalence of migraine is 18% for women, and 6% for men after puberty [29], suggesting that the huge hormonal changes that occur at puberty have a role in this change in prevalence. Clearly this is also a time when gender becomes more important. During pregnancy, migraine frequency decreases but increases postpartum as the oestradiol level declines [22]. Transsexuals experience a change in the incidence of pain as they undergo reassignment with hormonal medication [8]. One third of male-to-females taking oestradiol/antiandrogen treatment develop chronic pain and half of female-to-males treated with testosterone report a significant improvement in chronic headache. Low androgen levels have been thought to be a primary contributor to the incidence and anti-anabolic features of fibromyalgia and in women the prevalence of fibromyalgia in different age groups mirrors serum levels of dehydroepiandosterone (DHEA) suggesting that low androgen levels may be a risk factor for fibromyalgia [8].

These data might suggest that in general testosterone is somewhat 'protective' for pain, and the opposite seems true for high oestrogen states, but it is not that straight forward. After the menopause when oestrogen levels decrease, pain in areas such as the vagina and joints can increase.

Effects of Sex Hormones on Pain Modulation

This is a complex area and one where plenty of current research is focused, the main areas of interest being in the endogenous opioid system, dopamine, serotonin and NMDA receptor function. The role of hormones in inflammation is also substantial and outside the scope of this chapter.

Looking at the endogenous opioid system it would appear that preclinically, conditions characterised by high oestradiol are associated with reduced sensitivity to opioid agonists [10]. What is not clear is the effect of the sex hormones on responses to opioids in humans. A review chapter on brain imaging studies found that recent functional MRI studies suggest 'at least some of the sex differences in pain arise from activation of the endogenous opioid system', and that they also 'demonstrate different receptor availability at baseline, potentially underlying sex differences in the response to opioid analgesia' [31]. This work concluded that there is evidence to suggest that women focus on the affective component of the pain experience in response to a somatic stimulus to a greater extent than men and that the prefrontal cortex appears to play a central role in generating sex differences in pain in adults.

Dopamine has a role in modulating pain perception and evidence suggests sex-specific differences in dopaminergic function but additional research is needed to determine these. Oestrogens are also involved in maintaining the integrity and functional activity of the dopamine system [10]. Oestrogenic enhancement of NMDA (N-Methyl-D-Aspartate) receptor excitability might also contribute to more robust central sensitisation among women than men [17]. Serotonin's peripheral effects are thought to contribute to sex-related pain conditions like migraine and IBS. Serotonin's central function is modulated by ovarian hormones and greater brain serotonin synthesis in females with IBS may explain the female preponderance for this condition [10].

Gender Roles

Peoples' expectation of men and womens' response to pain exerts a strong influence on that pain experience and behaviour. Despite common attestations from both sexes about men not being able to withstand the pain of labour for example, in studies, both men and women consider women to be more sensitive to pain, less enduring of pain and more willing to report pain compared with men [15]. High masculinity and high femininity scores predict higher and lower pain sensitivity respectively in experimental pain [10]. The sex of the experimenter is also important, with male subjects enduring more pain in the presence of a female researcher. Clinical pain findings are more limited and less consistent. Do these findings merely reflect gender-related response bias that is men report less, women more, or might there be a difference in endogenous pain modulation?

Gender Bias in Pain Treatment

We should be very aware of gender bias that may impact on treatment of APP. Numerous studies indicate that women's pain may be under-treated. In a study of emergency room care, women with abdominal pain were less likely to receive analgesics and wait longer to receive them [6]. Another study showed that women were more likely to receive sedatives whereas men received analgesia after cardiac surgery [5]. Both male and female doctors were more likely to provide non-specific somatic diagnoses, address psychosocial variables in the history and prescribe analgesic and psychoactive medications for female patients with neck pain[16]. The authors concluded that 'physicians' gendered expectations are involved in creating gender differences in medicine'. They recommended the inclusion of gender theory and discussions about gender attitudes into medical school curricula to bring about awareness of the problem.

Stress, Coping, and Catastrophising

Differences in the response to acute and chronic stress and pain are sexually dimorphic with men's diurnal variation in cortisol levels influenced more [30]. In general, women use more behavioural coping strategies and social or emotional support than men and men are more likely to effectively use distraction. Catastrophising is more prevalent in healthy women than men, but is also more strongly related to negative mood in women. Most studies of people in pain show women report higher levels of catastrophising, and in some studies this mediates sex differences in pain [10].

Anxiety and Depression

It is well established that higher anxiety is associated with increased pain both clinically and in the laboratory. Women may report higher levels of anxiety so it is perhaps surprising that anxiety is more strongly related to experimental, clinical and to treatment-related pain in men [20]. In one study, male participants scoring above the median on the Trait Anxiety Inventory reported significantly greater pain intensity, unpleasantness. and showed lower pain tolerance compared to males scoring below the median on the cold pressor pain procedure, while no such differences in cold pressor pain report were found between high and low anxious women [19]. One could postulate that because women are more likely to express anxiety, this can be attended to or treated, thus reducing the anxiety enhanced component of pain.

Pain and depression are highly related and depression is more common in women.

Among those with depression, women are more likely to report pain complaints than men. Whether depression influences pain perception differently in men and women is not known.

PRACTICAL IMPLICATIONS

It is important to consider that both sexes with abdominal and pelvic pain are under referred for painful conditions. The author would urge the reader to be very aware of one's own and colleagues' gender biases and how this may impact on the expectations and treatment of those with APP. Women are more likely to be labelled as anxious or depressed, men more likely to continue to be treated for 'prostatitis' or varicoceles; both miss out on effective treatment for their pain. Practically, one should also consider if hormone treatment might help or is contributing to pain. Is your patient (male or female) lacking in testosterone? Is the opioid they are on inducing a hypogonadic state by suppressing their hypothalamic-pituitary-gonadal axis resulting in low testosterone levels?

Another practical consideration is whether one can minimise pain sensitisation via treating dysmenorrhoea or any other acute pain well. If you are a gynaecologist or urologist, early referral to a pain team is essential even if all investigations may not be complete. Although the reader is likely to be part of a group who understands this well, education of colleagues is of vital importance as part of an inter-disciplinary team. Finally, consider if there are any sex related predictors of treatment outcome that might be useful – are you running a program that is more likely to be successful in certain men or women?

LOOKING AT THE FUTURE

Until 1993, women were excluded from clinical phase I and early phase II trials due to risk of studying women with child-bearing potential. Thus, there is a paucity of data on sex differences in pharmacokinetics, dose-response, and adverse effects. In 1993, the United States' Food and Drug Administration (FDA) guidelines emphasized that trials of new drugs should address:

- The effects of the menstrual cycle and menopausal status on the pharmacokinetics of a drug
- The effect of oestrogens and oral contraceptives on the pharmacokinetics of a drug
- The influence of oral contraceptives on the effectiveness of a drug

IASP SIG on Sex, Gender and Pain's Consensus report [14] concluded the following as issues for future investigation of sex differences:

- Identifying hormonal versus chromosomal contributions
- Understanding the contribution of local versus gonadal hormone effects
- Elucidating the role of psychological factors
- Understanding whether pain chronicity contributes
- Role in ascending and descending modulation
- Cellular and molecular bases in pain and analgesia
- Across the lifespan
- Consideration of sex-specific diagnostic criteria for some pain disorders

One hopes that continued research in sex and gender differences will aid our understanding and treatment of APP.

TAKE HOME MESSAGES

- Women are at greater risk of abdominal and pelvic pain even when accounting for dysmenorrhoea is taken into account.
- Females exhibit greater pain sensitivities for most experimental pain modalities.
- Sex differences occur in clinically relevant pain models such as temporal summation and in functional MRI.
- The interplay between hormonal influences, endogenous pain modulation, and psychosocial factors is complex and not fully understood.
- There has been limited clinical impact of new knowledge from sex, gender and pain research.
- It is essential that future research controls the hormonal profile of women.

FURTHER READING

Craft RM, Mogil JS, Aloisi AM. Sex differences in pain and analgesia: the role of gonadal hormones. Eur J Pain 2004 8(5): 397–411.

Fillingim RB, King CD, Ribeiro-Dasilva MC, et al. Sex, gender, and Pain: A review of Recent Clinical and Experimental Findings. J Pain 2009;10(5):447–485.

Fillingim RB. Sex, gender and pain. IASP Press, 2000.

Greenspan JD, Craft RM, LeResche L, et al; Consensus Working Group of the Sex, Gender, and Pain SIG of the IASP. Studying sex and gender differences in pain and analgesia: a consensus report. Pain. 2007;132(Suppl 1): S26–45. Epub 2007 Oct 25.

Vincent K, Tracey I. Brain Imaging: Sex Differences in Cerebral Responses to Pain. In: Chin ML, Fillingim RB, Ness TJ (eds). Pain in women. New York: Oxford University Press, 2013.

Definitions

Sex = either of the two main categories (male and female) into which humans and most other living things are divided on the basis of their reproductive functions.

Gender = the state of being male or female (typically used with reference to social and cultural differences rather than biological ones).

REFERENCES

1. Adeyemo M, Spiegel B, Chang L. Do irritable bowel syndrome symptoms vary between men and women? Aliment Pharmacol Ther. 2010;32(6):738–755.
2. Aloisi AM, Bachiocco V, Constantino A, et al. Cross-sex hormone administration changes pain in transsexual women and men. Pain 2007; 132 (Suppl 1): S60-S67.

3. Berkley KJ. Vive la difference. Trends Neurosci.1992 15:331–332.
4. Brandner B, Bromley L, Blagrove M. Influence of psychological factors in the use of patient controlled analgesia. Acute Pain 2002: 4(2) 53–56.
5. Calderone KL. The influence of gender on the frequency of pain and sedative medication administered to postoperative patients. *Sex Roles*. 1990;23(11–12):713–725.
6. Chen EH, Shofer FS, Dean AJ, et al. Gender disparity in analgesic treatment of emergency department patients with acute abdominal pain. Acad Emerg Med 2008; 15(5):414–8.
7. Ciftci H, Savas M, Yeni E, et al. Chronic Orchalgia and Associated Diseases. Curr Urol 2010;4:67–70.
8. Craft RM, Mogil JS, Aloisi AM. Sex differences in pain and analgesia: the role of gonadal hormones. Eur J Pain 2004 8(5): 397–411.
9. Edwards RR, Doleys DM, Lowery D, Fillingim RB. Pain tolerance as a predictor of outcome following multidisciplinary treatment for chronic pain: differential effects as a function of sex. Pain 2003;106(3):419–426.
10. Fillingim RB, King CD, Ribeiro- Dasilva MC, et al. Sex, gender, and Pain: A review of Recent Clinical and Experimental Findings. J Pain 2009;10(5): 447–485.
11. Fillingim RB, Edwards RR, Powell T. The relationship of sex and clinical pain to experimental pain responses. Pain 1999; 83:419–25.
12. George SZ, Fritz JM, Childs JD, Brennan GP. Sex differences in predictors of outcome in selected physical therapy interventions for acute low back pain. J Orthop Sports Phys Ther. 2006;36(6):354–63.
13. Gerdel B, Jonas B, Coster L, et al. Prevalence of widespread pain and associations with work status: a population study. BMC Musculoskelet Disord 2008; 9:102.
14. Greenspan JD, Craft RM, LeResche L, et al; Consensus Working Group of the Sex, Gender, and Pain SIG of the IASP. Studying sex and gender differences in pain and analgesia: a consensus report. Pain. 2007;132(Suppl 1): S26–45. Epub 2007 Oct 25.
15. Hadjistavropoulos T, McMurty B, Craig KD. Beautiful faces in pain: Biases and accuracy in the perception of pain. Psychol Health. 1996;11(3):311–420.
16. Hamberg K, Risberg G, Johansson EE, Westman G. Gender bias in physicians' management of neck pain: a study of the answers in a Swedish national examination. J Womens Health Gend Based Med. 2002;11(7):653–66.
17. Herrero JF, Laird JM, Lopez-Garcia JA. Wind-up of spinal cord neurones and pain sensation: much ado about something? Prog Neurobiol. 2000;61(2):169–203.
18. Isacson D, Bingefors K. Epidemiology of analgesics use: a gender perspective. Eur J Anaesthesiol Suppl 2002; 26:5–15.
19. Jones A, Zachariae R, Arendt-Nielsen L. Dispositional anxiety and the experience of pain: gender-specific effects. Eur J Pain. 2003;7(5):387
20. Jones A, Zachariae R. Gender, anxiety, and experimental pain sensitivity: an overview. J Am Med Womens Assoc. 2002;57(2):91–4.
21. Kreiger JN, Riley DE, Cheah PY, et al. Epidemiology of prostatitis: new evidence for a world-wide problem. World J Urol 2003; 21(2):70–74.
22. LeResche L, Sherman JJ, Huggins K, et al. Musculoskeletal orofacial pain and other signs and symptoms of temporomandibular disorders during pregnancy: a prospective study. J Orofac Pain 2005; 19:193–201.
23. Malone M, Lee J. Epidemiology of Urogenital Pain. Baranowski, Abrams P, Fall M (eds). Urogenital Pain in Clinical Practice. New York: Informa Healthcare, 2008:18–2.
24. Miaskowski C, Levine JD. Does opioid analgesia show a gender preference for females? Pain Forum 1999;8:34–44.
25. Oxford English Dictionary www.oed.com/
26. Quallich SA, Arslanian-Engoren C. Chronic testicular pain in adult men: an integrative literature review. Am J Mens Health. 2013;7(5):402–13.
27. Sax, Leonard "How common is intersex? a response to Anne Fausto-Sterling." J Sex Res 2002;39(3): 174–178.
28. Shetty P, Holdcroft A. Gender and Pain. In: Baranowski, Abrams P, Fal M (eds). Urogenital Pain in Clinical Practice. New York: Informa Healthcare, 2008:71–76.
29. Stewart WF, Lipton RB, Celentano DD, Reed ML. Prevalence of migraine headache in the United States: Relation to age, income, race and other sociodemographic factors. JAMA 1992; 267:64–69.
30. Turner-Cobb JM, Osborn M, da Silva L, et al. Sex differences in hypothalamic-pituitary-adrenal axis function in patients with chronic pain syndrome. Stress. 2010;13(4):292–300.
31. Vincent K, Tracey I. Brain Imaging: Sex Differences in Cerebral Responses to Pain. In: Chin ML, Fillingim, RB, Ness TJ (eds). Pain in women. New York: Oxford University Press, 2013.
32. Vincent K, Warnaby C, Stagg C, et al. Dysmenorrhoea is associated with central changes in otherwise healthy women. *Pain*, 2011;152(9):1966–75. www.efic.org/userfiles/EFIC_EYAP_Bladder%20pain.pdf
33. Zondervan K, Yudkin P, Vessey M, et al. The prevalence of chronic pelvic pain in women in the United Kingdom: a systematic review. Br J Obstet Gynaecol 1998; 105 (1):93–8.

PART 2

Phenotyping Aspects

MUSCULOSKELETAL

Chapter 6 **Body, Mind, and Brain in Pelvic Pain**

Chapter 7 **Referred Soft Tissue Phenomena**

Chapter 8 **Pelvic Floor Muscle Pain and Trigger Points**

PSYCHOLOGICAL/SEXOLOGICAL

Chapter 9 **Understanding the Psychological Components of Pain**

Chapter 10 **Sexual Dysfunctions**

Chapter 11 **Addressing Psychosexual Components of Pelvic Pain**

Chapter 12 **Research, Assessment, and Treatment of Sex Related Pain**

UROLOGICAL

Chapter 13 **Bladder pain**

Chapter 14 **Male genital pain**

GYNECOLOGICAL

Chapter 15 **Gynaecological Aspects of Chronic Pelvic Pain**

Chapter 16 **Mechanisms and Treatment of Endometriosis Associated Pain**

Chapter 17 **Diagnosis and Treatment of Female Genital Pain**

GASTRO-INTESTINAL

Chapter 18 **Functional Disorders of The Gastro-intestinal Tract**

Chapter 19 **Anorectal dysfunction and chronic pain**

CHAPTER 6

Body, Mind, and Brain in Pelvic Pain

Carolyn Vandyken and Sandra Hilton

INTRODUCTION

Mind-body connection has been a popular topic over the past decade when looking at persistent pain states in the clinical setting. Despite this shift, the lens used for assessing patients still employs a dominating filter of biomedicalism instead of biopsychosocialism. This chapter will look at historical perspectives, current trends and research to support a significant shift in treatment for persistent pelvic pain towards a biopsychosocial model. Historically, treatment of persistent pelvic pain has been mired in the tissues, and realistically, the tissues should not be ignored. Educating patients about the neurophysiology of pain will allow practitioners to make the shift towards a more comprehensive approach where the biological, psychological and social contributors are all given appropriate consideration. However, we should also exercise caution so that the pendulum does not swing so far in the opposite direction that we only consider the psychosocial characteristics of persistent pain.

BASIC ASPECTS

Mechanisms

Mechanisms underlying persistent pain differ from those underlying acute pain states, and yet from a therapeutic and medical perspective, they are often treated in a similar fashion [21]. In the absence of anatomical causes in persistent pain states, medical subspecialties have historically applied various labels including fibromyalgia, irritable bowel syndrome, interstitial cystitis or somatization [21]. Patients have often been made to feel that their pain is all "in their head" as if they are imagining their symptoms, causing untold despair and frustration. Recent evidence has suggested central pain mechanisms play a considerable role in many patients with persistent pain, even in those that were traditionally thought to have strong peripheral mechanisms, such as rheumatoid arthritis and osteoarthritis [21]. Therefore, the role of central pain mechanisms needs to be considered in all persistent pain states, not as a default diagnostic consideration but as a primary diagnostic indicator in pain that lasts longer than 3–6 months. "The medical profession has unwittingly created a form of mental imprisonment that I call medicalization, when diagnosis and treatment (of pain) causes an increase in pain and suffering"[13].

Definitions

Central Sensitization

As early as 1883, Dr. Sturge envisaged a possible central nervous system "commotion passed up from below" that contributed to the clinical features of ischemic cardiac pain [32]. Indeed, the spinal gate control theory by Melzack and Wall in 1965 highlighted that this sensory relay system could be modulated in the spinal cord by inhibitory controls [15]. Woolf first described central sensitization in the early 1980's and operationally defined central sensitization 30 years later as an amplification of neural signaling within the CNS that elicits pain hypersensitivity [32]. The structural changes that occur in the nervous system are complex and are the subject of ongoing extensive basic science research. When pain persists, reorganization of the brain may contribute to persistent pain [17]. Central sensitization is a real phenomenon that can contribute to inflammatory, neuropathic and dysfunctional pain disorders. In other words, people experiencing these symptoms are not crazy, and the structural changes that occur in the nervous system in persistent pain are as tangible as the changes that occur in the tissues in acute pain.

DESCRIBING THE SUBJECT

Biopsychosocial Perspective

Thirty years ago, Dr. Waddell introduced the biopsychosocial model of disability for chronic low back pain [31]. Waddell recommended taking a three-pronged approach to the management of chronic low back pain, including the assessment of tissue involvement (biological perspective), illness behavior (psychological perspective) and socio-economic factors (social perspective) as they affect persistent pain. He defined non-organic signs of pain, which have been used extensively in the last thirty years to describe malingers and patients with perceived secondary gain issues. What Waddell put forward as non-organic signs are now recognized as significant factors that suggest central sensitization [25]. Cogwheeling (seen as an absence of smooth movement around a joint) is a classic non-organic sign that presents as a lack of coordination in the sensori-motor cortex, leading to jerky movements within agonist and antagonist muscle groups. Cogwheeling represents an organic change within the central nervous system rather than a poor effort put forth by a patient. Waddell emphasized taking a biopsychosocial approach with patients who demonstrate non-organic signs and symptoms. These patients should be identified as having organic nervous system changes, as defined by central pain mechanisms. Woolf has created a list of syndromes and conditions that have been shown to have a strong basis in central pain mechanisms, and many of those conditions are familiar to the persistent pelvic pain practitioner [32]. These include:

- Fibromyalgia
- Irritable Bowel Syndrome and other functional GI disorders
- Idiopathic Low Back Pain (LBP)
- Primary Dysmenorrhea
- Bladder Pain Syndrome/ Interstitial Cystitis/ Chronic Prostatitis
- Chronic pelvic pain and endometriosis
- Myofascial Pain Syndrome/Regional Soft Tissue Pain Syndrome [21].

Biomedical versus Biopsychosocial Perspective

A biopscychosocial approach is not neurocentric, focusing only on the brain and central processing. Peripheral pathology certainly needs to be considered, and a careful assessment of the balance of peripheral and central drivers should be completed for the person experiencing persistent pelvic pain. It is reasonable to assume that central pain mechanisms play a part in persistent pelvic pain, just as they do in all pain, even though we do not have the growing body of evidence underpinning other complex pain states such as Complex Regional Pain Syndrome (CRPS).

It can be challenging to change paradigms. We have identified 3 likely barriers to adopting a biopshycosocial approach to persistent pelvic pain.

First, the diagnostic terminology for persistent pelvic pain remains biomedical. Diagnostic labels include such conditions as levator ani syndrome, piriformis syndrome, coccydynia, vaginismus, vulvodynia, vestibulodynia and pudendal neuralgia. The labelled anatomical parts in these diagnoses encourage the clinician to consider the anatomical tissues as the main driver of the pain state. It may be sensible to follow the lead of other complex pain syndromes, such as Complex Regional Pain Syndrome, which was renamed from Reflex Sympathetic Dystrophy, in recognition that this syndrome is more complex and not limited to the autonomic nervous system. This re-labeling approach is beginning to occur in persistent pelvic pain as evidenced by renaming Interstitial Cystitis to Bladder Pain Syndrome (BPS). Phenotyping is the next logical step in this identification process, which would then help to direct appropriate treatment within the syndrome. This phenotypic approach is currently being studied in BPS [27]. Perhaps a change from the biomedical labels of pelvic pain as described previously to Chronic Pelvic Pain Syndrome would emphasize the need to approach this complex population from a biopsychosocial framework. Within Chronic Pelvic Pain Syndrome, it would then be prudent to determine if the predominant expression of the pain presentation is urological, gynaecological, gastrointestinal, sexual, or orthopaedic in order to direct treatment efforts and team member involvement.

Second, educational and training programs are biomedical. Domenech compared biomedical training versus biopsychosocial training of second-year physiotherapy (PT) students in the treatment of chronic LBP and how it drove their beliefs and clinical reasoning [2]. When trained in the commonly held biomedical approach, PT student interactions with chronic LBP patients were more limiting with regards to fear avoidance beliefs and had weaker return to work recommendations than those trained in a biopsychosocial approach [2]. Dr. Goldstein reports that gynaecologists are not taught a biopsychosocial perspective either in their residency programs [6]. He reports that in his training, he had one hour of education in a 20,000-hour residency on the nature of pelvic pain. It should also be noted that many patients hold very strong biomedical beliefs even before their visit to a physiotherapist or physician. Research has shown treatment expectancy and credibility to be of significant prognostic value to rehabilitation outcomes in patients with chronic low back pain [26]. The clinicians' beliefs and attitudes account for the communication between the clinician and patient, including patient education, which in turn modulates treatment expectancy and credibility. The patient's expectancy and beliefs of treatment credibility can be positively influenced by the clinician, but focusing on the biomedical model will result in inadequate illness perceptions in patients, which in turn leads to more negative initial response to treatment [29].

Third, randomized clinical trials (RCT) published in persistent pelvic pain are biomedical. Clinical RCT's are not common in pelvic pain. However, Fitzgerald published a RCT looking at tissue-based treatment for urological pain including connective tissue massage, internal trigger point massage and external trigger point massage vs. generalized whole body massage [3]. Tissue-based physical therapy produced a 59% response rate in the female participants compared to a 26% response rate in the general whole body massage control group. The American Urological Association heralded this important study as the first study in the preceding ten years to demonstrate a positive effect to an intervention for chronic urological pain. This Fitzgerald study provides high quality evidence for manual therapy intervention in the treatment of urogynecological syndromes, since this has not been established to date. It is important to note that this study did not include the use of a biopsychosocial perspective in its treatment approach nor did it include the use of neurophysiology based pain education. The question remains: What happened to the other 41% in the study? Would a program including neurophysiology based pain education and a biopsychosocial approach have improved the outcomes of this study?

There is a developing body of research that supports the use of a biopsychosocial framework in the treatment of persistent pelvic pain. Dr. Pukall, a psychologist and sex therapist, has completed a series of studies over the past ten years to answer the questions:

- Is the pain of provoked Vestibulodynia in the vulva?
- Does the pain of provoked Vestibulodynia exist outside the vulva?
- Is the pain of provoked Vestibulodynia "in the head"?

In a 2002 study, Pukall tested tactile and pain thresholds of women with Vulvar Vestibulitis Syndrome (VVS) compared to matched pain-free controls [22]. Stimuli to the vulvar tissues that evoked tactile sensations in the control group produced pain responses in women with VVS. Tactile threshold tolerance levels were 95 mg for the VVS group compared to 371 mg in the control group. Interestingly, pain thresholds were also statistically significantly lower for women with VVS in the tibia, forearm, deltoid and thigh suggesting an overall generalized sensitivity in women with VVS versus controls. This study suggests there may be a general sensory disturbance given the widespread pain and tenderness.

Further research by Pukall in the chronic vulvar pain population looked at the structural correlates and cortical changes in the brain [23,24]. These findings support a biopsychosocial perspective for the treatment of chronic vulvar pain given the consistency of central sensory dysregulation and correlation to pain catastrophization as well as tactile and pain thresholds. Gray matter density was significantly increased in women with chronic vulvar pain in the hippocampus, parahippocampus and basal ganglia vs matched controls [24]. These areas are conceptually linked to involvement in pain modulation, stress and emotional assessment. Apkarian has also demonstrated white matter changes that predict the transition from acute to chronic low back pain [14]. These nervous system changes provide further momentum for the need to take a biopsychosocial approach to the management of persistent pelvic pain, at least in the vulvar pain syndromes.

PRACTICAL IMPLICATIONS

When utilizing a biopsychosocial approach to the treatment of persistent pain, both clinicians and patients alike must have an accurate understanding of pain. Pain is defined as an unpleasant sensory and emotional experience associated with actual or potential tissue damage, or described in terms of such damage [11]. Pain can exist without any anatomical tissue damage. The tenacious use of phrases such as "pain receptors" and "pain pathways" provide examples of common misconceptions surrounding the pain system. Nociceptors include temperature, pressure and chemical sensors. There are no "pain" sensors. The information carried by the nerves is not pain; it is a neuro-chemical message. Pain exists only when the brain concludes that the body is in danger (or potential danger) and that action is required. There are no pain pathways that have been identified. The central nervous system can enhance, delay or cancel the messages it receives from nociceptive input. Neurophysiology-based pain education accurately explains the biology of pain and the pain system. Neurophysiology-based pain education as a treatment intervention has been extensively studied with consistent positive results [12]. Good communication skills are required when providing pain education, and clinicians need to practice this approach with patients [19]. Pain education reinforces the fact that pain is not "in their head"; instead, pain is understood to be a biological response to actual or potential threat. In this vein, persistent pain is explained as the result of central pain mechanisms and adaptive changes within the patient's nervous system. This approach contributes to hope and transforms the despair and frustration often seen in people suffering from persistent pain states. In his research, George proposed that it is almost "unethical" to not provide accurate pain education to patients [5].

Two factors need to be considered when determining who requires pain education as an intervention:

The clinical picture is characterized and dominated by central sensitization. This includes those conditions identified in research by Woolf as well as those patients who demonstrate specific characteristics identified by Smart including disproportionate, non-mechanical pain, hypersensitivity, allodynia, pain persisting beyond normal healing time frames (12–16 weeks), and diffuse pain [25,32].

The presence of maladaptive illness perceptions including catastrophization and fear avoidance. It is important to use standardized validated questionnaires to measure these important and predictive psychological factors, which are strong predictors of chronicity [18].

Nijs outlines five steps, which need to be incorporated by clinicians in order to move from a biomedical to a biopsychosocial approach [18]. They are:

The assessment of the clinician's beliefs and attitudes: It is important to assess one's beliefs with regards to pain and the nervous system. Nijs recommends filling out self-report questionnaires as if you are a patient with persistent pain and evaluate your responses. In order to change interventional strategies, one needs to broaden the illness beliefs held by the clinician [11]. Outcomes improved for patients who had a high risk of developing long-term disability and had higher levels of catastrophization or depression, but only if the attitude and beliefs of their treating clinicians changed [21]. Outcomes did not improve with clinical training courses unless the learned information translated into a change in the clinician's belief system [21].

The assessment of the patient's attitudes and beliefs: Disability at six months is predicted by the patient's perception that the problem will persist for a long time, an expanding array of symptoms, weak beliefs about self-control and the patient's low confidence in their own ability to perform activities despite the pain [4].

The reconceptualization of pain into clinical reasoning: A deep understanding of the pain system by the patient and therapist is required in order to change behaviors. Education is necessary to close the gap between the clinician's beliefs and patient expectations and should form the basis of clinical decision making.

The assessment of social support is critical: It is essential to understand the patient's social support system and the interplay of attitudes and beliefs of the members in that system towards the patient's problem.

The intervention provided should not be focused on targeting the tissues alone: When planning interventions for the patient it is crucial that the patient understands the clinical reasoning behind each of the therapeutic interventions. They need to be actively engaged in the process. There is little or no difference between behavioral therapy and group exercises for improving pain or depressive symptoms in persistent pain [7]. Interventions such as supervised or individualized exercise therapy and self-management techniques enhance exercise adherence and improve self-efficacy [10]. Self-efficacy is one of the main predictors of treatment outcome for patients with chronic musculoskeletal pain [16].

Translating theoretical knowledge into clinical practice remains challenging despite basic science and clinical evidence to support the use of a biopsychosocial approach in the treatment of persistent pelvic pain. A framework has been presented previously to guide the assessment of individual patients regarding the balance of their unique contribution of tissue dysfunction and central pain mechanisms (see Appendix A) [8]. The use of this framework can help to direct treatment to the appropriate structures early in the rehabilitation process [28]. This framework employs the use of validated measures to assess the presence of psychosocial risk factors such as fear avoidance and catastrophization [8]. The Pain Catastrophization Scale and the Tampa Scale of Kinesiophobia are good predictors of central pain mechanisms as one potential driver of the pain expression in persistent pain states. Evidence exists for the use of pain education as an effective intervention for persistent pain [12]. Despite the preponderance of evidence supporting pain education, many health professionals are unsure how to incorporate this into practice in a way that the patient will accept and that does not sound as if the pain is "in your head". Resources are available for the health professional including Explain Pain by Butler and Moseley [1], and Understand Pain, Live Well again by Pearson [20].

Appropriate pharmacological interventions for the identified pain state are part of an effective inter-disciplinary approach [14,21]. Acute pain often responds well to nonsteroidal anti-inflammatories while central pain states respond best to neuromodulating agents [21]. Phillips and Clauw reinforce that most chronic pain conditions are likely a mixed pain state with peripheral and central factors playing a role. Pharmacological intervention can influence the immunological cascades, which contribute to the facilitation or inhibition of persistent pain and central sensitivity [21]. Research does not support the use of opioids in persistent pain. The strongest evidence for appropriate medication in persistent pain states is for Dual Uptake Inhibitors such as:

- Tricyclic compounds (amitryptilline, cyclobenzaprine)
- SNRI's and NSRI's (milnacipran, duloxetine)
- Anticonvulsants (pregabalin, gabapentin) [21]

Effective rehabilitation involves the targeting of cortical structures for those patients who present with indications of centrally driven pain states as described previously. Strategies for targeting cortical structures include Cognitive Behavioral Therapy and Sensory Discrimination Training of the involved body part. It is reasonable to re-establish ownership and accurate sensory/motor awareness of the affected areas in order to retrain accurate body mapping. Moseley and Flor discussed this issue with the use of Graded Motor Imagery involving three distinct components of 1) Laterality (right/left discrimination) 2) Imagined movements and 3) Mirror Therapy [17]. The application of these techniques to pelvic pain is pre-evidence, but it is reasonable to conclude that an accurate representation of sensation and movement in the sensori-motor cortex would be beneficial in the effort to reestablish efficient control and coordination. Focused treatment at the brain level should include purposeful attention to the affected area during functional movements and activities. Movement therapies such as Feldenkrais, the Franklin Method, Yoga, Tai Chi, or Qi Gong can provide graded exposure with a mind towards integrating function to the pelvic floor in a nonthreatening way.

LOOKING AT THE FUTURE

To help clinicians integrate a biopsychosocial model in their treatment approach of patients with persistent pelvic pain, the following changes need to occur:

The role of central pain mechanisms needs to be considered in all persistent pain states, not as a default diagnostic consideration but as a primary diagnostic indicator in pain that lasts longer than 3–6 months.

It is critical that the initial assessment of each patient utilizes a biopsychosocial approach to identify the appropriate phenotype (peripheral or central pain mechanisms) in order to generate a proper target for intervention.

The literature supports distinguishing between peripheral tissue triggers and cortically driven central pain states. Clinicians should utilize validated assessments including but not limited to the Tampa Scale of Kinesiophobia and the Pain Catastrophization Scale for consistency and accuracy.

Clinicians should target interventions to cortical structures through Mind/Body awareness techniques such as Cognitive Behavioural Therapy, Movement Therapies, Graded Motor Imagery, and Graded Exposure.

There is strong evidence that pain education assists in the recovery of normal function; therefore, Health Care Practitioners should speak about pain clearly and accurately in accordance with the literature.

TAKE HOME MESSAGES

- The biopsychosocial model suggests that not only is pain a complex biomedical, psychological, and social phenomenon, but that it can also be changed through each of these aspects.
- It is imperative that we continue to recognize that treatments of the physical body may be equally valuable in people with persistent pelvic pain. The central nervous system is altered by inputs from the physical body.
- Treating people with persistent pelvic pain with psychosocial interventions only is likely to lead to as poor outcomes as when we historically have tried to fix the tissues, which the patient states are painful.

FURTHER READING

Explain Pain by Butler DS, Moseley GL. *Explain pain.* Adelaide, South Australia: Noigroup Publications; 2013.
Therapeutic Neuroscience Education by Adriaan Louw and Emilio Puentedura. Minneapolis, MN: OPTP; 2013
Chronic Pain. An Integrated Biobehavioral Approach. Herta Flor and Dennis C. Turk. Seattle WA, IASP Press 2011.

REFERENCES

1. Butler DS, Moseley GL. Explain pain. Adelaide, South Australia: Noigroup Publications; 2013.
2. Domenech J, Sánchez-Zuriaga D, Segura-Ortí E, et al. Impact of biomedical and biopsychosocial training sessions on the attitudes, beliefs, and recommendations of health care providers about low back pain: a randomised clinical trial. Pain. 2011;152(11):2557–63. doi: 10.1016/j.pain.2011.07.023.
3. FitzGerald MP, Payne CK, Lukacz ES, et a;; Interstitial Cystitis Collaborative Research Network. Randomized multicenter clinical trial of myofascial physical therapy in women with interstitial cystitis/painful bladder syndrome and pelvic floor tenderness. J Urol. 2012;187(6):2113–8. doi: 10.1016/j.juro.2012.01.123.
4. Foster NE, Thomas E, Bishop A, et al. Distinctiveness of psychological obstacles to recovery in low back pain patients in primary care. Pain. 2010;148(3):398–406. doi: 10.1016/j.pain.2009.11.002.
5. George SZ, Teyhen DS, Wu SS, et al. Psychosocial education improves low back pain beliefs: results from a cluster randomized clinical trial (NCT00373009) in a primary prevention setting. Eur Spine J. 2009;18(7): 1050–8. doi: 10.1007/s00586-009-1016-7.
6. Goldstein T. Forward. In: Stein A (ed). Healing Pelvic Pain. New York, NY: McGraw-Hill; 2009: vii – x.
7. Henschke N, Ostelo RW, van Tulder MW, et al. Behavioural treatment for chronic low-back pain. Cochrane Database Syst Rev. 2010;(7):CD002014. doi: 10.1002/14651858.CD002014.pub3.
8. Hilton S, Vandyken C. The puzzle of pelvic pain – a rehabilitation framework for balancing tissue dysfunction and central sensitization I: pain physiology and evaluation for the physical therapist. J Women's Health PT. 2011;35(3):103–113.
9. International Association of the Study of Pain. Taxonomy. http://www.iasp-pain.org/Content/NavigationMenu/GeneralResourceLinks/PainDefinitions/default.htm. Accessed 29 September 2013.
10. Jordan JL, Holden MA, Mason EE, Foster NE. Interventions to improve adherence to exercise for chronic musculoskeletal pain in adults. Cochrane Database Syst Rev. 2010;(1):CD005956. doi: 10.1002/14651858.CD005956.pub2.
11. Laekeman MA, Sitter H, Basler HD. The pain attitudes and beliefs scale for physiothera- pists: psychometric properties of the German version. Clin Rehabil. 2008;22(6):564–75. doi: 10.1177/0269215508087485.
12. Louw A, Diener I, Butler DS, Puentedura EJ. The effect of neuroscience education on pain, disability, anxiety, and stress in chronic musculoskeletal pain. Arch Phys Med Rehabil. 2011;92(12):2041–56. doi: 10.1016/j .apmr.2011.07.198.
13. Lumley MA, Cohen JL, Borszcz GS, et al. Pain and emotion: a biopsychosocial review of recent research. J Clin Psychol 2011;67(9):942–68. doi: 10.1002/jclp.20816.
14. Mansour AR, Baliki MN, Huang L, et al. Brain white matter structural properties predict transition to chronic pain. Pain. 2013;154(10):2160–8. doi: 10.1016/j.pain.2013.06.044.
15. Melzack R, Wall PD. Pain mechanisms: a new theory. Science. 1965; 150(3699): 971–979.
16. Miles CL, Pincus T, Carnes D, et al. Can we identify how programmes aimed at promoting self-management in musculoskeletal pain work and who benefits? A systematic review of sub-group analysis within RCTs. Eur J Pain. 2011;15(8):775.e1–11. doi: 10.1016/j.ejpain.2011.01.016. Epub 2011 Feb 26.
17. Moseley GL, Flor H. Targeting cortical representations in the treatment of chronic pain: a review. Neurorehabil Neural Repair. 2012;26(6):646–52. doi: 10.1177/1545968311433209.
18. Nijs J, Roussel N, Paul van Wilgen C, et al. Thinking beyond muscles and joints: therapists' and patients' attitudes and beliefs regarding chronic musculoskeletal pain are key to applying effective treatment. Man Ther. 2013;18(2):96–102. doi: 10.1016/j.math.2012.11.001.
19. Overmeer T, Boersma K, Denison E, Linton SJ. Does teaching physical therapists to deliver a biopsychosocial treatment program result in better patient outcomes? A randomized controlled trial. Phys Ther. 2011;91(5): 804–19. doi: 10.2522/ptj.20100079.
20. Pearson N. Understand Pain, Live Well Again. Penticton, British Columbia, Canada: Life Is Now, 2007.
21. Phillips K, Clauw DJ. Central Pain mechanisms in chronic pain states-maybe it is all in their head. Best Pract Res Clin Rheumatol 2011; 25(2): 141–154 doi: 10.1016/j.berh.2011.02.005.
22. Pukall CF, Binik YM, Khalifé S, et al. Vestibular tactile and pain thresholds in women with vulvar vestibulitis syndrome. Pain. 2002;96(1–2):163–75.
23. Pukall CF, Strigo IA, Binik YM, et al. Neural correlates of painful genital touch in women with vulvar vesibulitis syndrome. Pain 2005;115(1–2):118–27.
24. Schweinhardt P, Kuchinad A, Pukall CF, Bushnell MC. Increased gray matter density in young women with chronic vulvar pain. Pain. 2008;140(3):411–9. doi: 10.1016/j.pain.2008.09.014.

25. Smart KM, Blake C, Staines A, Doody C. Clinical indicators of 'nociceptive', 'peripheral neuropathic' and 'central' mechanisms of musculoskeletal pain. A delphi survey of expert clinicians. Man Ther. 2010;15(1): 80–87. doi: 10.1016/j.math.2009.07.005.
26. Smeets RJ, Beelen S, Goossens ME, et al. Treatment expectancy and credibility are associated with the outcome of both physical and cognitive-behavioral treatment in chronic low back pain. Clin J Pain. 2008;24(4):305–15. doi: 10.1097/AJP.0b013e318164aa75.
27. Tripp DA, Nickel JC, Wong J, et al. Mapping of pain phenotypes in female patients with bladder pain syndrome/ interstitial cystitis and controls. Eur Urol. 2012;62(6):1188–94. doi: 10.1016/j.eururo.2012.05.023.
28. Vandyken C, Hilton S. The puzzle of pelvic pain – a rehabilitation framework for balancing tissue dysfunction and central sensitization II: A review of treatment considerations. J Women's Health PT. 2012;36(1):34–54.
29. Van Wilgen CP, van Ittersum MW, Kaptein AA. Do illness perceptions of people with chronic low back pain differ from people without chronic low back pain? Physiotherapy. 2013;99(1):27–32. doi: 10.1016/j.physio.2011.09.004.
30. Waddell G, McCulloch JA, Kummel E, Venner RM. Nonorganic physical signs in low-back pain. Spine 1980;5(2):117–25.
31. Woolf CJ. Central sensitization: implications for the diagnosis and treatment of pain. Pain 2011;152(3 Suppl):S2–15. doi: 10.1016/j.pain.2010.09.030. Epub 2010 Oct 18. Review.

CHAPTER 7

Referred Soft Tissue Phenomena

Stephanie Prendergast

INTRODUCTION

Patients with abdominal and pelvic pain (APP) are often evaluated by numerous clinicians in an inconclusive search for a source of their symptoms. Diagnostic confusion arises because organic disease, peripheral and central nervous system dysfunction, and psychological and musculoskeletal impairments can all contribute to a patient's pain syndrome. Common symptoms of APP include intermittent or constant burning, aching, stabbing, or pressure-like sensations in the abdomen, pelvis, genitals, anus, perineum, buttocks, and tailbone region in both men and women. Patients with APP may also report a combination of urinary, bowel, and sexual symptoms, including urinary urgency, frequency, dysuria as well as constipation, difficulty with evacuation or incomplete bowel emptying, dyspareunia, anorgasmia, and post-ejaculatory pain. The single clinician is not prepared to evaluate all of the possible involved systems in APP; therefore, the ideal management of APP occurs within an interdisciplinary evaluation and treatment model. While a review article of 69 journal entries about APP reported considerable inconsistency in clinical trials on how APP is evaluated, the consensus of the article did illuminate the fact that myofascial structures are clearly defined sources of APP. The article concluded by stating that patients warrant a musculoskeletal examination as part of an interdisciplinary management approach [9]. Physical therapists are trained to evaluate and treat musculoskeletal structures; therefore, they are well positioned to play this role within the APP team. When evaluating for APP, a physical therapist must consider the muscles of the pelvic floor and pelvic girdle. All muscles attached to the pelvic girdle can create APP as well as symptoms of urinary, bowel, and sexual dysfunction. While a number of musculoskeletal impairments contribute to APP, two that are extremely common are myofascial trigger points (MTrPs) and connective tissue restrictions (CTRs). This chapter will focus on the evaluation and treatment of these two musculoskeletal causes of APP as well as the associated dysfunctions.

DESCRIBING THE SUBJECT

Myofascial Trigger Points

Active MTrPs spontaneously create local pain at the MTrP site and referred pain in distant sites. This same local and referred pain is often created when the MTrP is manually compressed. Active MTrPs develop as a result of motor endplate dysfunction when muscle fibers are overloaded creating taut, unrelaxing band within a muscle. Muscle fibers can be overloaded in a few different ways [3]. One instance occurs as a result of the viscerosomatic reflex, a phenomenon where disturbances or disease in organs refer pain along the distribution of the somatic nerves that share the same spinal segment as the sympathetic fibers to the affected organ. Organ-based stressors such as endometriosis and repetitive urinary tract and vaginal infections are instances where the viscerosomatic reflex comes into play [14]. Eccentric mechanical stressors, such as excessive straining from constipation or childbirth, or heavily weighted squatting exercises create MTrPs via the same mechanism. Conversely, concentric mechanical stressors such as ongoing, forceful core strengthening programs or ongoing "holding" of the pelvic floor muscles in activities such as dance and gymnastics can also overload muscle fibers and create MTrPs. In addition, psychological distress can contribute to repetitive "guarding" of the pelvic floor muscles, creating a low-load prolonged stress that can also result in active MTrPs [10].

To evaluate a MTrP, the clinician applies pressure perpendicular to the direction of the muscle fibers using the pad of his or her finger. The clinician is looking to identify a taut band of muscle fibers that is tender upon compression and may cause local allodynia or referred hyperalgesia in a distant site. Patients may also report a replication of one or more of their chief complaints with palpation [3]. Additionally, palpation may result in a local twitch response. This is a spinal cord reflex that is characterized by an involuntary contraction of the contractured, taut band when mechanically stimulated [15].

It is important to note that a patient's APP symptoms may be due to multiple MTrPs that exist in several different muscles groups in combination with dysfunction in other systems of the body.

The problems that MTrPs cause extend beyond peripheral and local referred pain. Indeed, MTrPs are peripheral sources of nociceptive input thereby influencing the central nervous system. As a result, individuals with MTrPs demonstrate abnormal central pain processing mechanisms showing enhanced brain activity in the somatosensory and limbic regions, suppressed activity in the hippocampus, and hyperalgesia in response to electrical stimulation and compression of the MTrPs. MTrPs are involved in almost all pain syndromes and are a major contributing factor to central sensitization [4]. In addition to local and referred pain and central sensitization, active MTrPs cause an increase in cutaneous and subcutaneous hypersensitivity and contribute to the development of connective tissue restrictions, as described later in the chapter [3].

When it comes to eradicating MTrPs, a variety of different treatment options exist. Manual therapy techniques, dry needling, and MTrP injections have all shown efficacy in eradicating MTrPs [3,13].

Manual Therapy

Once a MTrP has been identified, a physical therapist can use the manual therapy technique of direct pressure to the MTrP with his or her finger. The therapist sustains the pressure on the MTrP for 60–90 seconds. In addition, the patient can be directed to perform slight concentric contractions of the muscle that the therapist is applying pressure to [3]. The combination of the pressure and a small contraction can result in mechanical interruption and eradication of the trigger point.

Dry Needling

Dry needling is performed with a solid filiform needle in a tube. The term "dry needling" refers to both superficial and deep dry needling. With deep dry needling, the needle is tapped through the tube and skin to elicit a local twitch response from the MTrP. Similar to the abovementioned manual techniques, the intent of the needle is to disrupt the MTrP and allow the taut muscle fibers to return to normal resting tone. The deep dry needling technique is repeated until the muscle stops eliciting a twitch response and the muscle fibers return to normal tone. When executing superficial needling, the needle is injected into a muscle close to the MTrP; however, a local twitch response is not elicited. The needle is then kept in for about 30 seconds with the intent to decrease the sensitivity of the MTrP [13]. Dry needling can be administered by physical therapists, acupuncturists, chiropractors, and medical doctors in most countries.

MTrP Injections

Similar to manual therapy and dry needling, the intent of a trigger point injection is to mechanically interrupt the MTrP. Typically a local anesthetic and possibly a corticosteroid are used to mitigate the effects of a larger, hollow needle and reduce the tissue sensitivity associated with the insertion of the larger needle into a MTrP. Complete or partial resolution of the patient's symptoms immediately following the injection can be diagnostic of the role this impairment plays in their pain presentation. The second benefit of this procedure is that the needle itself serves as treatment for the trigger point. Trigger point injections are typically administered by physicians.

Manual therapy, dry needling, or MTrP injections should eliminate a particular MTrP, which in turn causes the elimination of the local twitch response resulting in the alleviation of spontaneous motor endplate noise, a reduction of nociceptive, inflammatory and immune system related chemicals, and a reduction of the taut band. Collectively, these responses will reduce or eliminate the pain associated with the MTrP in questions [8,11].

Interpreting the Response to MTrP Interventions

In certain situations a MTrP may be eradicated with one session of either manual therapy, dry needling, or trigger point injections. However, It is not uncommon to use the above-listed interventions over a series of sessions to eradicate chronic, active MTrPs. When treating a patient with APP, communication and skilled physical examination techniques are imperative. Often a patient may report feeling "no change" from the procedure. If this is the case it is important for the clinician to ask him or herself several questions, such as: *Is the trigger point still present?* If the trigger point persists, the symptoms may persist as well. Therefore, the MTrP needs to be treated until it resolves. *Has the MTrP been eliminated?* If the MTrP has been eliminated and symptoms are unchanged, that particular MTrP may not have been as involved in the patient's APP as the provider initially thought. Symptoms may be slightly altered but not eradicated with the resolution of a trigger point. In this case, the MTrP was likely meaningful but there are other contributing factors that need to subsequently be addressed. Excellent communication can help create realistic patient expectations and guide the clinician towards effective clinical reasoning.

Connective Tissue Restrictions

A connective tissue restriction, otherwise known as "subcutaneous panniculosis," is defined as a dense thickening of the subcutaneous tissue that is sensitive upon pinch rolling due to ischemia in the tissue [16]. Dysfunctional connective tissue causes muscular impairment in the underlying muscles and local and referred pain and dysfunction. Connective tissue can become dysfunctional via four general mechanisms:

Viscerosomatic Reflex

The tissues can remodel as a resultant effect of organic disturbance via the viscerosomatic reflex, which was described above. These reflexes are called Head's zones, Chapman's reflexes, or Mackenzie's zones [1]. In a sophisticated animal study, pseudorabies virus was injected into the abductor caudaedorsalis tail model of the rat. This resulted in hemorrhagic changes in the bladder in the absence of a viral infection. Denervation of the bladder prevented the cystitis, suggesting the cystitis is neurogenic in nature. In a second animal study, the uterus of the rat was injected with Evans Blue Dye. The resultant effect was dye extravasation in the skin over the abdomen, groin, lower back, thighs, proximal tail and perineum. [18]. Forty-nine patients with urogynecological symptoms had connective tissue restrictions in these same regions [7]. Two later studies repeated and confirmed the same findings [5,6]. Similar to MTrPs, connective tissue restrictions are found in patients with Bladder Pain Syndrome/Interstitial Cystitis, Vulval pain syndrome, Prostate Pain Syndrome, irritable bowel syndrome, and endometriosis. As the above-mentioned studies show, the connective tissue of the abdomen, low back, lower extremities and vulvar/scrotal area warrants evaluation in patients with APP.

Active MTrPs

Researchers Travell and Simons reported a strong association between active MTrPs and subcutaneous connective tissue restrictions. They suggest that the formation of the connective tissue restrictions may be related to sympathetic nervous system activity involving mechanisms operating in the underlying MTrPs. Therefore, connective tissue should be evaluated superficial to any identified MTrPs in the trunk, bony pelvis, and lower extremities [17].

Neurotrophic Reflexes

Connective tissue restrictions may also develop as a result of the initiation of neurotrophic reflexes stemming from intervertebral joint dysfunction. For example, thoraco-lumbar junction syndrome is known to cause referred pain and subcutaneous panniculosis in the ipsilateral groin [12].

Peripheral Nerve Inflammation

Connective tissue restrictions develop in response to repetitive stimuli from inflamed peripheral nerves. For example, patients with pudendal neuralgia may present with a thickening of the connective tissue in the perianal tissue, medial to the ischial tuberosities, and/or in the vulva [2].

Locally, dysfunctional connective tissue is ischemic and allodynic. Connective tissue restrictions can contribute to clothing intolerance, genital and perianal itching, feelings of foreign objects in the pelvis, vaginal and anal fissures, neural ischemia, and therefore neuralgia, pain at the ischial tuberosities when sitting (mechanical compression upon an ischemic area), and referred disturbance to create dysuria and uterine discomfort via the somatic-visceral refelex. Visually, the tissues may look discolored or have a peau' d'orange appearance [14]. In addition to the associated symptomatology, dysfunctional connective tissue causes other problematic musculoskeletal impairments. For instance, the ischemic tissues cause underlying muscle dysfunction, which can lead to MTrPs. Also, connective tissue restriction can cause an impairment called "neural ischemia" thus creating symptoms of neuralgia on peripheral nerves [14].

Connective tissue can be evaluated by grasping the tissue between a thumb and forefinger and pushing the thumb through the created tissue roll. The physical therapist uses this technique to assess for tension and mobility impairments. If the connective tissue is impaired, the physical therapist will feel a thickening of the tissue, decreased mobility and increased tension. The patient will usually report an uncomfortable scratching sensation in the areas of restriction secondary to the ischemia [14].

Connective Tissue Manipulation (CTM)

CTM is the technique used to treat connective tissue restrictions. It is performed by grasping the connective tissue between the thumb and forefingers creating a "roll" as the therapist pushes through the tissue. The technique is uncomfortable if connective tissue restrictions are present, and the patient will often report a scratching, nail-like sensation during the initial treatments. This may be surprising to the patient, as he or she may not feel pain in the areas where the tissue is restricted without the provocation of CTM. The level of discomfort the patient experiences correlates with the severity of the impairments [14]. Similar to the treatment of MTrPs, the eradication of connective tissue restrictions occurs over a series of subsequent treatments. The discomfort decreases over the course of time during a treatment session as well as with subsequent sessions. The connective tissue of patients with APP should be evaluated in the trunk, pelvis, and lower extremities. The intent of treatment is to improve blood flow, restore mobility, and decrease the density of impaired tissues. The technique is applied to areas of restriction and will decrease tissue hyperalgesia and allodynia as well as have a positive effect on distal structures via the somatic-visceral reflex [14].

PRACTICAL IMPLICATIONS

Evidence of Clinical Benefit of Physical Therapy Treatment for APP

Two recent studies were conducted to determine the efficacy of myofascial physical therapy for the treatment or urologic pelvic pain syndromes [5]. In a prospective, randomized feasibility trial 48 subjects were recruited and randomized to myofascial physical therapy or global therapeutic massage in six clinical centers in the United States. The myofascial physical therapy group received 10 weekly, one-hour, skilled physical therapy sessions that included connective tissue manipulation, myofascial trigger point release, and internal pelvic floor manual therapy. The control group received 10 weekly, one-hour Swedish massage sessions. A total of 94% of the patients completed the study, and the adherence of the physical therapist to the treatment protocol was excellent. The group that received skilled physical therapy demonstrated a 57% response rate, which was significantly higher than the 21% response rate in the group that received massage. The conclusion was that myofascial physical therapy offers a conservative and meaningful treatment option for patients suffering with APP [5].

The results of the feasibility trial warranted a full-scale clinical trial of similar design. In this trial, 81 subjects were recruited and randomized into the same two groups, skilled myofascial physical therapy and Swedish massage [6]. Both groups received 10 weekly, one-hour sessions in 11 different clinical centers in the United States. The global response rate was 26% in the group receiving massage, and 57% in the group receiving physical therapy. In both groups, pain, urinary urgency and frequency rates decreased.

In conclusion, myofascial causes of pelvic pain can be found in the majority of patients suffering from APP. Two defined cause of APP, MTrPs and connective tissue restrictions, both cause local and referred pain as well as contribute to the formation of other impairments, which in turn can also cause pelvic pain and dysfunction. Patients suffering from APP will benefit from a musculoskeletal examination and assessment addressing the muscles and connective tissue of the trunk, lower extremities, bony pelvis, and pelvic floor. When impairments are identified manual physical therapy techniques are a reasonable, conservative treatment that demonstrates clinical efficacy in managing APP.

LOOKING AT THE FUTURE

Our knowledge about the diagnosis and management of chronic pelvic pain has increased substantially over the last 5 years. It is now commonly accepted that the majority of patients with complaints of abdominal and pelvic pain present with musculoskeletal impairments, including myofascial trigger points and connective tissue restrictions, that may be a primary or secondary source of their pain and dysfunction. Concurrently, the number of medical professionals involved in the management of patients with pelvic pain is also increasing. This is evidenced by the increasing number of members to societies committed to pelvic pain, the number of conferences on the topic, and finally the increasing volume of attendees at these specialty meetings. It is our job as specialists to continue to educate the general medical community about abdominal and pelvic pain. Screening tools and treatment algorithms have been developed and will be increasingly utilized in the coming years.

TAKE HOME MESSAGES

- Myofascial Physical Therapy is a conservative and effective treatment for abdominal and pelvic pain syndromes.
- Evidence demonstrates that dry needling and myofascial trigger point injections are also useful treatments to eradicate myofascial trigger points.
- Physical Therapists treating pelvic pain can be found through the International Organization of Physical Therapists in Women's Health (http://www.ioptwh.org), the American Physical Therapy Association's Section on Women's Health (http://www.womenshealthapta.org), and the International Pelvic Pain Society (www.pelvicpain.org).

FURTHER READING

Chronic Pelvic Pain and Dysfunction: Practical Physical Medicine. Edited by Leon Chaitow and Ruth Lovegrove Jones

REFERENCES

1. Beal MC. Vicerosomatic reflexes, a review. J Am Osteopath Assoc 1985; 85: 786–801.
2. Beco J. Pudendal nerve decompression in perineology: a case series. BMC Surg 2004; 4: 1–17.
3. Dommerholt J. Dry needling - peripheral and central considerations. J Man Manip Ther 2001;19:223–37.
4. Dommerholt J, Adler T. Intramuscular manual therapy: Dry needling. In: Chaitow, L. Chronic Pelvic Pain and Dysfunction: Practical Physical Medicine. Edinburgh: Churchill Livingstone; 2012: 363–376.
5. Fitzgerald MP. Randomized multicenter feasibility trial of myofascial physical therapy for the treatment of urologic chronic pelvic pain syndromes. J Urol 2009; 182: 570–580.
6. Fitzgerald MP. Randomized multicenter clinical trial of myofascial physical therapy in women with Interstitial Cystitis/Painful Bladder Syndrome and pelvic floor tenderness. J Urol 2012; 187: 2113–2118.
7. Fitzgerald MP, Kotarinos RK. Rehabilitation of the short pelvic floor. I : Background and patient evaluation. Int Urogynecol J 2003; 14: 261–267.
8. Ge HY, Fernandez-de-Las-Penas C, Yue SW. Myofascial trigger points: spontaneous electrical activity and its consequences for pain induction and propagation. Chinese Med 2011; 6: 13.
9. Kaavadias T, Baessler K, Schuessler B. Pelvic pain in urogynaecology. Part I: evaluation, definitions and diagnoses. Int Urogynecol J 2011;22:385–93.
10. Kotarinos K. Myofascial Pelvic pain. Curr Pain Headache Rep 2012;16: 433–438.
11. Kuan TS, Hseih YL, Chen SM, et al. The myofascial trigger point region: correlation between the degree of irritabilty and the prevalence of endplate noise. Am J Phys Med Rehabil 2007; 86:183–189.
12. Maigne R. Thoracolumbar junction syndrome: a source of diagnostic error. J Ortho Med 1995; 17: 84–89.
13. Mense S. Morphology of myofascial trigger points: what does a trigger point look like? In: Mense S, Gerwin RD (eds). Muscle pain, diagnosis and treatment. Heidelberg: Springer; 2010: 85–102.
14. Prendergast SA, Rummer EH. Connective Tissue Manipulation. In: Schleip R (ed). Fascia: The Tensional Network of the Human Body. Edinburgh: Churchill Livingstone, 2012: 327–334.
15. Rha DW, Shin JC, Kim YK, et al. Detecting local twitch response of myofascial trigger points in the lower-back muscles using ultrasonography. Arch Phys Med Rehabil 2011;92:1576–1580.
16. Stecco C, Stern R, Porzinonato A. Hyaluronan within fascia in the etiology of myofascial pain. Surg Radiol Anat 2011; 66: 1074–7.
17. Travell D, Simons J. In: Myofascial pain and dysfunction, the trigger point manual. Philadelphia: Lippincott Williams & Wilkins; 1993: 11–82.
18. Wesselmann U, Burnett AL, Heinberg LJ. The urogential and rectal pain syndromes. Pain 1997; 73: 269–294.

CHAPTER 8

Pelvic Floor Muscle Pain and Trigger Points

Helena Frawley

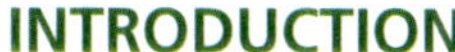

INTRODUCTION

Pelvic floor muscle (PFM) pain and PFM tension are often implicated in the complex presentation of chronic pelvic pain. The etiology of this is not well understood, however a model has been proposed to explain the interconnected relationships between the viscera, pelvic floor muscles/myofascial structures, and the central nervous system, which create the multisymptom presentation of chronic pelvic pain (CPP), as illustrated in Figure 1 [1].

Terminology

Pelvic Floor Muscle Pain

Muscle pain or tenderness may be a symptom of many diseases or disorders [2]. Muscle pain can be described as per below, however the distinctions between these definitions may be arbitrary:

A trigger point is defined as a tender, taut band of muscle that can be painful spontaneously or when stimulated [3]. Local or referred pain may be reproduced. An active trigger point is said to have a characteristic 'twitch' response when stimulated, however the twitch response to palpation has been shown to be unreliable [4]. The most reliable sign is sensitivity to applied pressure; however, due to the limited number of studies available and significant methodological problems, physical examination is not currently recommended as a reliable test for the diagnosis of trigger points [4]. There have been no reports of reliability testing of trigger points in the PFM.

Myofascial pain is localized pain or tender spots within the muscles or their fascial linings, with or without trigger points being identified. For an excellent overview of myofascial pain syndromes and their evaluation, the reader is directed to Giamberadino et al. [5].

Fibromyalgia, which refers to the constellation of widespread pain and muscle tenderness, affecting multiple body sites, accompanied by fatigue, unrefreshed sleep and cognitive problems [6]. Trigger points found in fibromyalgia may have specific body localization.

Pelvic floor muscle pain or tenderness may be present in either the perineal or levator ani muscles.

Pelvic Floor Muscle Tension

Resting muscle tension is determined as the resistance to stretch, passive movement, or deformation when the tissue is digitally palpated. Mense et al. [7] suggest this can be

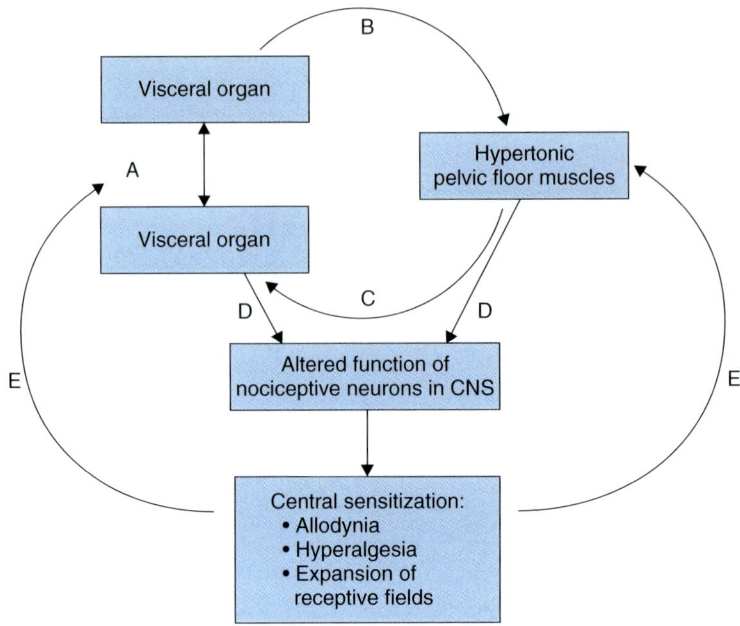

FIGURE 1 Viscerovisceral, viscerosomatic, and somatovisceral convergence are depicted by pathways A, B, and C. D represents nociceptive inputs from viscera and/or myofascial sources leading to central sensitization. E represents central sensitization creating pain perception in either myofascial structures or a visceral organ. All can occur in a single patient, contributing to multiple seemingly unrelated symptoms.

Reprinted from Hoffman D. Understanding multisymptom presentations in chronic pelvic pain: *the inter-relationships between the viscera and myofascial pelvic floor dysfunction. Curr Pain Headache Rep. 2011;15(5):343.*

determined by the compliance (compressibility) of a muscle. This is assessed by pressing a finger into a muscle belly to determine how easily it indents and how 'springy' it is. Normal PFM function includes the ability to remain in a 'normal' rested state when required, the ability to contract when required, and the ability to relax fully following a contraction. The difficulty with interpreting and measuring these states is that little normative data exists on 'normal' PFM activity, hence it is difficult to describe and quantify deviations from normal.

Pelvic floor muscle 'overactivity' is a term applied by Messelink et al. [8, 9] to a condition in which the PFM do not relax, or may even contract when relaxation is functionally needed (for example, during micturition, defecation or sexual intercourse). Initially the term 'overactivity' was based on a symptom (such as pain) plus a physical examination sign (such as inability to relax the PFM or an increased resting level of tension). Various terms can be found throughout the literature referring to altered muscle tension, including: tone, tension, stiffness, firmness, hardness, rigidity, compliance, resting pressure, compressibility, elasticity; with the terms hypertonic, high-tone, shortened pelvic floor, overactive, non-relaxing and spasm used to refer to the finding of increased activity in the PFM. It is important to note that the term 'tone' has a very specific neurological meaning in upper (hypertonic: rigidity) and lower (hypotonic: flaccidity) motor neurone lesions [10] and as such, would seem incorrect when applied to muscle tension in a patient without a neurogenic condition.

The relationship between the symptom (pain) and the sign (increased tension at rest) in the PFM is not well understood, but the co-occurrence of these two features is frequently observed in patients presenting with chronic pelvic floor pain, both in women [11] and men [12]. Indeed the terms 'muscle hyperalgesia' and 'muscle hypertonicity' are often used interchangeably in the literature, however the validity of this equivalence has not been established. It is not known if the relationship between PFM pain and PFM tension is causal and if so, in which direction the causality lies. Increased tension may occur without pain and pain may be present with no abnormality of muscle property, therefore independent assessment of the symptom and the sign are required.

As pain and altered tension in the PFM appear implicated in Chronic Pelvic Pain Syndromes (CPPS), it is important to define these terms accurately, and to reliably measure these aspects of peripheral tissue dysfunction. This chapter focuses on the steps required to effectively evaluate the PFM in a patient who presents with PFM pain

DESCRIBING THE SUBJFECT

The subjective history and objective physical assessment of PFM pain should be comprehensive and relevant to the presenting symptoms and signs. A thorough biopsychosocial history should be taken, to include assessment of all biological, medical, psychological, and social factors known to affect pelvic floor dysfunction and pain. This also assists the clinician to evaluate the relative contribution of peripheral tissue dysfunction, peripheral sensitisation and central sensitization to the patient's condition. The clinical process of peripheral tissue assessment does not distinguish between acute and chronic PFM pain, as assessment of the peripheral tissues should be undertaken with the same degree of methodological rigor and clinical sensitivity, regardless of chronicity.

Confirmation of Primary Pain Generator

If the clinician suspects the PFM as the source of the pain the patient describes, the PFM must be fully evaluated to confirm the primary tissue pain generator. You may be the first clinician whom the patient consults, hence adequate clinical investigation is still required to exclude serious pathology, avoid missing obvious visceral dysfunction and to 'rule in' or 'rule out' local tissues as primary pain generators, so that treatment is effectively targeted. This is the biomedical part of the biopsychosocial model of Chronic Pelvic Pain (CPP) evaluation. Tissue assessment does not mandate a tissue-based treatment approach, but may provide the clinician with symptoms and signs to use in re-assessment and management planning.

Subjective Assessment: Symptoms

Pain History

As pain is usually the predominant symptom the patient presents with, a thorough pain history should include: the site and duration of pain, nature of onset or precipitating event, pain characteristics, response of pain to activity, and associated symptoms [13]. The clinician must be aware of the terminology the patient uses to describe his or her 'pain' symptom(s), which may include: discomfort, tenderness, pressure, sensitivity, soreness and refer to this terminology accordingly. Pelvic floor muscle pain may be present at rest or appear mechanical in nature, (altered with change of posture, movement, activity or state of muscle activity). The clinician needs to determine factors that suggest peripheral dysfunction, such as a mechanical onset or trauma as the precipitating initial event. The clinician should be aware of the clinical state the patient presents in at the time of consultation. From the pain history, factors that suggest central sensitization include patient description of disproportionate and non-mechanical pain, fear avoidance and catastrophisation, poor sleep and multiple system involvement. Pain history may also include evaluation utilising pain rating scales, pain mapping, pain checklists, and pain questionnaires.

Objective Assessment: Signs

Examination

Firstly, obvious pathology which may present with primary or referred PFM pain or altered tension should be assessed and excluded. Following this, much information may be gathered by objective assessment of the PFM, but the validity, reliability, responsiveness and generalizability of this information is limited by a lack of normative data especially in patients with increased PFM tension. Despite this, the information that is gathered by careful assessment is of prime clinical utility, and may lead the way to the development of robust assessment tools and normative values of PFM activity in the future. Basic PFM observation and objective assessment should be performed as per routine pelvic floor assessment.

The distinguishing features of chronic PFM pain syndrome are pain and altered tension (with or without trigger points) in the PFM [14]. Hence in the assessment of a patient with pelvic pain, particular emphasis is placed on assessment of pain and muscle resting tension, contractile activity and the ability to relax. Sensitive and careful examination is vital. A suggested process to elicit useful information regarding pain and muscle tension from the internal pelvic floor physical assessment is outlined below.

Assessment of the internal vagina / rectum. This should always be performed gently and sensitively. In patients presenting with CPP, careful attention is required to assess the symptom of muscle pain and the signs of altered tension (at rest, on contraction and relaxation), and trigger points.

PFM Pain

Digital evaluation should always be performed very gently, with a single, well lubricated digit. The clinician should evaluate: the presence of pain and specifically PFM pain, identifying and recording the site, nature and whether it is localized or diffuse. The aim is to reproduce the patient's pain, at a mild intensity only. Pain may also be assessed on PFM contraction and on relaxation following contraction. Pain in the PFM should be assessed and recorded bilaterally. It is uncommon to find pain on digital palpation of the PFM in asymptomatic women [15–17], whereas PFM tenderness is commonly observed in women [11] and men [12] with CPP. Hence pain on palpation of the PFM should be considered a positive finding.

- Four studies have tested the reliability of a scale designed to record patient-reported pain on clinician's digital palpation of the PFM, as shown in the Table 1. Differences in reliability findings may be explained by variance in populations tested (age, parity, symptom status), pelvic muscle topographical sites assessed, pressure applied by tester(s), scales and scoring methods, resulting in large differences in reliability found within and between studies. Only one scale reported results for levator ani alone, however the reliability values varied widely between anterior and posterior, and left and right levator ani. Furthermore, this study investigated only pain-free women, therefore this scale requires further testing in a symptomatic cohort.

TABLE 8–1 **Reliability of Digital Palpation Scales to Assess Pelvic Floor Muscle Pain**

Study	Population	Scale Tested	Tissue Assessed	Method of Measurement	Scaling and Score	Reliability
Kavvadias et al [14]	17 asymptomatic, nulliparous women	'pelvic muscle tenderness'	levator ani (anterior; posterior), obturator internus, piriformis	"pressure was steadily applied"	0–10 VAS	ICC = 0.28–0.87 for levator ani
Montenegro et al [15]	48 asymptomatic and 108 women with 'chronic pelvic pain'; mixed parity	'pelvic muscle tenderness'	levator ani, obturator internus, piriformis	"as comfortable and delicate a manner as possible"	no pain; painful discomfort; intense pain; maximum total score of 12	$\kappa = 0.91$ for tenderness (levator ani not assessed independently)
Slieker-ten Hove et al [17]	41 women, with and without pelvic floor disorders; mixed parity	'pain scale'	Vaginal walls: anterior, posterior, left and right	Amount of pressure not stated	Dichotomous pain scale: present *vs* absent	Intra-reliability: $\kappa_w = 0.79$; inter-reliability: $\kappa_w = 0.85$
Tu et al [18]	20 asymptomatic and 19 women with 'chronic pelvic pain'; mixed parity	'muscle hyperalgesia scale'	iliococcygeus, pubococcygeus, coccygeus, obturator internus	"small rotating movements of the index finger"	4-point pain scale, 8 sites = composite score 0–24	$\kappa = 0.02–0.35$. (collapsed to 2-pt pain scale, $\kappa = 0.04–0.63$)

Muscle Tension

Pelvic floor muscle tension may be present during the examination, and may be associated with pain. Tension may be invoked by overly-vigorous examination, therefore it is paramount to assess the PFM carefully. Increased tension may be present at rest, or be provoked by a voluntary PFM contraction attempt, and thus confound measurement of the voluntary contraction. Tension may be detected generally throughout the PFM, or concentrated in discrete areas, or taut bands (which may themselves harbor a trigger point). The location and type of altered tension should be described as clearly as possible; marking on an anatomical sketch may assist accuracy. It is important to use a valid and reliable scale for assessing muscle tension, as this sign is often the target of treatment, in order to effect a reduction in pain.

- While many studies have observed increased PFM tension in patients with pelvic floor pain, only one study has investigated the reliability of a scale for measuring levator ani tension: Kavvadias et al [15] investigated the intra- and inter-rater reliability of PFM tension in 17 nulliparous asymptomatic women, using 3-point digital palpation scale (high-, normal- or low-tone). Exact description of pressure applied when assessing 'tone' was not stated. Their results revealed very low (poor) and non-significant scores for reliability (ICC $= -0.36, p=0.92 - 0.03, p=0.45$). Dietz and Shek [18] tested the reliability of a 6-point scale they devised to test the elasticity of the PFM in women with Pelvic Organ Prolaps (POP). The method of assessment involved passive distension of the levator hiatus. While their scale demonstrated moderate reliability ($\kappa_w = 0.55$, 95% CI 0.44–0.66), it has not been tested in a population with pain.
- Trigger points: the sign of increased resting tension in the PFM may be accompanied by the presence of a trigger point.
- Contractile activity of the PFM. This is well documented elsewhere [19].
- Relaxation of the PFM. Pelvic floor muscle relaxation has been defined as the diminution or termination of PFM contraction [8] and is always tested after a contraction. The International Continence Society proposed qualitative rating scale has three levels: absent (no relaxation palpable), partial (return to resting state), complete (relaxation beyond the resting level). Reliability testing of this scale by Slieker-ten Hove at al [20] revealed substantial intra-rater reliability ($\kappa_w = 0.76$; 95% CI: $0.59 - 0.87$), however inter-rater reliability was only fair ($\kappa_w = 0.39$; 95% CI: $-0.01 - 0.38$) indicating further refinement of the scale is required. These authors proposed an improvement to the scale may occur with an additional level of relaxation added to the scale, to be termed 'incomplete', which indicates relaxation that does not (quite) reach the resting level. Another scale for PFM relaxation in a neurogenic population has been described as: 3 for active (good) relaxation after active contraction, 2 denotes hypertonic muscle with temporary relaxation after elongation, and 1 indicates a spastic muscle, unable to relax even after passive elongation [21]. This scale has been reported to be reliable in a population of Multiple Sclerosis patients. It is assumed that elongation is achieved by stretching the PFM, however the technique to perform this assessment has not been described.

Further Evaluation and Investigations

Instrumented methods of measuring PFM pain, sensitivity and PFM tension have been described, and potentially offer more promise as objective measures of these aspects than digital scales.

Pressure-Pain Thresholds

- Vulval tissue: a vulvalgesiometer has been reported to reliably measure the genital pressure-pain threshold in the vulval tissues of women with urogenital pain [22], however this device is available in the research setting only.
- Vaginal pressure algometer: Tu et al [23] investigated the reliability of vaginal pressure-pain thresholds in 19 asymptomatic women, using a prototype vaginal pressure algometer. Validity and reliability proved acceptable in this study and suggest this could be a promising method of objectively measuring PFM pain, however the tool is available in the research setting only at present.

Pelvic Floor Muscle Tension

- Pressure manometry: while this method has established reliability in an asymptomatic population [24] and has been used in CPP intervention studies to measure pre- and post-treatment values of resting pressure [25–27], reliability of the tool in a pain population has not been established. Thomson et al [28] used a cut-off value of 40cm H_2O to determine 'high' resting tension in their cohort of pelvic pain participants, however there are no published normative resting pressure values of levator ani, so the threshold for resting tension is not known.
- Surface EMG: this tool provides a potentially useful surrogate measure of muscle tension as myoelectrical activity is a component of the definition of muscle tone. However despite proposed cut-off values reported for determining the threshold of normal *versus* increased muscle resting tension [29, 30], no widely accepted 'normal' resting values of EMG of the PFM exist. Further, this tool has only poor-fair reliability in a non-pain population [31].
- Real-time ultrasound: trans-perineal ultrasound has been used by Davis et al [32] to assess anorectal angle (ARA) and levator plate angle (LPA) in men with urological chronic pelvic pain syndromes (UCPPS) compared with controls. They found men with UCPPS had more acute ARAs than controls both at rest and during contraction. The two groups did not differ in LPA at rest; however, men with UCPPS had significantly more acute angles during contraction and levator plate excursion. Reliability testing and normative data is required using real-time ultrasound in a PFM pain population.
- Dynamometry: Morin et al [33] have investigated passive properties of the PFM using a dynamometer, by stretching the vaginal tissues and recording passive resistance and elastic stiffness. Values from a pelvic pain population, reliability testing and normative data are required for further application of this tool, however at present, dynamometry is only available in a research setting.
- Elastometry: a further device, an elastometer, is also in early testing phases as a measurement tool of the passive properties of the PFM [34]. Reliability in this small cohort was reported (ICC = 0.92; 95% CI 0.89 – 0.93; ICC = 0.86; 95% CI 0.82 – 0.89).

PRACTICAL IMPLICATIONS

Assessment of PFM tension and pain requires a comprehensive biopsychosocial assessment. For the peripheral tissue evaluation, reference data of normal PFM activity against which abnormalities may be compared is lacking. Useful clinical information of the presence and extent of local tissue dysfunction in a patient presenting with suspected PFM pain or altered tension can be gained from a careful and comprehensive perineal and levator ani evaluation.

LOOKING AT THE FUTURE

Unfortunately at present, valid and reliable scales for measuring PFM pain, tension or trigger points are scarce. The clinician should choose the most robust scale available for the parameter under measure, and carefully record assessment findings.

TAKE HOME MESSAGES

- Pelvic floor muscle dysfunction is often present in chronic pelvic pain presentations. Whether it is a primary pain generator or a secondary consequence is not well understood and indeed may vary between individuals.
- Clinicians need to be able to evaluate both peripheral and central pain drivers to fully understand complex pain presentations. In the case of pelvic floor pain syndromes, PFM pain and altered tension are often present, hence requiring careful evaluation.

FURTHER READING

Bø K, Berghmans LCM, Van Kampen M, Morkved S (eds). Evidence-Based Physical Therapy for the Pelvic Floor: Bridging Science and Clinical Practice. 2nd ed. Elsevier: London, 2014.

Baranowski AP, Abrams P, Fall M. Urogenital Pain in Clinical Practice. Informa Healthcare, 2008.

REFERENCES

1. Hoffman D. Understanding multisymptom presentations in chronic pelvic pain: the inter-relationships between the viscera and myofascial pelvic floor dysfunction. Curr Pain Headache Rep 2011;**15**(5): 343.
2. Mense S, Simons DG, Russell IJ, Pain associated with increased muscle tension. In: Mense S, Simons DG, Russell IJ (eds). Muscle pain: understanding its nature, diagnosis and treatment. Philadelphia: Lippincott Williams & Wilkins, 2001: 99–130.
3. Gerwin RD. Myofascial Pain Syndrome. In: Mense S, Gerwin RD (eds). Muscle Pain: Diagnosis and Treatment. New York: Springer, 2010: 15–83.
4. Lucas N, et al. Reliability of physical examination for diagnosis of myofascial trigger points: a systematic review of the literature. Clin J Pain 2009;**25**(1):80.
5. Giamberardino MA, et al. Myofascial pain syndromes and their evaluation. Best Pract Res Clin Rheumatol 2011;**25**(2):185–198.
6. Woolf CJ. Windup and central sensitization are not equivalent. Pain 1996;**66**(2–3):105–8.
7. Mense S, Simons DG. Pain referred from and to muscles. In: Mense S, Simons DG, Russell IJ (eds). Muscle pain: understanding its nature, diagnosis and treatment. Philadelphia: Lippincott Williams & Wilkins, 2001: 84–98.
8. Messelink EJ, et al. Standardization terminology of pelvic floor muscle function and dysfunction: report from the pelvic floor clinical assessment group of the International Continence Society. Neurourol Urodyn 2005;**24**:374–380.
9. Messelink EJ. Pelvic Floor Muscle Dysfunction and Pelvic Pain. In: Baranowski A (ed). Urogenital Pain in Clinical Practice. New York: Informa Healthcare, 2007: 327–340.
10. Bhidayasiri R, Water MF, Giza CC. Neurological Differential Diagnosis: a prioritized approach. Massachusetts, USA: Blackwell Publishing Ltd, 2005.
11. Fitzgerald CM, et al. Pelvic Floor Muscle Examination in Female Chronic Pelvic Pain. J Reprod Med 2011;**56**(3–4):117–122.
12. Shoskes DA, et al. Muscle tenderness in men with chronic prostatitis/chronic pelvic pain syndrome: The chronic prostatitis cohort study. J Urol 2008;**179**(2):556–560.
13. Hopwood MB. Collection of historical data. In: Abram SE, Haddox JD (eds). The Pain Clinic Manual. Philadelphia: Lippincott Williams & Wilkins, 2000: 33–36.

14. Engeler D, et al. EAU Guidelines on chronic pelvic pain. 2012; Available from: http://www.uroweb.org/guidelines/online-guidelines/ Accessed July 16, 2014.
15. Kavvadias T, et al. Pelvic floor muscle tenderness in asymptomatic, nulliparous women: topographical distribution and reliability of a visual analogue scale. Internat Urogynecol J 2013;**24**(2):281–286.
16. Montenegro MLLdS, et al. Importance of pelvic muscle tenderness evaluation in women with chronic pelvic pain. Pain Med 2010;**11**(2):224–8.
17. Tu FF, et al. Physical therapy evaluation of patients with chronic pelvic pain: a controlled study. Am J Obstet Gynecol 2008;**198**(3):7.
18. Dietz HP, Shek KL. The quantification of levator muscle resting tone by digital assessment. Internat Urogynecol J Pelvic Floor Dysfunct 2008;**19**(11):1489.
19. Bø K, Sherburn M. Evaluation of female pelvic-floor muscle function and strength. Phys Ther 2005;**85**(3):269–82.
20. Slieker-ten Hove MCP, et al. Face validity and reliability of the first digital assessment scheme of pelvic floor muscle function conform the new standardized terminology of the International Continence Society. Neurourol Urodyn 2009;**28**(4):295–300.
21. De Ridder D, et al. Clinical assessment of pelvic floor dysfunction in multiple sclerosis: urodynamic and neurological correlates. Neurourol Urodyn 1998;**17**(5): 537–42.
22. Pukall CF, et al. The vulvalgesiometer as a device to measure genital pressure-pain threshold. Physiol Measure 2007;**28**(12): 1543–1550.
23. Tu FF, et al. Vaginal pressure-pain thresholds: Initial validation and reliability assessment in healthy women. Clin J Pain 2008;**24**(1):45–50.
24. Frawley HC, et al. Reliability of pelvic floor muscle strength assessment using different test positions and tools. Neurourol Urodyn 2006;**25**(3): 236–42.
25. Palsson OS, Heymen S, Whitehead WE. Biofeedback treatment for functional anorectal disorders: a comprehensive efficacy review. Appl Psychophysiol Biofeedback 2004;**29**(3):153–74.
26. Abbott JA, et al. Botulinum toxin type A for chronic pain and pelvic floor spasm in women: a randomized controlled trial. Obstet Gynecol 2006;**108**(4):915–923.
27. Rogalski MJ, et al. Retrospective chart review of vaginal diazepam suppository use in high-tone pelvic floor dysfunction. Internat Urogynecol J 2010;**21**(7): 895–9.
28. Thomson AJ, et al. The use of botulinum toxin type A (BOTOX) as treatment for intractable chronic pelvic pain associated with spasm of the levator ani muscles. BJOG 2005;**112**(2):247–9.
29. Tu FF, et al. Physical therapy evaluation of patients with chronic pelvic pain: a controlled study. Am J Obstetr Gynecol 2008;**198**(3):272.
30. Voorham-van der Zalm PJ, et al. "Diagnostic investigation of the pelvic floor": A helpful tool in the approach in patients with complaints of micturition, defecation, and/or sexual dysfunction. J Sex Med 2008;**5**(4):864–71.
31. Auchincloss CC, McLean L. The reliability of surface EMG recorded from the pelvic floor muscles. J Neurosci Methods 2009;**182**(1): 85.
32. Davis SN, et al. Use of pelvic floor ultrasound to assess pelvic floor muscle function in Urological Chronic Pelvic Pain Syndrome in men. J Sex Med 2011;**8**(11):3173–80.
33. Morin M, et al. Application of a new method in the study of pelvic floor muscle passive properties in continent women. J Electromyogr Kinesiol 2010;**20**(5): 795–803.
34. Kruger J, et al. Test - Retest reliability of an Instrumented Elastometer for Measuring Passive Stiffness of the Levator Ani Muscle. Neurourol Urodyn 2011;**30**(6):865–867.

CHAPTER 9

Understanding the Psychological Components of Pain

Dean A. Tripp and J. Curtis Nickel

INTRODUCTION

The diagnosis/management of pelvic pain is challenging. As noted at the recent 1st World Congress on Abdominal and Pelvic pain (2013, Amsterdam, the Netherlands), pelvic pain may be considered a type of visceral pain, which promoted the inclusion of abdominal pain in that scientific program. As a combined entity, abdominal and pelvic pain in women and men can be perplexing. Diagnosis and treatment recommendations are based on clinical history, with the qualified accuracy of diagnosis often supported with imaging techniques, physical exams [pelvic and abdominal] and laboratory findings. Unfortunately, the examination and treatment of the patient's psychological state has been traditionally ignored.

Urological Chronic Pelvic Pain Syndromes (UCPPS) have been identified as a non-gender specific set of illnesses that are a significant health care issue. This chapter provides a review and management perspective on two prominent Urological chronic pelvic pain conditions [Chronic Pelvic Pain Syndrome/Chronic Prostatitis/Prostate Pain Syndrome and Bladder Pain Syndrome/Interstitial Cystitis]. Research has highlighted the important role that psychosocial risk factors have in determining both UCPPS symptom severity and quality of life. As discussed in recent urogenital pain research, and proposed at the 1st World Congress on Abdominal and Pelvic Pain, practitioners must recognize and act upon the psychosocial risk factors to optimize therapeutic strategies for UCPPS cases, that in reality apply to many diagnoses of chronic abdominal and pelvic pain.

BASIC ASPECTS

Abbreviations:

CPPS/CP/PPS (Chronic Pelvic Pain Syndrome/Chronic Prostatitis/Prostate Pain Syndrome), CPCI (Chronic Pain Coping Inventory), BPS/IC (Bladder Pain Syndrome/Interstitial Cystitis), NIH (National Institutes of Health), QoL (Quality of Life), UCPPS (Urological Chronic Pelvic Pain Syndromes).

Pain, although an unwelcomed occurrence, is essential for facilitating medical diagnoses and treatment. Pain is a complex union of sensation, emotions, and thoughts. Pain is a motivating factor for physician consultations [50], emergency room visits, and increased

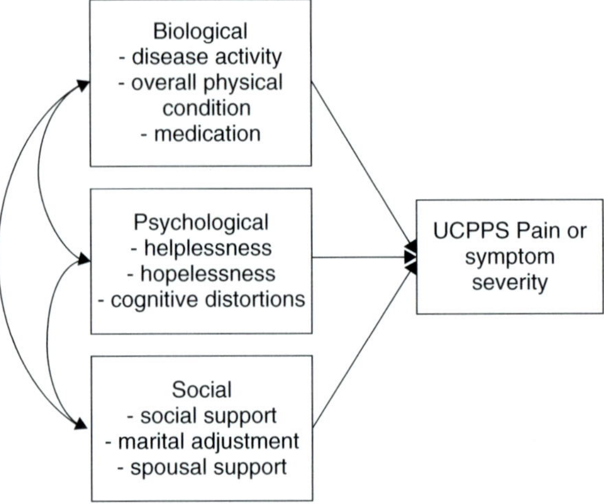

FIGURE 1 A Biopsychosocial Model for UCPPS Outcomes.

healthcare utilization [11]. The International Association for the Study of Pain defines pain as, "an unpleasant sensory and emotional experience associated with actual or potential tissue damage, or described in terms of such damage" [1]. Pain is often described in terms of its sensory components (burns, throbs), but pain expression and impact vary substantially by the cognitive and biological traits of the individual and their environment [42] (see Fig. 1). Cognitive-behavioral pain models are commonly used to guide interventions for chronic pain, where the role, and often the absence of coping proficiencies are emphasized. Regardless of the management framework, patient self-regulation is a key process. Indeed, the patient's self-awareness and problem solving ability shape their pain interpretation and thus management attempts [15,48]. For example, when patients believe they suffer an inability to self-manage a situation or physical sensation and their environment is not supportive, such combinations result in various degrees of anxiety and appraisals of helplessness, which can exacerbate pain.

DESCRIBING THE SUBJECT

Urologic Chronic Pelvic Pain Syndromes?

UCPPS are characterized by pelvic pain. Chronic Pelvic Pain Syndrome/Chronic Prostatitis/Prostate Pain Syndrome (CPPS/CP/PPS) and Bladder Pain Syndrome/Interstitial Cystitis (BPS/IC) are two such syndromes, with similar symptom profiles and unknown etiologies [22,33]. The shared symptoms include dysuria, pain (perineal, suprapubic, bladder and sexual), and diminished QoL [4]. High prevalence rates exist for CPPS/CP/PPS in men, with symptoms severely impacting patient QoL [26]. Fifty percent of BPS/IC patients report work-related disability [34] and QoL is rated worse than persons' receiving hemodialysis [12]. CPPS/CP/PPS QoL is comparable to those suffering severe congestive heart failure, diabetes, recent myocardial infarction, unstable angina, hemodialysis dependent end stage renal disease or active Crohn's disease [20,53]. It is suggested that diminished QoL in UCPPS may partially stem from physician powerlessness within a curative medical framework [13].

Chronic Pelvic Pain Syndrome/Chronic Prostatitis/ Prostate Pain Syndrome

Acute and chronic bacterial prostatitis (i.e., Category 1 & Category 2 respectively) are the best known and least common of the prostatitis syndromes. CPPS/CP/PPS, with or without inflammation, is the third category of prostatitis syndrome with type 3A manifesting noted inflammation, but no evidence of infection. Type 3B, which has no noted inflammation, is regarded as the most common but least understood of the categories and is highlighted in this chapter [25]. The fourth category is asymptomatic inflammatory prostatitis in which white blood cells are present in semen but with no associated pain.

CPPS/CP/PPS symptoms can vary [27], with most men reporting acute pain, long-standing persistent pain, or some combination of the two pain features. CP/CPPS/PPS pain is localized mostly to the urogenital regions (perineum, pelvic area, genitalia) [15,36]. Similar to other chronic pain, CPPS/CP/PPS pain does not correspond strongly with medical findings [6] and no medical findings exist for confirmatory diagnosis, making CPPS/CP/PPS a set of symptoms rather than specific disease [23,24]. The National Institutes of Health define CPPS/CP/PPS with pelvic pain for 3 of the previous 6 months, with or without voiding symptoms and with no evidence of uropathogenic bacterial infection [27]. A prostatitis diagnosis is common, accounting for 8% of urology outpatient visits in the United States and 3% in Canada [27]. The North American prevalence of CPPS/CP/PPS symptoms varies between 2–16% [15,36]. Although symptoms peak at 35–65 years [5], they range widely [36]. Research on North American male adolescents are alarming, suggesting as many as 8.3% report CPPS/CP/PPS [46]. Similarly, rates in African adolescents were 13.3% [45].

CPPS/CP/PPS may not routinely remit, with 66% of community-based samples reporting symptoms 1-year later [27], and Urology outpatients showing no drop in pain, disability, or catastrophizing over a multi-year assessment [47]. CPPS/CP/PPS cure successes are rather bleak, with monotherapy methods considered less than optimal [25]. CPPS/CP/PPS QoL is diminished to levels comparable with severe illnesses [21,54] and reviews of QoL outcomes suggest psychiatric disorders strongly coexist [16]. Research supports a biopsychosocial model for CPPS/CP/PPS pain and QoL, with psychosocial risk factors such as pain catastrophizing given a prominent position [29,48].

Catastrophizing in CPPS/CP/PPS

Pain-related "catastrophizing" is a negative, exaggerated cognitive schema engaged in when a patient is in, or anticipates, pain [39]. Catastrophizing is assessed using the Pain Catastrophizing Scale [39], capturing three interrelated factors: rumination, magnification, and helplessness (see Fig. 2). Rumination and magnification tend to be reactionary or proximal cognitive responses to pain, whereas helplessness may develop following ruminative thoughts and or protracted pain. There is little doubt that helplessness about one's pain and your perceived ability to manage it is associated with feelings of despair.

Catastrophizing is long known in the pain literature as a robust pain predictor in clinical and nonclinical samples [39]. The first CPPS/CP/PPS catastrophizing study found it associated with greater disability, depression, urinary symptoms, and pain [48]. Further, helplessness was the strongest pain predictor, even when urinary symptoms and depression were controlled. Diminished CPPS/CP/PPS mental QoL has also been predicted by greater helplessness and lower support from friends and family, even when demographics, medical status, and other utilized psychosocial variables where controlled [29]. Helplessness is

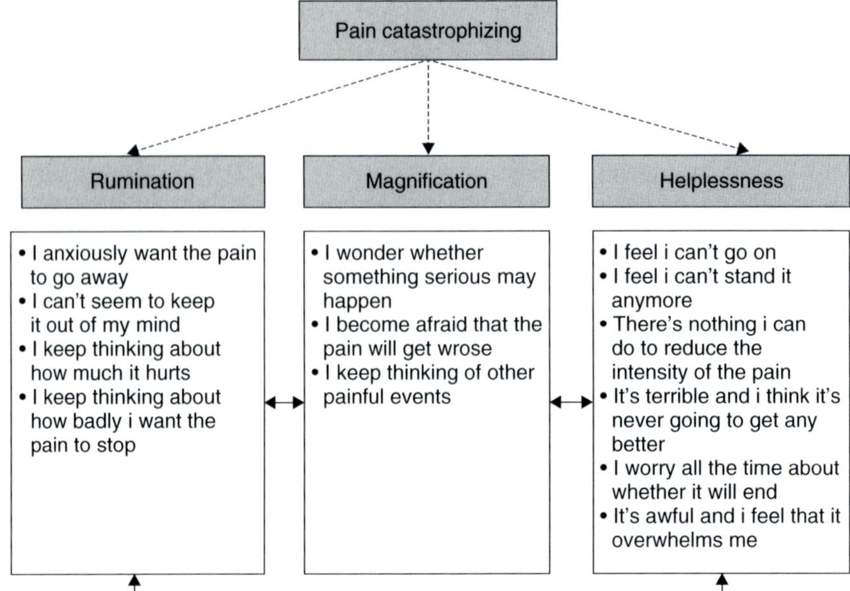

FIGURE 2 The items, subscales and interrelations of the Pain Catastrophizing Scale.

a predominant pain and QoL predictor in CPPS/CP/PPS, commonly reported by patients with longer pain duration (4–7 years) [40]. Interestingly, in the Canadian adolescent sample reporting prevalent CPPS/CP/PPS symptoms, the magnification subscale for catastrophizing (e.g., "I keep thinking of other painful events") was the lone predictor of diminished QoL after controlling urinary status and pain [46]. Magnification was likely a predictor in these young males due to the relatively acute disease onset and duration these younger males experienced compared to older males.

Evaluations of CPPS/CP/PPS QoL, pain, and psychosocial factors, indicated stability in significant depression and anxiety and that pain, disability, and catastrophizing did not lessen over this 2-year period [47]. Further, catastrophizing was comparable to patients with whiplash [41], BPS/IC [31], and CPPS/CP/PPS [48]. Thus, in the absence of a psychosocial or catastrophizing intervention or a reduction in pain, CPPS/CP/PPS patients are likely to exhibit alarmingly steady negative affect and catastrophic thinking about pain for extended periods. Catastrophizing and its helplessness is most likely a product of feeling unable to affect positive changes in pain.

Social Relations in CPPS/CP/PPS

By investigating spousal support for pain behaviour as buffering agents to poor patient outcomes such as pain or disability, research has provided some appreciable insights in UCPPS and how social support from spouses may be important intervention targets. The supportive spousal coping behaviours are operationalized into couples' interactions in the form of positive and negative responses to pain behaviour by significant others. Three categories of spousal responses include: *solicitous* (tries to get me to rest), *distracting* (tries to get me involved in some activity), and *negative* (gets angry with me) [14]. When examined in men with CPPS/CP/PPS, solicitous responses from spouses were associated with poorer patient adjustment [8]. Basically, at higher spouse solicitousness, patient pain was more highly associated with disability than at lower levels of solicitousness, indicating that greater solicitousness from a spouse should be avoided [8]. However, these results could also mean that spouses may be responding solicitously as a reaction to the patient's pain and level of disability, where patients are physically incapable of completing certain tasks, and thus require the help of their spouse. These results may also suggest that spousal responses may be differentially associated with patient adjustment in men and women with chronic pain [7] and may be influenced by a series of inter- and intrapersonal variables [17,18].

Bladder Pain Syndrome/Interstitial Cystitis

BPS/IC presents with pressure or pain related to the bladder, with at least one or more other urinary symptom, such as urinary urgency or frequency, with no demonstrable infection or other confusable diseases [51]. BPS/IC pain is suprapubically localized, radiating to the groin, vagina, rectum, or sacrum [10], but patients also report multiple pain locations external to the pelvic-abdominal region with greater pain locations associated with worse outcomes [49]. BPS/IC pain may be mild-severe and can be constant, usually associated with bladder filling and voiding. BPS/IC patients also often suffer multiple comorbid abdominal-pelvic region conditions that have pain as a common symptom (e.g. irritable bowel syndrome) [31]. Painful BPS/IC voiding frequency can reach 10–25+ times a day [2], and prevalence is estimated at 3300–11,200/100,000 [2], with symptom onset between 20–40 years [2]. Biomedical treatments that primarily target the bladder are often ineffective [32]. Although men are diagnosed with BPS/IC, it is predominantly diagnosed in women with a female to male ratio of 9:1 [3]. This section focuses on female outcomes.

BPS/IC is associated with clinical phenotypes on the basis of their overlapping symptoms: 1) BPS/IC and no other symptoms, 2) BPS/IC and irritable bowel syndrome only, 3) BPS/IC and fibromyalgia only, 4) BPS/IC and chronic fatigue syndrome only, and multiple associated conditions [31]. Also, as comorbidity of conditions increased, patients presented a localized to systemic illness pattern, which also included greater pain, stress, depression, sleep disturbance, and deteriorating QoL. Both anxiety and catastrophizing remained a concern across such phenotypes [30] and longer symptom durations were associated with phenotypic progression.

In a study of BPS/IC pain mapping, using a full body diagram on which patients endorsed all areas of pain, patients reported more pain than controls in all reported body areas, and four pain phenotypes were created based on increasing counts of body locations [49]. When contrasted, patients reported more body pain locations, along with more pain, urinary symptoms, depression, catastrophizing, and diminished QoL than did the controls. This increasing-pain phenotype model was also found to be associated with poorer psychosocial adjustment and diminished physical QoL, with catastrophizing and scores for low mental QoL remaining stable across all groups [49]. These results suggest that clinicians carefully consider pain location distributions and the potential impact of body pain phenotypes during patient evaluation and treatment.

Catastrophizing in BPS/IC

Some of the earliest patient survey research to examine catastrophizing and BPS/IC showed that patients reporting the highest catastrophizing also reported greater depression, poorer mental health, worse social functioning, and greater pain [35]. Further, catastrophizing, but not age or symptom severity, was related to more severe symptoms for both depression and QoL, suggested similar associations to other pain samples. This finding would be repeated in part by several other future studies. For example, pain experience and catastrophizing have also been tested in a laboratory study examining generalized cutaneous hypersensitivity, which found that catastrophizing was correlated with duration of BPS/IC symptoms and with thresholds to warm stimuli at the T12 dermatome, suggesting habituation to somatic stimuli is impaired in patients. Though one should be cautious drawing conclusions from one study, the physical and psychological differences found in this study could potentially predispose patients with BPS/IC to chronic pain [19].

BPS/IC has also been examined for unique and shared associations between QoL, symptoms, catastrophizing, depression, pain, and sexual functioning [43]. Women recruited from North American centers completed a survey and regressions predicted the unique and combined factor effects on patient QoL. Poor physical QoL was predicted by longer symptom duration and greater pain. However, poor mental QoL was predicted by older age and greater pain catastrophizing, and in particular, the helplessness scale [43]. When considered together, these data indicated that longer duration of symptoms, pain, older age, and helplessness catastrophizing were predictors of poorer QoL over sexual functioning.

Social Relations

There has been research examining the potential for the spousal support manifest in the CPPS/CP/PPS research and also with women suffering from BPS/IC [9]. In this study, the association between pain and all outcome variables did not vary as a function of levels of solicitous and negative spousal responses. However, the association between pain and mental QoL was stronger at lower levels of distracting responses than it was at moderate and higher levels of such responses from spouses (tries to get me involved in some activity)(See Fig. 3). In principle, it seems that the distracting spousal responses of a spouse act to "buffer" the deleterious effects of pain on mental QoL in BPS/IC. Although this study also scrutinized

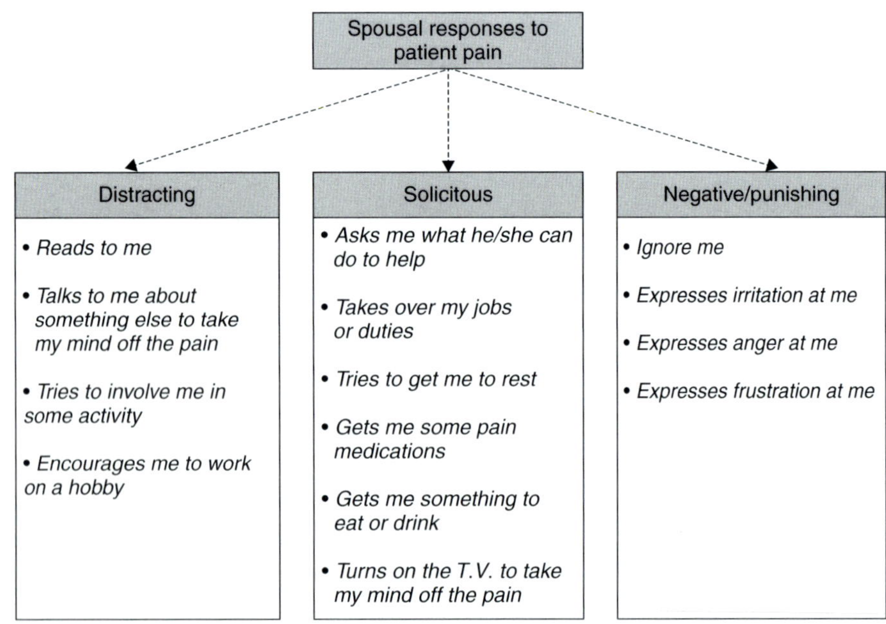

FIGURE 3 The items and subscales for spousal support.

the effects of "negative" spousal responses as well as "solicitous" spousal responses, no significant relationships were established. Interestingly, the findings that distracting responses act to buffer the relationship between pain and QoL, are in contrast to the spousal findings in CPPS/CP/PPS, where distracting spouse responses did not affect relations between pain and mental QoL.

PRACTICAL IMPLICATIONS

Catastrophizing in CPPS/CP/PPS

Practical implications for the management in the CPPS/CP/PPS patient must include discussions of patient catastrophizing and its "meaning" to the patient. There are basic therapy models to be applied to the practitioner-patient relationship [44]. Such modes of patient engagement can provide exceptionally valuable insights that can assist practitioners in managing patients fears and feelings of despair. As in Figure 2, the subscales and the items of the Pain Catastrophizing Scale can be reviewed with patients, with the practitioner leading a conversation concerning pain catastrophizing. A practitioner might initiate by saying:

> "What is clear is that everyone experiences pain at some point in their lives. We know that such experiences may include headaches, tooth pain, joint or muscle pain. Some people also have pain that can be chronic or pain that repeat without warning overtime, making that pain chronic.
>
> We want to look at what fits for you and your experience? This is an exercise that will help you and I find patterns in your life that your pain creates. That is important to your treatment because if we know when and how your pain makes you feel and think, we can start to look at possible solutions to battle these negative effects of your pain... understanding these patterns will help us with both medical and self-management and we can work together to come up with suggestions that will provide you with concrete things to do for your pain.
>
> What I am most interested in today are the types of thoughts and feelings that you experience when you are in pain, whether that is a burst of pain or a chronic aching pain. Look at this diagram [present Figure 2], here are some statements describing different thoughts and feelings that many patients in pain say are related to them being in pain. Let's read through these statements and please tell me how often you believe you have these thoughts when you are in pain."

Using a similar therapy method as above, patient baseline scores showed significant linear reductions across 8-weeks for pain, disability and catastrophizing [44]. CPPS/CP/PPS symptoms and QoL were also significantly improved. Further analyses also showed that the change in symptoms and psychosocial risk factors from baseline to 8-week termination were predicted by associated reductions in catastrophizing. Although these findings were not statistically significant that was due to the small sample size. Referent to these findings, management for CPPS/CP/PPS risk factors is feasible and practitioner engagement is important. Catastrophizing can be reduced.

Relations in CPPS/CP/PPS

The practical implications for the findings above will also focus on conversations of the patient's social interactions. As was suggested for the patient experiencing catastrophizing, opportunities to consider, reflect and problem solve potential issues in regard to spousal support is recommended. As shown in Figure 3, the items of spousal reactions to patient pain are listed for easy reading. As with the catastrophizing items, these can be reviewed or discussed by the patient and practitioner to initiate or lead a discussion into the types of support experienced and benefit of spousal support. A practitioner could lead a discussion as suggested below:

> "Many patients have reported that pain has affected their relationships with people close to them. If we take a look at various ways a partner responds to a patient's pain, you can see there are some positive and some not-so positive reactions. What I am most interested in knowing is how your partner responds to you when they know you are in pain. Now, I understand that this can vary from day-to-day so I am looking for the average type of response you think you might get from your spouse when you are in pain. [Showing Figure 3] Look at these listings of some potential responses from a partner. They are listed here under three categories. After reading these, let's discuss how often your significant other responds to you in that particular way when you are in pain."

Catastrophizing in BPS/IC

As promoted for men suffering CP/CPPS, the practical implications of the BPS/IC findings focus on discussion of catastrophizing and the introduction of this risk-factor for reflection and problem solving. Indeed, it would seem that both men and women report catastrophizing that is associated with UCPPS outcomes, making it a patient risk factor that should be targeted for reduction regardless of gender. As suggested earlier, a key feature of the practitioner-patient relationship might be the discussion of catastrophizing, and in particular helplessness in managing pain. Anecdotal reports from the therapy trial targeting catastrophizing [44] suggest that patients are often unaware of the extent to which they engage in such illness-focused thinking and associated behavior (i.e., feeling sad, giving up hope, not feeling loved). As shown in Figure 2, the subscales and the items of the Pain Catastrophizing Scale can be discussed with the patient in an interactive model, enforcing catastrophizing "recognition" leading to discussions on how to problem solve such appraisals [44]. Problem solving can take the initial format of asking a simplified series of questions, such as

> "What is the evidence that that thought [referring to the catastrophizing statement on Figure 2] is actually true of you? Maybe you feel that way sometimes but are there other times when you do not have that thought? If you had a best friend thinking that way, what advice would you give to them? What thought would you suggest to replace the sense of helplessness?"

This conversation can take many turns but the driving notion of getting the patient to approach and improve self-regulation is the primary goal and an open-ended discussion is to ensue.

The UCPPS catastrophizing findings have directed current efforts in the area of clinical assessment and management of psychosocial factors for improving patient adjustment. Utilizing the UPOINT classification system for patients diagnosed with BPS/IC [30,38] the psychosocial domain, which emphasizes catastrophizing, identified patients with BPS/IC who also reported more severe pain and greater urinary urgency and frequency [28]. Although the determination of cause-and-effect in these associations (i.e., pain, BPS/IC symptoms, psychosocial parameters) are not possible in cross-sectional research, psychosocial factors and catastrophizing in particular significantly affect BPS/IC outcomes.

Relations in BPS/IC

As was suggested for the BPS/IC patient reporting catastrophizing, providing the patient with yet another opportunity to consider, reflect and problem solve potential issues in regard to spousal support is recommended. You can use Figure 3 and its items of spousal reactions to patient pain to direct attention and discussion. This Figure and its items can be reviewed with your patient as was suggested for the men previously. It is important that you do not hold gender-based stereotypes during such conversations. As stated earlier the studies are not conclusive on differences between men and women, which may result in many various responses. Again, the aim is to get the patient discussing social support in an interactive model, enforcing support "recognition" leading to discussions on how to problem solve perceived social support deficits.

LOOKING TO THE FUTURE

Urogenital illnesses that are associated with persistent or sporadic spikes of acute pain are more than a physical phenomenon and must be conceptualized as a complex physical, emotional, cognitive and interpersonal synthesis of factors associated with negative patient QoL. The research herein strongly suggests that psychosocial risk factors and the regulation of such thinking styles may play a significant role in patients' responses to symptoms like pain. This "self-response" can be life-altering and must be considered in all new research on patient UCPPS outcomes. Indeed, patient's who perceive their environment as a potential source of pain, suffer diminished life satisfaction and emotional adaptation. However, there is hope because even the simple insertion of walking and social engagement is associated with improved QoL [52].

The narrative from this chapter compels the practitioner to consider and act upon the influences of a prior history with pain, catastrophizing, and social milieu in which the pain occurs [37]. If we are striving to help patients endeavor for more health promoting self-regulation, we must understand our collective relationship with our patients sets the tone for patient change. Indeed, the term self-regulation refers to the application of control over oneself by oneself, which involves altering the manner in which a person feels, thinks, and behaves in order for them to pursue short or long-term wellness. What is also intriguing is that the last 30 years of science has shown us that much of our thought processes occur without conscious awareness of the triggers and cues that promote certain responses, in some way regulating our behavior. Thus, treatment that allows a patient to reflect upon such processes, to deliberate and consider such events and the usefulness of such thinking in their attempt to reclaim their life in spite of pain, is an important step.

TAKE HOME MESSAGES

- Pain catastrophizing and social support can levy heavy impact on UCPPS patient outcomes like QoL.
- Psychological therapies in UCPPS are feasible, demanding that adjunctive psychosocial interventions should be considered and expanded in existing patient care maps.
- Discussions about catastrophizing (e.g., helplessness) with our patients may be a critical step in improving outcomes and the basic therapy guidelines proposed [44] are amenable to the practitioner-patient relationship providing a broader set of disease management strategies.

SUGGESTED READINGS

Nordling J, Wyndaele JJ, Van de Merwe JP, et al (Eds). Bladder Pain Syndrome: A Guide for Clinicians. London UK: Springer, 2013.

Shoskes D (Ed). Urological Men's Health: A Guide for Urologists and Primary Care Physicians. London, UK: Springer, 2012.

Preedy VR, Watson RS (Eds). Handbook of Disease Burdens and Quality of Life Measures. London UK: Springer, 2010.

DEFINITIONS

Urologic Chronic Pelvic Pain Syndromes [UCPPS] is an umbrella term referring to pain syndromes associated with the male and female pelvises. The UCPPS include Bladder Pain Syndrome/Interstitial Cystitis in men and women, and Chronic Pelvic Pain Syndrome/Chronic Prostatitis/Prostate Pain Syndrome in men that have common symptoms include dysuria, perineal, suprapubic, bladder, and/or sexual pain, and diminished QoL.

Bladder Pain Syndrome/Interstitial Cystitis [BPS/IC] Bladder pain syndrome is the occurrence of persistent or recurrent pain perceived in the urinary bladder region, accompanied by at least one other symptom, such as pain worsening with bladder filling and day-time and/or night-time urinary frequency. There is no proven infection or other obvious local pathology. Bladder pain syndrome is often associated with negative cognitive, behavioral, sexual, or emotional consequences as well as with symptoms suggestive of lower urinary tract and sexual dysfunction. Bladder pain syndrome is believed to represent a heterogeneous spectrum of disorders. There may be specific types of inflammation as a feature in subsets of patients.

*Chronic Pelvic Pain Syndrome/Chronic Prostatitis/Prostate Pain Syndrome [*CPPS/CP/PPS*]* is a pelvic pain condition in men, and should be distinguished from other forms of prostatitis such as chronic bacterial prostatitis and acute bacterial prostatitis. The cause of CPPS/CP/PPS is currently unknown and the condition is considered using a diagnosis of exclusion. CPPS/CP/PPS is characterized primarily by pelvic or perineal pain without evidence of urinary tract infection, greater than 3 months duration. Pain ranges from mild to severe and can radiate to the back and rectum, making sitting positions difficult to maintain or achieve. Pain can be present in several areas, such as the perineum, testicles, penis, or the pubic or bladder area. Other pain features such as dysuria, myalgia, abdominal pain may all be present with post-ejaculatory pain common, and a noted reduction in patient quality of life. If the pain is localized to the prostate the IASP classification would use the term Prostate Pain Syndrome.

REFERENCES

1. Bonica JJ. The need of a taxonomy. Pain 1979;6:247–8.
2. Clemens JQ, Joyce GF, Wise M, Payne CK. Interstitial cystitis and painful bladder syndrome. In: Litwin MS, Saigal CS (eds). Urologic diseases in America. Washington, DC: US Government Printing Office, 2007: 125–154.
3. Clemens JQ, Meenan RT, O'Keeffe J, et al. Prevalence of interstitial cystitis symptoms in a managed care population. J Urol 2005;174:576–580.
4. Clemens JQ, Meenan RT, O'Keefe F, et al. Prevalence of prostatitis-like symptoms in a managed care population. J Urol 2006;176:593–596.
5. Collins MM, Stafford RS, O'Leary MP, Barry MJ. Distinguishing chronic prostatitis and benign prostatic hyperplasia symptoms: results of a national survey of physician visits. Urology 1999;53:921–925.
6. Deyo RA, Weinstein JN. Low back pain. N Engl J Med 2001;344:363–70.
7. Fillingim RB, Doleys DM, Edwards RR, Lowery D. Spousal responses are differentially associated with clinical variables in women and men with chronic pain. Clin J Pain 2003;19:217–224.
8. Ginting JV, Tripp DA, Nickel JC. Self-reported spousal support modifies the negative impact of pain on disability in men with chronic prostatitis/chronic pelvic pain syndrome. Urology 2011;78:1136–1141.
9. Ginting JV, Tripp DA, Nickel JC, et al. Spousal support decreases the negative impact of pain on mental quality of life in women with interstitial cystitis/painful bladder syndrome. BJU Int 2010;31:1–5.
10. Hanno PM, Burks DA, Clemens JQ, et al. AUA guideline for the diagnosis and treatment of interstitial cystitis/bladder pain syndrome. J Urol 2011;185:2162–2170.
11. Hasselstrom J, Liu-Palmgren J, Rasjo-Wraak G. Prevalence of pain in general practice. Eur J Pain 2002;6:375–385.
12. Held PJ, Hanno PM, Wein AJ. Epidemiology of interstitial cystitis. In: Hanno PM, Staskin DR, Krane RJ, et al. Interstitial Cystitis. New York: Springer-Verlag, 1990: 29–48.
13. Kaye J, Moldwin RM. Interstitial cystitis in men: diagnosis, treatment, and similarities to chronic prostatitis. In: Preedy VR, Watson RS. Handbook of Disease Burdens and Quality of Life Measures. London: Springer, 2009.
14. Kerns RD, Turk DC, Rudy TE. The West Haven-Yale Multidimensional Pain Inventory (WHYMPI). Pain 1985;23:345–356.
15. Krieger JN, Nyberg L Jr, Nickel JC. NIH consensus definition and classification of prostatitis. JAMA 1999;282:236–247.
16. Ku JH, Kim SW, Paick JS. Quality of life and psychological factors in chronic prostatitis/chronic pelvic pain syndrome. Urology 2005;66:693–701.
17. Lakey B. Social support: basic research and new strategies for intervention. In: Maddux JE, Tangney JP (eds). Social psychological foundations of clinical psychology. New York: Guilford, 2010: 177–194.
18. Lakey B, Orehek E. Relational regulation theory: a new approach to explain the link between perceived social support and mental health. Psychol Rev 2011;118:482–495.
19. Lowenstein L, Kenton K, Mueller ER, et al. Patients with painful bladder syndrome have altered response to thermal stimuli and catastrophic reaction to painful experiences. Neurourol Urodyn 2009;28:400–403.
20. McNaughton CM, Pontari MA, O'Leary MP. Quality of life is impaired in men with chronic prostatitis: the Chronic Prostatitis Collaborative Research Network. J Gen Intern Med 2001;16:656–659.
21. McNaughton-Collins M, Pontari MA, O'Leary MP, et al. Quality of life is impaired in men with chronic prostatitis: the Chronic Prostatitis Collaborative Research Network. J Gen Intern Med 2001;16:656–662.
22. Moldwin RM. Similarities between interstitial cystitis and male chronic pelvic pain syndrome. Curr Urol Rep 2002;3:313–318.
23. Nickel JC. Chronic prostatitis/chronic pelvic pain: the syndrome. J Urol 2009;182:18–9.
24. Nickel JC. Words of wisdom. Re: Clinical phenotyping in chronic prostatitis/chronic pelvic pain syndrome and interstitial cystitis: a management strategy for urologic chronic pelvic pain syndromes. Eur Urol 2009;56:881.
25. Nickel JC, Downey J, Ardern D, Clark J, Nickel K. Failure of a monotherapy strategy for difficult chronic prostatitis/chronic pelvic pain syndrome. JUrol 2004;172:551–4.
26. Nickel JC, Downey J, Hunter D, Clark J. Prevalence of prostatitis-like symptoms in a population based study using the National Institutes of Health chronic prostatitis symptom index. J Urol 2001;165:842–845.
27. Nickel JC, Downey JA, Nickel KR, Clark JM. Prostatitis-like symptoms: one year later. BJU Int 2002;90:678–81.
28. Nickel JC, Shoskes DA, Irvine-Bird K. Clinical phenotyping of women with interstitial cystitis/painful bladder syndrome: a key to classification and potentially improved management. J Urol 2009;182:155–157.
29. Nickel JC, Tripp DA, Chuai S, et al. NIH-CPCRN Study Group. Psychosocial variables affect the quality of life of men diagnosed with chronic prostatitis/chronic pelvic pain syndrome. BJU Int 2008;101:59–64.
30. Nickel JC, Tripp DA, Pontari M, et al. Psychosocial phenotyping of women with IC/PBS: a case control study. J Urol 2010;183:167–170.

31. Nickel JC, Tripp DA, Pontari M, et al. Interstitial cystitis/painful bladder syndrome and associated medical conditions with an emphasis on irritable bowel syndrome, fibromyalgia and chronic fatigue syndrome. J Urol 2010;184:1358–1362.
32. Peters KM. Interstitial cystitis: is it time to look beyond the bladder? J Urol 2012;187:381–382.
33. Pontari MA. Chronic prostatitis/chronic pelvic pain syndrome and interstitial cystitis: are they related? Curr Urol Rep 2006;7:329–334.
34. Ratner V, Slade D, Green G. Interstitial cystitis: A patient's perspective. Urol Clin North Am 1994;21:1–4.
35. Rothrock NE, Lutgendorf SK, Kreder K. Coping strategies in patients with interstitial cystitis: relationships with quality of life and depression. J Urol 2003;169:233–235.
36. Schaeffer AJ, Datta NS, Fowler JE, et al. Overview summary statement. Diagnosis and management of chronic prostatitis/chronic pelvic pain syndrome (CP/CPPS). Urology 2002;60(6 Suppl):1–4.
37. Shoskes DA, Nickel JC, Dolinga R, Prots D. Clinical phenotyping of patients with chronic prostatitis/chronic pelvic pain syndrome and correlation with symptom severity. Urology 2009;73:538–542.
38. Shoskes DA, Nickel JC, Rackley RR, Pontari MA. Clinical phenotyping in chronic prostatitis/chronic pelvic pain syndrome and interstitial cystitis: a management strategy for urologic chronic pelvic pain syndromes. Prostate Cancer Prostatic Dis 2009;12:177–183.
39. Sullivan MJL, Bishop SR, Pivik J. The Pain Catastrophizing Scale: development and validation. Psych Assess 1995;7:524–532.
40. Sullivan MJ, Stanish W, Sullivan ME, Tripp D. Differential predictors of pain and disability in patients with whiplash injuries. Pain Res Manag 2002;7:68–74.
41. Sullivan MJL, Thibault P, Simmonds MJ, et al. Pain, perceived injustice and the persistence of post-traumatic stress symptoms during the course of rehabilitation for whiplash injuries. Pain 2009;145:325–331.
42. Sullivan MJ, Thorn B, Haythornthwaite JA, et al. Theoretical perspectives on the relation between catastrophizing and pain. Clin J Pain 2001;17:52–64.
43. Tripp DA, Nickel JC, FitzGerald MP, et al. Sexual functioning, catastrophizing, depression and pain as predictors of quality of life in women suffering from interstitial cystitis/painful bladder syndrome. Urology 2009;73:987–990.
44. Tripp DA, Nickel JC, Katz L. A feasibility trial of a cognitive-behavioural symptom management program for chronic pelvic pain for men with refractory chronic prostatitis/chronic pelvic pain syndrome. Can Urol Assoc J 2011;5:328–332.
45. Tripp DA, Nickel JC, Pikard JL, Katz L. Chronic prostatitis-like symptoms in African males aged 16–19 years. Can J Urol 2012;19:5343–5349.
46. Tripp DA, Nickel JC, Ross S, et al. Prevalence, symptom impact and predictors of chronic prostatitis-like symptoms in Canadian males aged 16–19 years. BJU Int 2009;103:1080–4.
47. Tripp DA, Nickel JC, Shoskes D, Koljuskov A. A 2-year follow-up of quality of life, pain, and psychosocial factors in patients with chronic prostatitis/chronic pelvic pain syndrome and their spouses. World J Urol 2013;31(4):733–9.
48. Tripp DA, Nickel JC, Wang Y, et al. National Institutes of Health-Chronic Prostatitis Collaborative Research Network (NIH-CPCRN) Study Group. Catastrophizing and pain-contingent rest predict patient adjustment in men with chronic prostatitis/chronic pelvic pain syndrome. J Pain 2006;7:697–708.
49. Tripp DA, Nickel JC, Wong J, et al. Mapping of pain phenotypes in female patients with bladder pain syndrome/interstitial cystitis and controls. Eur Urol 2012;62:1188–1194.
50. Turk DC, Dworkin RH. What should be the core outcomes in chronic pain clinical trials? Arthritis Res Ther 2004;6:151–154.
51. van de Merwe JP, Nordling J, Bouchelouche P, et al. Diagnostic criteria, classification, and nomenclature for painful bladder syndrome/interstitial cystitis: an ESSIC proposal. Eur Urol 2008;53:60–67.
52. Webster DC, Brennan T. Self-care effectiveness and health outcomes in women with interstitial cystitis: implications for mental health clinicians. Issues Ment Health Nurs 1998;19:495–498.
53. Wenniger K, Heiman JR, Rothman I. Sickness impact of chronic nonbacterial prostatitis and its correlates. J Urol 1996;155:965.
54. Wenninger K, Heiman JR, Rothman I, et al. Sickness impact of chronic nonbacterial prostatitis and its correlates. J Urol 1996;155:965–968.

CHAPTER 10

Sexual Dysfunctions

Ellen Laan, Lisa B.A. Bloemendaal, and Rik van Lunsen

INTRODUCTION

Chronic Pelvic Pain (CPP) in women and "Chronic Prostatitis"/ Chronic Pelvic Pain Syndrome (CP/CPPS) in men, is chronic or persistent pain perceived in structures related to the pelvis. It is often associated with negative cognitive, behavioral, sexual and emotional consequences as well as with symptoms suggestive of lower urinary tract, sexual, bowel, pelvic floor or gynaecological dysfunction [38,97,98]. In men, there is considerable overlap between CPP, unexplained genital pain, bladder outlet obstruction and irritable bowel syndrome (IBS), interfering with sexual function [3,36,37,51,60,85]. In women, CPP overlaps with Bladder Pain syndrome/Intersistial Cystitis (BPS/IC), IBS, and with sexual conditions such as dyspareunia and Provoked Vulvodynia (PVD), as defined by the International Society for the Study of Vulvovaginal Disease (ISSVD) [13,30,60,61,69,70]. The IASP taxonomy on female genital pain is based on their general pain term rule: localization-pain-syndrome. Therefore, the term Vulvar Pain Syndrome (VPS) is used instead of vulvodynia. VPS is subdivided into generalized and localized vulvar pain syndrome.

In this chapter, sexual problems comorbid with CPP in women and men will be discussed, focusing on terminology, prevalence, etiology, and treatment.

DESCRIBING THE SUBJECT

Sexual Dysfunction Related to CPP in Women

Terminology and Assessment

Dyspareunia, VPS/vulvodynia, and vaginismus are common pain problems in women interfering with sexuality. Because differentiation between these problems using clinical tools has proven difficult, these disorders were recently merged in the Diagnostic and Statistical Manual of Mental Disorders 5th edition (DSM-5) under the heading of Genito-Pelvic Pain/Penetration Disorder [2]. The disorder refers to four commonly comorbid symptom dimensions: (1) difficulty with intercourse/penetration; (2) vulvovaginal or pelvic pain during vaginal intercourse/penetration attempts; (3) fear or anxiety about vulvovaginal or pelvic pain or vaginal penetration; and (4) tensing or tightening of the pelvic floor muscles during attempted vaginal penetration. Because difficulty in any one of these symptom dimensions may result in clinically significant distress, a diagnosis can also be made if only one of these dimensions is present. Symptoms should persist for a minimum duration of approximately 6 months and cause clinically significant distress in the individual. Subtypes of Genito-pelvic pain/penetration disorders are early-onset (lifelong) or late-onset (acquired), and symptoms can be generalized (occurring in each and every sexual situation) or situational. To make a diagnosis, somatic explanations for all symptom dimensions should be ruled out.

The first symptom dimension, *difficulty with vaginal penetration,* is comparable to what was formerly called vaginismus, and can vary from a complete inability to experience vaginal penetration in any situation (generalized) to the ability for vaginal penetration in one situation (e.g., tampon insertion, gynaecological examination, sexual intercourse) but not in another (situational).

Vulvovaginal or pelvic pain during vaginal intercourse or penetration attempts is related to the Diagnostic and Statistical Manual of Mental Disorders 4th edition (DSM-IV) diagnosis of dyspareunia [1], and to VPS, which is not mentioned in DSM-IV. This symptom dimension refers to pain in different locations in the genito-pelvic area. Pain can be characterized as superficial (vulvovaginal or occurring during penetration) or deep (pelvic; i.e., not felt until deeper penetration). The intensity of the pain is often not linearly related to distress or interference with sexual intercourse or other sexual activities. Some genito-pelvic pain only occurs when provoked (i.e., by intercourse or mechanical stimulation); other genito-pelvic pain may be spontaneous as well as provoked. Genito-pelvic pain can also be characterized qualitatively (e.g., "burning," "cutting," "shooting," "throbbing"). The pain may persist for a period after intercourse is completed and may also occur during urination. The next two symptom dimensions can be considered to be emotional and behavioural consequences of sexual pain that may be more or less salient.

Fear or anxiety about vulvovaginal or pelvic pain, whether in anticipation of, during, or following vaginal penetration is associated with avoidance of sexual situations and is often reported by women who have regularly experienced pain during intercourse, but is also seen in women who have not yet had much experience with painful intercourse.

Tensing or tightening of the pelvic floor muscles can vary from an involuntary, reflex-like reaction of the pelvic floor in response to attempted vaginal entry, to voluntary muscle guarding in response to the anticipated or the repeated experience of pain.

To support diagnosis, a number of associated features should be investigated. First, genito-pelvic pain/penetration disorder is often associated with reduced sexual interest and arousal, but arousal and desire can be preserved in sexual situations that are not painful or in which penetration is not anticipated. Five other factors should be considered during assessment as they may be relevant to etiology and/or treatment: (1) partner factors (e.g., partners sexual problems or health status); (2) relational factors such as poor communication and discrepancies in desire; (3) individual vulnerability factors (e.g., poor body image, a history of sexual or emotional abuse), psychiatric comorbidity or stressors; (4) cultural and religious factors that may restrain sexual activity or pleasure; and (5) medical factors relevant to prognosis, course, or treatment. Each of these factors may contribute differently to the presenting symptoms [2].

For painful orgasm in women, no publications in Pubmed are available, nor is this type of pain acknowledged in DSM 5, even though it is not an uncommon clinical phenomenon [94].

Headaches associated with sexual activity is another type of sexual pain. The International Classification of Headache Disorders (2nd Ed) differentiates between preorgasmic (sexual arousal related) headaches, and orgasmic headaches, sudden and severe explosive pain as soon as orgasm starts [48].

All sexual pain disorders associated with CPP are frequently comorbid with DSM-IV sexual dysfunctions such as inhibited sexual desire, female arousal disorder and female orgasm disorder [92]. Anticipation of painful intercourse, painful orgasm or headache after sexual activity will seriously impede sexual arousal, which in itself reduces the likelihood of experiencing orgasm [20]. Even though reduced sexual desire is still conceptualized by many as a biological deficit, as a problem of sexual 'drive', incentive-motivation models of sexual desire propose that sexual desire is the consequence rather than the cause of rewarding sexual experiences [50]. It is highly unlikely that the prospect of painful sex, whatever its nature, will evoke much sexual desire.

Prevalence

The prevalence of this new genito-pelvic pain/penetration disorder is currently unknown, but sexual pain problems are common. Prevalence estimates for dyspareunia range from 14–34% in younger women to 6.5–45% in older women [53,65,92,99]. Women with VPS vary in ages from 16 to 80 years, with the majority between the ages of 20 to 50 years [44], even though VPS is also seen in children [22]. The incidence of VPS is approximately 10 to 15% [44,75], and the lifetime prevalence of VPS is estimated between 10 and 20% 8,44,52,75]. Prevalence estimates of vaginismus vary between 1–6% [57]. The prevalence of orgasmic pain in women is unknown, the lifetime prevalence of sexual headaches is less than 1%, with prevalence rates in women being one-fourth of that in men (72,89].

Etiology

The etiology of all sexual pain problems in women is much debated. Several monocausal factors and mechanisms have been proposed. However, sexual pain, of whatever kind, is progressively regarded as a multifaceted problem with medical, psychological, sexual, and relational sequalae [40,94], the most important of which are discussed below. Recently, the hypothesis that pelvic floor overactivity may be an integrating causal and/or maintaining mechanism involved in sexual pain as well as CPP is becoming more important [30,62,69,76,94].

- **Biomedical mechanisms.** Past research has focused predominantly on (genetic vulnerability for) vulvovaginal infections, hormonal influences, tissue abnormalities and immune system function [39,92]. Even though the human papillomavirus, bacterial vaginosis and candida have often been labeled as causal mechanisms underlying chronic vulvar pain, systematic studies have not supported this [92]. The prevalence of candida in the general population may be as high as 75 to 80% [81], but a US study showed that of all women who had bought an over-the-counter antimycotic agent, only one-third were found to actually have candida [83]. Women may have had a history of candida or bacterial vaginosis, but in most cases, treatment of those conditions does not alleviate the chronic pain problems. Even though oral contraceptive use has been associated with the risk for VPS, the most recent study in the largest sample to date found no evidence of an increased risk for VPS in oral contraceptive users [74].
- **Psychological mechanisms.** Women with vulvar pain report higher rates of depression and anxiety disorders [92]. Evidence is emerging that chronic sexual pain involves problems in information processing, with attentional bias, hypervigilance to pain and catastrophizing thoughts about the pain, and stronger disgust associations

being among the most important factors discriminating between women with and without sexual pain [15,43,67]. A history of a sexual abuse in women with dyspareunia is associated with increased sexual impairment [54]. Significant associations have been found between sexual abuse and chronic pelvic pain (OR, 2.73). When the definition of abuse was restricted to rape, the OR for chronic pelvic pain increased (3.27) [66]. Another recent study found the effect between documented childhood victimization and pain in adulthood to be moderated by the presence of posttraumatic stress disorder (PTSD) in adulthood, such that only individuals who had experienced childhood abuse/neglect and who had PTSD in adulthood were at significantly increased risk for adult pain [71].

- **Sexual mechanisms.** Women with sexual pain are less satisfied with their sex life and experience more negative feelings during sexual activity [e.g.,17]. Dyspareunia is not associated with a reduced capacity to become (genitally) aroused with adequate sexual stimulation [18], but pain-related fear does reduce subjective and genital sexual responding [20]. Often women do not have arousal problems or orgasm problems with masturbation, but become only moderately sexually aroused as of their first coital attempts. Pain during intercourse frequently is associated with a limited noncoital sexual repertoire, adding to the likelihood of sexual arousal being insufficient for pain free intercourse [19].
- **Relational mechanisms.** Characteristically, women with dyspareunia do not cease sexual activity that is painful for them. They ignore the primary function of pain as signaling damage to the body [30]. While intercourse frequency of women with dyspareunia is lower than that of women without sexual pain [73], not engaging in sexual intercourse is, by definition, not a behavioural choice that women with dyspareunia make [33,34]. The wish to be 'normal' seems to be an important underlying mechanism [35]. In heterosexual partnered sex, many women forego their own needs for fear of the negative impact this might have on the male partner's ego [77]. A very recent study found that women with dyspareunia exhibited more mate-guarding and duty/pressure motives for engaging in intercourse and had more maladaptive penetration-related beliefs than women without sexual pain. The factor that best predicted continuation of painful intercourse (attempts) was the partner's negative response to pain [19]. Many women with vaginismus, in contrast, avoid any form of vaginal penetration because of negative cognitions and expectations about vaginal penetration. As a consequence, anxiety-inducing penetration related thoughts cannot be disconfirmed and thereby maintain the condition [56,86,87].
- **Pain perception.** It has been proposed that vulvar pain represents a chronic local inflammatory condition, starting with tissue injury releasing inflammatory mediators, which may lead to neurogenic inflammation and peripheral sensitization with lowered pain thresholds [40]. There is also evidence of a central sensitization mechanism with enhanced systemic pain response [14].
- **Pelvic floor overactivity.** As also recently acknowledged in DSM 5, pelvic floor overactivity is considered to be an important causal and/or maintaining factor of dyspareunia as well as VPS [30,62,94]. The pelvic floor consists of a deep and a superficial layer [76,95]. The deep layer is stretched over the bones of the pelvis and consists of the puborectalis muscle, musculus pubococcygeus, iliococcygeus muscle, musculus ischiococcygeus and the external urethral sphincter. The main functions of this deep layer are the support of the abdominal organs, sustaining genital vasocongestion during sexual arousal and orgasm, and maintaining a good posture. Underrecognized, but very

relevant in sexual pain problems as well as in CPP, is the fact that the pelvic floor also has an emotional function. In situations of imminent physical or mental pain the pelvic floor contracts involuntarily and often unconsciously [16,90]. In a number of psychophysiological studies in which pelvic floor muscle tone was measured using electromyography, exposure to threatening film excerpts resulted in a significant increase in pelvic floor muscle activity relative to neutral film exposure, both in women with [90,91] and without sexual pain problems [16]. Activity in the shoulder muscles was also significantly enhanced during these film excerpts, suggesting that pelvic floor overactivity in threatening situations should be regarded as part of a general defense mechanism [91].

An elevated pelvic muscle tone reduces vasocongestion in sexual situations [16], resulting in a weakened genital response and diminished lubrication. Repetitive friction between the vulvar skin and the penis may cause vulvar tissue damage, irritation of the skin and possibly secondary hypersensitivity [101]. Anticipation of pain in future sexual encounters may further decrease sexual arousal and increase pelvic floor muscle tension, adding to the friction between vulvar skin and penis [20,30]. Repetitive painful intercourse without adequate genital arousal and a tense pelvic floor aggravates vulvar burning [94]. In women with vaginismus, pelvic floor relaxation is absent in sexual situations and there are reflexogenic involuntary contractions of the perivaginal musculature upon attempts of vaginal penetration. Women whose first sexual pain problem consisted of painful intercourse may develop an anticipatory protective vaginistic response (secondary vaginismus). Women who continue with intercourse despite pain may acquire chronic pelvic floor overactivity, with a pattern of obstructive micturition- and defecation consisting of hesitancy and problems with initiating voiding, urgency and frequency, slow or intermittent stream and straining, dysuria and vulvar burning after micturition, feelings of incomplete emptying, nocturia, obstructed defecation, constipation, symptoms of IBS and CPP.

For women with experiences of sexual abuse, even consensual sexual situations can be negative and threatening [90]. Therefore, it is not surprising that chronic pelvic floor overactivity is more common in women with negative sexual experiences, such as rape or incest [10,66,68].

Orgasm pain in women may also be related to pelvic floor overactivity. Van Lunsen and Ramakers depict painful orgasm as being related to the involuntary clonic pelvic floor contractions associated with orgasm, which become painful in women with a chronic overactive pelvic floor [94].

Patients with complaints associated with pelvic floor overactivity often have other stress-related complaints, particularly in the neck/shoulder area, possibly related to (tension) headache [94]. Women with dyspareunia suffer from tension headache more often than women without sexual pain [63]. Sexual arousal headaches are a type of tension headache. The most prevalent type of sexual headache is orgasmic headache, which may be related to a temporary increase of intracranial pressure during sexual activity [12].

Sexual Dysfunction Related to CPP in Men

Terminology, Assessment, and Prevalence

Relatively new research concerning pelvic pain syndrome in men is starting to emerge [26,27,28,29]. According to the DSM 5 Working Group for the sexual dysfunctions, research and clinical experience are not yet sufficiently developed to justify the application of this diagnosis to men [2].

Male pelvic pain has traditionally been the domain of urologists who have paid limited attention to its associated sexual dysfunction [28]. Until the past decade, male pelvic pain which had no identifiable cause was diagnosed as prostatitis, hypothesizing that pain throughout the pelvic region radiated from infection and inflammation of the prostate [28]. However, in many of the reported cases, no evidence for bacterial prostatitis was found. The National Institute of Health (NIH) characterized CPP in men by symptoms of chronic pelvic pain and possibly symptoms of voiding in the absence of urinary tract infection [49].

Research suggests that 5–15% of men have pelvic pain [23,24]. A growing body of literature suggests a high prevalence of sexual dysfunction in men with CPP. Men with CPP have reported sexual problems such as ejaculatory pain, pain during or after intercourse, partial or complete erectile dysfunction (ED), decreased sexual desire, and premature ejaculation (PE) [84]. Painful ejaculation appears to be the most common sexual symptom in men with CPP [55]. The prevalence of pain on ejaculation is about 1% in healthy men, but up to 58% in men with pelvic pain [58], about 90% of whom consider it a serious problem [47].

Ejaculatory pain may cause distress associated with sexual activity [28], which may be one of the mechanisms through which men with CPP develop ED. ED is the most investigated sexual dysfunction in men with CPP [see 28, for a comprehensive review]. Reported ED prevalence findings for these men range from 15% to 41% [83]. PE is another common sexual dysfunction associated with CPP. PE prevalence rates vary widely as well, ranging from 26.2% to 77.3% [42,84].

Etiology

Of cases that were formerly diagnosed as prostatitis, 90% fall within the CPP category established by NIH (chronic pelvic pain syndrome type III), indicating that the majority of cases have no known etiology [64,78]. As in women with CPP, many men with CPP also suffer urinary symptoms, including dysuria, frequent urination, the sensation of incomplete urination [28], and IBS [3]. A study that examined physiological factors associated with ED in men with CPP, using Doppler ultrasonography, found no evidence of vascular deficiency [42]. There is a lack of research focusing on other organic factors associated with sexual functioning in men with CPP.

- **Psychological mechanisms.** In a sample of 253 men with CPP from tertiary-care clinical centers in North America, quality of life was compromised and found to be related to pain catastrophizing, pain-contingent resting, and a lack of social support 64,88]. In two other North American studies, frequency of sexual activity in men with CPP was found to be negatively related to depressive symptoms and sexual arousal was lower in men who experienced more pain and distress [9,80]. In addition, men with CPP reported higher levels of fear and distress and had higher cortisol levels than men without CPP [4,5].
- Sexual abuse appears to be more prevalent in men with CPP [46]. In two recent Dutch studies investigating the association between pelvic floor overactivity and problems in the domain of micturation, defecation and sex in men, elevated rates of sexual abuse were found relative to prevalence figures in the Dutch male population [36,37]. As in women, (early) sexual abuse experiences in men may have generated an involuntary, unconscious protective response of the pelvic floor musculature, as part of a general defense mechanism, leading to an increased likelihood of CPP and sexual dysfunction later in life.

- **Relational mechanisms.** In men with CPP relational satisfaction, sexual pleasure and sexual satisfaction do not appear to be compromised by experienced pain [e.g., 9]. Interestingly, female partners of men with CPP appear to have a somewhat higher prevalence of vaginismus [32,80].
- **Pain perception.** Compared to controls, men with CPP were found to have lower pressure pain thresholds in the genital area [29], more muscle tenderness [79] and higher pain reports and increased sensitization to thermal stimuli on the perineum, suggestive of hyper excitability of dorsal horn neurons [100].
- **Pelvic floor overactivity.** A number of empirical studies have recently been published suggesting a role for pelvic floor overactivity in men with sexual pain-related sexual dysfunction [e.g., 11]. Up to 50% of men with CPP were found to have signs of pelvic floor overactivity on physical exam [79]. Other recent studies also supported the role of pelvic floor overactivity as an underlying mechanism in men with CPP. Pelvic floor physical therapy with myofascial release was found to significantly improve pelvic pain, urinary symptoms, as well as sexual dysfunction in these men [3]. In two separate studies, Elsevier and colleagues [36,37] investigated pelvic floor overactivity in men with problems in three domains: micturation problems, defecation problems and/or sexual problems. The second study focused specifically on men with CPP. The majority of men in both studies had complaints on all three domains and exhibited enhanced pelvic floor basal tone. Davis and colleagues [29] found lower pelvic and nonpelvic pressure pain thresholds in men with CPP, using pelvic floor ultrasound. Andersen and colleagues studied the relationship between myofascial trigger points and pain symptoms in 72 men with CPP [6]. The most prevalent myofascial trigger point pain sites were the penis, the perineum and rectum, and palpation of trigger points reproduced the pain in most cases. Decreased arterial inflow associated with ED may also be related to extrinsic compression from chronic pelvic floor overactivity, which would indicate a similar mediating role of the pelvic floor in vasocongestion as in women. An increasing ability to contract and relax the pelvic floor improved sexual functioning in men with ED [25].

PRACTICAL IMPLICATIONS

As the above overview shows, evidence is emerging that pelvic floor overactivity may explain comorbidity of CPP symptoms and sexual problems, in women as well as in men. Researchers increasingly agree that the etiology of sexual pain is multifaceted [92,21], yet, to date, most treatment studies in women have only investigated efficacy of singular interventions [7]. Also in men, authors argue, further investigations into male CPP should focus on the mechanisms inducing and maintaining pain [100]. Given the fact that, for instance, a history of sexual abuse and other psychosocial stressors are more prevalent in both women and men with CPP, many inducing and maintaining mechanisms related to CPP, may be similar in both genders.

We hypothesize that in both men and women, pelvic floor overactivity may be the most important mechanism through which the relationship between (early) physical or psychological trauma, attachment problems, other psychological stressors on the one hand and CPP on the other, may be understood. Following (threats of) physical or mental pain, the pelvic floor will automatically, unconsciously, contract [16,90,91]. Therefore, pelvic floor overactivity should not be regarded as a musculoskeletal dysfunction, but as an emotional response, resulting from chronic activation of the defensive stress-system.

We therefore conceptualize pelvic floor overactivity to be a physical manifestation of emotional dysregulation.

With respect to sexual problems, gender differences do need to be addressed when treating CPP related sexual pain. Sexual pain problems in the general population are more prevalent in women than in men, and we hypothesize that this may be partly explained by differences in genital anatomy and gender differences in sexual behavior. With sexual intercourse probably being considered the most important type of sexual activity, the goal of heterosexual interactions, in most if not all cultures, it is important to realize that for women, in contrast to men, sexual intercourse is not the most sexually stimulating sexual activity, particularly when intercourse represents the sole source of sexual stimulation. Research clearly and consistently shows that vaginal intercourse without additional glans clitoris stimulation results in orgasm in only about 25 to 30% of heterosexual women [45,59]. This contrasts sharply with research suggesting that over 90% of heterosexual men always experience orgasm during sexual intercourse [31,96]. Unfortunately, women's genital anatomy allows for vaginal intercourse without sexual arousal, whereas for men, sexual arousal (producing an erection) is necessary for penetration. Many heterosexual women appear to prioritize their partner's sexual pleasure over their own [35,77], further reducing the likelihood that sexual intercourse takes place with sufficient sexual arousal. In many instances, vaginal intercourse without sexual arousal is painful, particularly with enhanced pelvic floor muscle activity, a protective response resulting from earlier painful sexual experiences, or from physical or psychological stressors that were present even before sexual debut. Thus, sexual problems in individuals with CPP require a gender-sensitive approach.

Our own treatment regimen of women with VPS and dyspareunia includes pain prohibition and cessation of intercourse to prevent further mechanical irritation by intercourse, but also a pleasure command aimed at lustful love making and improving women's confidence that they can become sexually aroused in a sexual context that takes into account their genital anatomy [93]. This tailored sexological and cognitive behavioural treatment also consists of stepwise exposure to sexual activities that were painful previously, and includes couple sessions aimed at improving communication and reinstatement of the sexual relationship. Referral to a pelvic floor physiotherapist for coordination of pelvic floor contraction and –relaxation is often a mandatory part of treatment, but not before underlying emotional/psychological and or behavioural causes of the pelvic floor overactivity are identified and addressed. It should be emphasized that a pain prohibition is not a prohibition to have sex, on the contrary, any sexual activity that is sexually arousing and that can lead to sexual pleasure is beneficial for breaking the cycle of (fear of) pain-muscle tension-pain. A retrospective evaluation of 300 women with sexual pain who underwent this treatment protocol showed that almost 90% significantly improved or recovered completely [41]. Another retrospective study using comparable treatment ingredients found a similar recovery rate [82].

LOOKING AT THE FUTURE

Pelvic floor overactivity is a multifaceted problem with medical, psychological, relational, and cultural sequalae. The view on sexual pain in individuals with CPP sketched above implies multidisciplinary collaboration, involving specialists in the field of urology, gynaecology, internal medicine, surgery, sexology, psychology/psychiatry, pain specialist, and pelvic floor physiotherapy. A gender-sensitive approach with respect to treatment of sexual pain is also necessary. Probably in many countries this multidisciplinary treatment of sexual pain and CPP requires changes in the organization of health care.

TAKE HOME MESSAGES

- Sexual problems are common in men and women with CPP.
- Pelvic floor overactivity may explain comorbidity of CPP and sexual problems. We conceptualize pelvic floor overactivity to be a physical manifestation of emotional dysregulation, which may explain the relationship between (early) attachment problems and trauma on the one hand, and sexual problems and CPP on the other.
- Treatment requires multidisciplinary collaboration and a gender-sensitive perspective.

FURTHER READING

Andrews JC. Vulvodynia interventions: systematic review and evidence grading. Obstet Gynecol Surv 2011;66:299–315.
National Vulvodynia Association website, https://www.nva.org/
Parks T. Teach us to sit still: a skeptic's search for health and healing. Emmaus USA: Rodale Books, 2011.

REFERENCES

1. American Psychiatric Association. Diagnostic and statistical manual of mental disorders 4th edition, text revision. Arlington, VA: American Psychiatric Publishing; 2013
2. American Psychiatric Association. Diagnostic and statistical manual of mental disorders 5th edition. Arlington, VA: American Psychiatric Publishing; 2013
3. Anderson RU, Chan CA, Sawyer T, Wise D. Sexual dysfunction in men with chronic prostatitis/chronic pelvic pain syndrome: improvement after trigger point release and paradoxical relaxation training. J Urol 2006;176:1534–9.
4. Anderson RU, Orenberg EK, Chan CA, et al. Psychometric profiles and hypothalamic-pituitary-adrenal axis function in men with chronic prostatitis/chronic pelvic pain syndrome. J Urol 2008;179:956–60.
5. Anderson RU, Orenberg EK, Morey A, et al. Stress induced hypothalamus-pituitary-adrenal axis responses and disturbances in psychological profiles in men with chronic prostatitis/chronic pelvic pain syndrome. J Urol 2009;182:2319–24.
6. Anderson RU, Sawyer T, Wise D, et al: Painful myofascial trigger points and pain sites in men with chronic prostatitis/chronic pelvic pain syndrome. J Urol 2009; 182: 2753–8.
7. Andrews JC. Vulvodynia interventions – systematic review and evidence grading. Obstet Gynecol Survey 2011;68:299–315.
8. Arnold L, Bachmann G, Rosen R, Rhoads GG. Assessment of vulvodynia symptoms in a sample of US women: a prevalence survey with a nested case control study. Am J Obstet Gynecol 2007;196:128.e1–6.
9. Aubin S, Berger RE, Heiman JR, Ciol MA. The association between sexual function, pain, and psychological adaptation of men diagnosed with chronic pelvic pain syndrome type III. J Sex Med 2008;5:657–67.
10. Beck JJH, Elzevier HW, Pelger RCM, et al. Multiple pelvic floor complaints are correlated with sexual abuse history. J Sex Med 2009;6:193–8.
11. Berger RE, Ciol MA, Rothman I, Turner JA. Pelvic tenderness is not limited to the prostate in chronic prostatitis/chronic pelvic pain syndrome (CPPS) type IIIA and IIIB: comparison of men with and without CP/CPPS. BMC Urol 2007;7:17.
12. Biehl K, Evers S, Frese A. Comorbidity of migraine and headache associated with sexual activity. Cephalalgia, 2007;27:1271–3.
13. Bodner DR. The urethral syndrome. Urol Clin North Am 19888;15:99–104.
14. Bohm-Starke N. Medical and physical predictors of localized provoked vulvodynia. Acta Obstet Gynecol Scand 2010;12:1504–10.
15. Borg C, Georgiadis JR, Renken RJ, et al. Brain processing of visual stimuli representing sexual penetration versus core and animal-reminder disgust in women with lifelong vaginismus. PLoS One 2014; doi: 10.1371/journal.pone.0084882
16. Both S, van Lunsen R, Weijenborg P, Laan E. A new device for simultaneous measurement of pelvic floor muscle activity and vaginal blood flow: a test in a nonclinical sample. J Sex Med 2012;9:2888–902.
17. Brauer M, de Jong PJ, Huijding J, et al. Automatic and deliberate affective associations with sexual stimuli in women with superficial dyspareunia. Arch Sex Behav 2009;38:486–97.
18. Brauer M, Laan E, ter Kuile MM. Sexual arousal in women with superficial dyspareunia. Arch Sex Behav 2006;35:191–200.

19. Brauer M, Lakeman M, van Lunsen RHW, Laan E. Predictors of task-persistent and fear-avoiding behaviors in women with sexual pain disorders. J Sex Med, *in press*.
20. Brauer M, ter Kuile MM, Janssen S, Laan E. The effect of pain-related fear on sexual arousal in women with superficial dyspareunia. Eur J Pain 2007;11:788–98.
21. Butrick CW. Pelvic floor hypertonic disorders: identification and management. Obstet Gynecol Clin North Am. 2009;36:707–22.
22. Clare CA, Yeh J. Vulvodynia in adolescence: childhood vulvar pain syndromes. J Pediatr Adolesc Gynecol. 2011;24:110–5.
23. Clemens JQ, Meenan RT, O'Keeffe et al. Incidence and clinical characteristics of National Institutes of Health type III prostatitis in the community. J Urol 2005;174:2319–22.
24. Collins MM, Meigs JB, Barry MJ, et al. Prevalence and correlates of prostatitis in the health professionals follow-up study cohort. J Urol 2002;167:1363–66.
25. Colpi GM, Negri L, Nappi RE, Chinea B. Perineal floor efficiency in sexually potent and impotent men. Int J Imp Res 1999;11:153–7.
26. Davis SN, Binik YM, Amsel R, Carrier S. Is a sexual dysfunction domain important for quality of life in men with urological chronic pelvic pain syndrome? Signs "UPOINT" to yes. J Urol 2013; 189:146–151.
27. Davis SN, Binik YM, Amsel R, Carrier S. A subtype based analysis of urological chronic pelvic pain syndrome in men. J Urol 2013; 190, 118–23.
28. Davis SNP, Binik YM, Carrier S. Sexual dysfunction and pelvic pain in men: a male sexual pain disorder? J Sex Marital Ther 2009;35:182–205.
29. Davis SN, Maykut CA, Binik YM, et al. Tenderness as measured by pressure pain thresholds extends beyond the pelvis in chronic pelvic pain syndrome in men. J Sex Med. 2011;8:232–9.
30. De Jong J, van Lunsen R, Robertson E, et al. Focal vulvitis: a psychosexual problem for which surgery is not the answer. J Psychosom Obstet Gynecol 1995;16:85–91.
31. Douglass M, Douglass L. Are we having fun yet? New York: Hyperion; 1997.
32. Drenth JJ. The tight foreskin: a psychosomatic phenomenon. J Sex Mar Ther 1991;297–306.
33. Elmerstig E, Wijma B, Berterö C. Why do young women continue to have sexual intercourse despite pain? J Adolesc Health 2008;43:357–63.
34. Elmerstig E, Wijma B, Swahnberg K. Young Swedish women's experience of pain and discomfort during sexual intercourse. Acta Obstet Gynecol Scand 2009;88:98–103.
35. Elmerstig E, Wijma B, Swahnberg K. Prioritizing the partner's enjoyment: a population-based study on young Swedish women with experience of pain during vaginal intercourse. J Psychosom Obstet Gynecol 2013;34:82–90.
36. Elzevier HW, Lyklama à Nijeholt AAB, et al. Diagnostic investigation of the pelvic floor: a helpful tool in the approach in patients with complaints of micturition, defecation, and/or sexual dysfunction. J Sex Med 2008;5:864–71.
37. Elzevier HW, Lycklama à Nijeholt AAB, Planken E, Voorham-van der Zalm PJ. Chronic testicular pain as a symptom of pelvic floor Dysfunction. J Urol 2010;183:177–81.
38. Engeler DS, Baranowski AP, Dinis-Oliveira P, et al. The 2013 EAU Guidelines on chronic pelvic pain: is management of chronic pelvic pain a habit, a philosophy, or a science? 10 years of development. Eur Urol 2013;64:431–9.
39. Farage MA, Galask RP. Vulvar vestibulitis syndrome: a review. Eur J Obstet Gynaecol Reprod Biol 2005;123;9–16.
40. Fugl-Meyer KS, Bohm-Starke N, Petersen CD, et al. Standard Operating Procedures for female genital sexual pain. J Sex Med 2013;10: 83–93.
41. Gaasterland CMW, Lunsen RHW, Laan E. Efficacy of a tailor-made, multifocal psychosexual treatment of vulvodynia: a retrospective study. Manuscript under revision.
42. Gonen M, Kalkan M, Cenker A. Ozkardes H. Prevalence of premature ejaculation in Turkish men with chronic pelvic pain syndrome. J Androl 2005;26:601–3.
43. Granot M, Lavee Y. Psychological factors associated with perception of experimental pain in vulvar vestibulitis syndrome. J Sex Marital Ther 2005;31:285–302.
44. Harlow B, Stewart EG. A population-based assessment of chronic unexplained vulvar pain: have we underestimated the prevalence of vulvodynia? J Am Med Women's Assoc 2003;58:82–8.
45. Hite S. The Hite report. New York: Dell, 1976.
46. Hu JC, Link CL, McNaughton-Collins M, et al. The association of abuse and symptoms suggestive of chronic prostatitis/chronic pelvic pain syndrome: results from the Boston Area Community Health Survey. J Gen Intern Med 2007;22:301–311.
47. Ilie CP, Mischianu DL, Pemberton RJ. Painful ejaculation. BJU Int 2007;99:1335–1339.
48. International Headache Society: International Classification of Headache Disorders, 2nd edition, Cephalalgia 2004; 24 suppl1–160.

49. Krieger JN, Nyberg L Jr, Nickel JC. NIH consensus definition and classification of prostatitis. JAMA 199;282:236–7.

50. Laan E, Both S. What makes women experience desire? Fem Psychol 2008;18:505–14.

51. Lackner KM, Chang-Xing MA, Keefer L, et al. Type, rather than number, of mental and physical comorbidities increases the severity of symptoms in patients with irritable bowel syndrome. Clin Gastroenterol Hepatol 2013;11:1147–57.

52. Landry T, Bergeron S. How young does vulvo-vaginal pain begin? Prevalence and characteristics of dyspareunia in adolescents. J Sex Med 1009;6:927–35.

53. Laumann EO, Paik A, Rosen RC. Sexual dysfunction in the United States: prevalence and predictors. JAMA 1999;281:537–44.

54. Leclerc B, Bergeron S, Binik YM, Khalifé W. History of sexual and physical abuse in women with dyspareunia: association with pain, psychosocial adjustment, and sexual functioning. J Sex Med 2010;7:971–80.

55. Lee SW, Cheah PY, Liong ML, et al, Northern Malaysia Prostatitis Study Group, Chronic Prostatitis Collaborative Research Network Group. Demographic and clinical characteristics of chronic prostatitis: prospective comparison of the University of Sciences Malaysia Cohort with the United States National Institutes of Health Cohort. J Urol 2007;177:153–7.

56. Leiblum SR. Vaginismus: a most perplexing problem. In Rosen RC, Leiblum SR (eds). Principles and practice of sex therapy, 3rd edition. New York: Guilford Press, 2000: 181–202.

57. Lewis RW, Fugl-Meyer KS, Bosch R, et al. Definition, classification, and epidemiology of sexual dysfunction. In Lue TF, Basson R, Rosen R, et al (eds). Sexual Medicine: Sexual Dysfunctions in men and women. Paris: Health Publications Limited, 2004: 37–72.

58. Litwin MS, McNaughton-Collins M, Fowler FJ. The national institutes of health chronic prostatitis symptom index: development and validation of a new outcome measure. J Urol 1999;162:369–75.

59. Lloyd EA. The case of the female orgasm: bias in the science of evolution. Cambridge, M.A.: Harvard University Press, 2005.

60. Maxton DG, Morris J, Whorwell PJ. More accurate diagnosis of irritable bowel syndrome by the use of "non-colonic" symptomatology. Gut 1991;32:784–6.

61. Monga AK, Marrero JM, Stanton SL, et al. Is there an irritable bladder in the irritable bowel syndrome? Brit J Obstet Gynaecol 1997;104:1409–12.

62. Morin M, Bergeron S, Khalifé S, et al. Morphometry of the Pelvic Floor Muscles in Women With and Without Provoked Vestibulodynia Using 4D Ultrasound. J Sex Med 2014;11:776–85.

63. Nappi RE, Terreno E, Tassorelli C, et al. Sexual function and distress in women treated for primary headaches in a tertiary university center. J Sex Med 2012;9:761–9.

64. Nickel JC, Tripp DA, Chuai S, et al. Psychosocial variables affect the quality of life of men diagnosed with chronic prostatitis/chronic pelvic pain syndrome. BJU Int 2008;101:59–64.

65. Oberg K, Fugl-Meyer AR, Fugl-Meyer KS. On categorization and quantification of women's sexual dysfunctions: an epidemiological approach. Int J Imp Res 2004;16:261–9.

66. Paras ML, Chen LP, Goranson EN, et al. Sexual abuse and lifetime diagnosis of somatic disorders. JAMA 2013;302:550–61.

67. Payne KA, Binik YM, Amsel R, Khalife S. When sex hurts, anxiety and fear orient attention towards pain. Eur J Pain 2005;9:427–36.

68. Postma R, Bicanic I, van der Vaart H, Laan E. Pelvic floor muscle problems mediate sexual problems in young adult rape victims. J Sex Med 2013;10:1978–87.

69. Ramakers MJ, van Lunsen RHW. (1997). Vulvodynia caused by vulvar vestibulitis syndrome. Ned Tijdsch Geneesk 1997;141:2100–05.

70. Randolph ME, Reddy DM. Sexual functioning in women with chronic pelvic pain: the impact of depression, support, and abuse. J Sex Res 2006;43: 38–45.

71. Raphael KG, Widom CS. Post-traumatic stress disorder moderates the relation between documented childhood victimization and pain 30 years later. Pain 2011;152:163–9.

72. Rasmussen BK, Olesen J. Symptomatic and nonsymptomatic headaches in a general population. Neurol 1992;42:1225–31.

73. Reed DB, Advincula AP, Fonde KR, et al. Sexual activities and attitudes of women with vulvar dysesthesia. Obstet Gynecol 2003;102:325–31.

74. Reed BD, Harlow SD, Legocki LJ, et al. Oral contraceptive use and risk of vulvodynia: a population-based longitudinal study. BJOG 2013;120:1678–1684.

75. Reed BD, Harlow SD, Sen A, et al. Prevalence and demographic characteristics of vulvodynia in a population-based sample. Am J Obstet Gynecol 2012;206:170.e1–9.

76. Rosenbaum TY, Owens A. The role of pelvic floor physical therapy in the treatment of pelvic and genital pain-related sexual dysfunction (CME). J Sex Med 2008;5:513–23.
77. Salisbury CM, Fisher WA. "Did you come?" A qualitative exploration of gender differences in beliefs, experiences, and concerns regarding female orgasm occurrence during heterosexual sexual interactions. J Sex Res 2014;51(6):616–631.
78. Schaeffer AJ. Clinical practice: chronic prostatitis and the chronic pelvic pain syndrome. N Engl J Med 2006;355:1690–8.
79. Shoskes DA, Berger R, Elmi A, et al. Muscle tenderness in men with chronic prostatitis/chronic pelvic pain syndrome: the chronic prostatitis cohort study. J Urol 2008;179:556–60.
80. Smith KB, Pukall CF, Tripp DA, Nickel JC. Sexual and relationship functioning in men with chronic prostatitis/chronic pelvic pain syndrome and their partners. Arch Sex Behav 2007;22:1532–7.
81. Sobel JD. Vulvovaginal candidosis. Lancet 2007;369:1961–71.
82. Spoelstra SK, Dijkstra JR, van Driel MF, Weijmar Schultz WC. Long-term results of an individualized, multifaceted, and multidisciplinary therapeutic approach to provoked vestibulodynia. J Sex Med 2011;8:489–96.
83. Steward EG. Developments in vulvovaginal care. Curr Opin Obstet Gynecol 2002;14:483–8.
84. Tran CN, Shoskes DA. Sexual dysfunction in chronic prostatitis/chronic pelvic pain syndrome. World J Urol 2013;31:741–6.
85. Trinchieri A, Magri V, Cariani L, et al. Prevalence of sexual dysfunction in men with chronic prostatitis/chronic pelvic pain syndrome. Arch Ital Urol Androl 2007;79:67–70.
86. Ter Kuile MM, van Lankveld JJ, Groot ED, et al. Cognitive-behavioral therapy for women with lifelong vaginismus: process and prognostic factors. Behav Res Ther 2007;45:359–7.
87. Ter Kuile MM, Melles R, de Groot HE, et al. Therapist-aided exposure for women with lifelong vaginismus: a randomized waiting-list control trial of efficacy. J Consult Clin Psychol 2013;81:1127–36.
88. Tripp DA, Nickel JC, Wang Y, et al; National Institutes of Health-Chronic Prostatitis Collaborative Research Network (NIH-CPCRN) Study Group. Catastrophizing and pain-contingent rest predict patient adjustment in men with chronic prostatitis/chronic pelvic pain syndrome. J Pain 2006;7:697–708.
89. Turner IM, Harding TM. Headache and sexual activity, a review. Headache 2008;48: 1254–6.
90. Van der Velde J, Everaerd W. The relationship between involuntary pelvic floor muscle activity, muscle awareness and experienced threat in women with and without vaginismus. Behav Res Ther 2001;39:395–408.
91. Van der Velde J, Laan E, Everaerd W. Vaginismus, a component of a general defensive reaction: an investigation of pelvic floor muscle activity during exposure to emotion-inducing film excerpts in women with and without vaginismus. Int Urogynecol J 2001; 12:328–31.
92. Van Lankveld JJDM, Granot M, Weijmar Schultz WCM, et al. Women's sexual pain disorders. J Sex Med 2010;7:615–31.
93. Van Lunsen RHW, Laan E, Brauer M. Sex, pleasure and dyspareunia in liberal Northern Europe. In: Hall K, Graham C (eds). The cultural context of sexual pleasure and problems: psychotherapy with diverse clients. New York: Routledge, 2012: 356–370.
94. Van Lunsen R, Ramakers M. The hyperactive pelvic floor syndrome (HPFS): psychosomatic and psycho-sexual aspects of hyperactive pelvic floor disorders with comorbidity of urogynecological, gastrointestinal and sexual symptomatology. Acta Endoscopia 2002;32:275–85.
95. Voorham-van der Zalm PJ, Lycklama á Nijeholt GAB, Elzevier HW, et al. Diagnostic investigation of the pelvic floor: a helpful tool in the approach in patients with complaints of micturition, defecation, and/or sexual dysfunction. J Sex Med 2008;5:864–71.
96. Wade LD, Kremer EC, Brown J. The incidental orgasm: the presence of clitoral knowledge and the absence of orgasm for women. Women Health 2005;42:117–38.
97. Walker EA, Gelfand AN, Gelfand MD, et al. Chronic pelvic pain and gynecological symptoms in women with irritable bowel syndrome. J Psychosom Obstet Gynaecol 1996;17:39–46.
98. Warren JW, Langenberg P, Clauw DJ. The number of existing functional somatic syndromes (FSSs) is an important risk factor for new, different FSSs. J Psychosom Res 2013;74:12–7.
99. Weijmar Schultz WW, Basson R, Binik Y, et al. Women's sexual pain and its management. J Sex Med 2005;2:301–16.
100. Yang CC, Lee JC, Kromm BG, et al. Pain sensitization in male chronic pelvic pain syndrome: why are symptoms so difficult to treat? J Urol 2003;170:823–6.
101. Zhang Z, Zolnoun DA, Francisco EM, et al. Altered central sensitization in subgroups of women with vulvodynia. Clin J Pain 2011;27:755–63.

CHAPTER 11

Addressing Psychosexual Components of Pelvic Pain

Talli Rosenbaum

INTRODUCTION

Chronic pelvic pain (CPP) is associated with psychological distress and decreased quality of life in both men and women. Pain itself is an emotional experience [32] and all chronic pain conditions can result in and be perpetuated by depression, anxiety, and sleep disturbances [13]. However, patients with CPP may deal with additional challenges. CPP affects functions that are intimate and difficult to discuss with others. There are generally no outward signs of disability, such as assisted walking devices and sufferers don't typically appear disabled. Furthermore, many individuals with symptoms of pelvic pain see several doctors before receiving an adequate diagnosis and this itself may be cause of psychological distress. CPP specifically involves areas intimately connected to sexuality which may negatively impact one's body image and sexual self-esteem [24]. The typical female pelvic pain patient may have suffered from painful periods upon menarche, experienced pain with sexual relations, and may have been challenged with infertility when attempting pregnancy. These challenges affect a woman's self perception in her role identity as a woman, leaving her feeling damaged, dysfunctional and disconnected from her body.

While all types of chronic pain affect functioning, CPP is most closely related to pelvic floor functioning that is associated with bothersome symptoms including urinary frequency, urgency and bowel complaints, that affect quality of life (QoL) in many emotional, physical and social dimensions [20]. Bladder symptoms affect social and recreational activities, limit exercise and physical activity, and have a negative impact on mental health, affecting self-esteem and mood [33]. Bothersome urogenital symptoms, in addition to pelvic pain, are particularly associated with distress related to sexual activity [50]. Women with sexual distress are more likely to report sexual difficulty related to pelvic floor symptoms, including sexual avoidance due to vaginal prolapse or sexual activity restriction due to fear of urinary incontinence [27]. Men with chronic pelvic pain have a higher incidence of lower urinary tract symptoms that affect their sexual functioning as well [41].

Overactive bladder (OAB) with or without incontinence negatively affects sexual health, reducing sexual desire and ability to achieve orgasm [14]. Bladder Pain Syndrome/Interstitial Cystitis (BPS/IC) characterized by a constellation of symptoms including urgency, frequency, dyspareunia, nocturia and pelvic pain and is also correlated with decreased sexual functioning [35].

Women and men with CPP struggle with associated sexual dysfunction. During sexual activity, pain can occur with arousal and with orgasm in both men and women. Painful intercourse affects over 40% of women with CPP[18]. Painful intercourse may be perceived deep in the pelvis secondary to endometriosis or pelvic adhesions. Painful intercourse in women can also be superficial due to several possible causes including vulvar pain syndrome/vulvodynia, the most common cause of superficial dyspareunia in women in their childbearing years, affecting 12–21% of women in this population [21]. Men with chronic pelvic pain have a higher incidence of erectile dysfunction and premature ejaculation [46]. Pelvic and genital pain syndromes, commonly associated with bladder symptoms, are highly correlated with decreased QoL and sexual dysfunction [47]. Sexual dysfunction in all domains, including desire, arousal, orgasm as well as painful intercourse is common in both men and women with CPP.

CPP conditions affect pelvic floor function, sexual function, and quality of life. Depression, anxiety and other psycho-social characteristics, are commonly associated with CPP and patients with CPP may present with these characteristics in the clinic [12]. Furthermore, patients who suffer with CPP will likely encounter challenges in their significant intimate relationships [43]. Often clients present to practitioners with their partners and challenging relationship dynamics may be observed in the clinic. Hence, medical practitioners, including physical therapists, must be able to address these psychosocial components in their management of patients with CPP.

BASIC ASPECTS

Female Sexual Pain Disorders: Classification

Sexual pain disorders (SPD) are common in both men and women with CPP. Sexual pain disorders in women have been traditionally divided into vaginismus and dyspareunia, with the former diagnosis implying a fear-based reactive inability to allow vaginal penetration and the latter implying a condition characterized by the essential experience of pain with sexual intercourse or other vaginal penetration [2]. The proposal to replace these two Diagnostic and Statistical Manual- IV (DSM-IV) sexual dysfunction categories with "genito-pelvic pain/penetration disorder" [7, 8] recognizes the significant overlap in these conditions, as well as their non-sexually related symptoms. Pain and anxiety are understood to be salient components of both vaginismus [49] and vulvar pain syndrome/vulvodynia (VPS/VVD) [26].

There are a variety of possible etiological causes for dyspareunia that may be hormonal, such as in atrophic vaginitis, dermatological, such as the various lichens conditions, infectious, inflammatory or mechanical, as with a thick or inflexible hymen. Therefore, women with symptoms of sexual pain should undergo a thorough vulvovaginal examination in order to determine the possible organic components and contributors to pain.

A recognized component of these chronic pelvic and sexual pain related conditions is overactivity of the pelvic floor muscles. Pelvic floor muscle therapy, which is aimed to normalize pelvic floor muscle function, has become a standard intervention [19, 37, 40, 44].

The Bio-Psycho-Social Paradigm

While the classic approach to sexual pain had been to treat medically if organic findings were present and consider psychological etiologies in the absence of physical findings, sexual pain disorders are currently understood to have multi-factorial components [51]. Therefore, we appreciate that treatment should follow the bio-psycho-social paradigm. Recognizing the multi-dimensional nature of SPDs, the current biopsychosocial treatment paradigm designates treatment of the medical aspects of SPD to physicians and the psychological aspects including anxiety and aversion, to mental health professionals such as psychologists or sex therapists. In this model, treatment of the overactive pelvic floor muscles, or what is referred to as "pelvic floor dysfunction" is designated to physical therapists. However, several problems exist with this model. The relaxing and containing atmosphere of the mental health environment, is not one in which the patient is likely to feel the most anxious. However, in the medical and physical therapy settings, where pelvic examination and treatment is a salient component of the intervention, it is most likely that the patient's anxiety will be most present. The patient may also experience a response of disassociation. Therefore, a treatment model that attributes treatment of anxiety only to the mental heath professional, and not to medical professionals who directly confront that anxiety, is insufficient.

Moreover, overactivity of the pelvic floor is not merely an isolated state, but is often related to emotional states. Pelvic floor muscle activity has been found to be reactive in response to anxiety, fear of penetration and fear of pain, and most recently has been found to be reactive to visual stimuli of even non-sexual related scary films [10]. Increased pelvic floor muscle tension may be a baseline state as well, related to early habits such as rigid toilet training. The experience of physical therapy, which involves internal examination and muscle treatment, or other potentially exposing treatments, may elicit significant emotional responses, trigger past traumatic episodes and if not properly identified, may result in dissociation which may be misinterpreted as cooperation.

DESCRIBING THE SUBJECT

From a Compartmentalized Biopsychosocial Model to an Integrative Approach

Addressing biopsychosocial components in medical and physical therapy practice is an important step to make.

Proposed biological and physiological mechanisms of CPP are understood to be related to visceral, musculoskeletal, hormonal and other processes and may be related to alteration in central pain processing, local tissue mast cell and nerve proliferation, and overactivity of the pelvic floor musculature. CPP is also associated with psychological, relational and sexual distress as mentioned previously.

Many women suffering from CPP also present with sexual pain disorders. The main psychological feature associated with sexual pain is anxiety. Higher catastrophizing, fears of pain, hypervigilance and lower self-efficacy have been associated with increased intercourse pain intensity [16, 36]. Vaginismus has been traditionally defined as a reflexive reaction of vaginal spasm in anticipation of intercourse and associated with increased levels of aversion and disgust [9]. The reflexive contraction associated with vaginismus has been understood to be related to fear and threat [48]. Doctors and physical therapists are typically examining patients with pelvic and sexual pain, and this reflexive response is observed in the clinic.

An additional psychological factor of relevance to medical practitioners and physical therapists is body image. When a woman perceives her body as damaged and dysfunctional, she may disconnect and detach herself from her physical self and in particular, her genitalia. There does not appear to be research that has examined efficacy of physical therapy interventions for pelvic pain, that also measure the patient's emotional presence and connection with her body during treatment. However, it is likely that patients may completely disconnect and disassociate during physical interventions such as internal trigger point massage therapy, particularly if the intervention feels painful or embarrassing.

The social component of the biopsychosocial paradigm should not be ignored. Social construction of gender and sexuality directly shape the fear and distress of women with sexual pain [17]. Social factors are related to women's perceptions of her role in society and include the perception that women must allow vaginal intercourse for satisfactory sex, to please her partner or fulfill his need for sex [5]. This perception is often related to feelings of guilt, responsibility for the lack of intimacy and lack of autonomy in her intimate relationships. These feelings of guilt and responsibility may compel her to engage in sexual intercourse when she is neither aroused nor interested. Furthermore, these feelings may compel her to undergo painful and difficult treatments while emotionally disconnecting. Medical and physical therapy practitioners should consider the possible affects of these social messages and consider whether clients may be undergoing painful treatment just to please their partner.

PRACTICAL IMPLICATIONS

Addressing Anxiety in Medical and Physical Therapy Treatment of CPP

History Taking

It is beyond the scope of this chapter to teach the various counseling skills that medical and physical therapy practitioners can learn in order to address the psychosocial and sexual aspects of clients with CPP. However, counseling skills should be utilized regularly in medical and physical therapy practice. These skills may come naturally to many practitioners, and others may need to learn them. These skills include actively listening to the patient's narrative, asking open ended questions, reflecting and mirroring what you heard the client say, and providing empathy. Allowing the patient to tell his or her personal narrative is therapeutic for the client and provides the practitioner with the opportunity to better appreciate the client's feelings and thoughts. The practitioner may look for opportunities to learn more by responding openly with questions such as "Can you tell me more about that?"

The PLISSIT model [3] (P: permission, LI: limited information, SS: specific suggestions, IT: intensive therapy) provides a framework for professionals who are not therapists to address psychosexual issues and counsel clients. Intensive therapy (IT) is reserved for psychotherapists, however, medical and physical therapy professionals may be trained and learn skills to provide permission to discuss the topic of sex, limited information, and specific suggestions.

Although medical practitioners may be hesitant to discuss sex with their clients, research indicates that clients want their health care workers to raise the issue.[4] The following guidelines may be helpful [42]:

- Mention that the presenting condition may impact sexual activity.
- Ask and give permission to discuss the topic
- Be direct, but appropriate with language
- Be aware of and consider client's body language
- Be personally comfortable with the subject matter or don't bring it up.

- Use simple and direct language
- Use compassionate, honest, and normalizing statements
- Demonstrate your lack of embarrassment
- Be aware of patient's cultural background
- Ensure confidentiality
- Avoid assumptions.
- Know how to ask about trauma and sexual abuse and know how to react when patients reveal abuse.

Pelvic Examination: Addressing Anxiety, Trauma, and Abuse

Women with SPD may be unable, or extremely anxious about undergoing internal pelvic examinations and internal ultrasounds. Physical and emotional discomfort with pelvic examination is common in women, and has been correlated with a negatively perceived first pelvic examination [51], a past history of sexual abuse [45], and a post-traumatic stress disorder [30, 52].

Studies of women's perceptions of pelvic examination have cited physician gender, informed communication, positioning, nakedness, and physician abruptness as factors influencing feelings of control and comfort [28, 55]. Pelvic examination can provoke many negative feelings such as fear of illness, pain, embarrassment and awkwardness [53]. There is little literature on perceptions of the pelvic examination specifically in women with SPD [11] though difficulty with, or inability to undergo an examination are defining features of vaginismus and dyspareunia.

Factors believed to decrease patients' anxiety during examination include trust in and ability to communicate with the examining practitioner [53].

Pelvic pain, and pelvic floor dysfunction, has been correlated with a history of sexual abuse [6]. Shame, lack of perception of safety, repression of painful memories and the inability to connect between present medical conditions and the abuse, often prevent women from disclosing sexual abuse, especially if not specifically queried [29]. Practitioners should inquire about trauma and abuse and know how to cope with post-traumatic exacerbations such as somatization, dissociative reactions, hypervigilance, and abuse flashbacks. The pelvic exam should always be stopped if the patient requests it [25].

Addressing Patient Anxiety and Fear Aversion

Medical practitioners are generally used to confronting the fears and anxieties of patients about to undergo painful or life altering experiences. Physical therapists in particular, are skilled in addressing anxiety and fear aversion in the clinical setting and many utilize models that do address the psychological components of pain and fear aversion. These models include the Fear Aversion Model (FAM) [31], the "Explain Pain" [34] model, and the Messendiak Cognitive Somatic Therapy [23] model. However, interventions that target psychological variables in women with CPP do not appear to be widely used by physical therapists to complement traditional physical therapy interventions [1]. In a study that investigated physical therapy interventions for vulvodynia, none targeted psycho social or psychological variables [22]. Furthermore, these models are generally cognitive and behavioral and do not directly address the clients emotional experience.

The mindfulness approach to women with SPD was initially developed to address in vivo anxiety with pelvic examination and physical therapy interventions [38]. The "Rosenbaum Protocol" was developed to assist practitioners in helping women recognize and contain, rather than battle with their growing anxiety, avoid disassociation and remain present during examination and treatment. However, the approach has expanded to explore and address the existential conflict between the cognitive desire that motivates women to allow exposure to penetration when they are emotionally unready and they perceive the anxiety, but are attempting to repress [39]. We may address this by understanding the patient's experience on a cognitive, emotional, sensory, and behavioral level. For example, a woman about to undergo a pelvic examination may experience the following:

- Cognitive: "I have to allow this examination because I have to get better "
- Emotional (Anxiety manifested by catastrophizing): "If I don't fix this, my husband is going to leave me."
- Sensory: "My heart is beating fast and I feel tightness in my chest and my pelvic muscles"
- Behavior: "I am withdrawing and disconnecting 'going through the motions'"

Applying mindfulness in treatment, allows the client to focus on and accept feelings and perceptions, whether they refer to physical perceptions of pain, the physical manifestations of anxiety, such as tightness in the chest or increased heart rate, or emotional feelings such as of shame, exposure, sadness and frustration. Once she stays present and attentive to her feelings and refrains from self-judgment, she becomes capable of holding herself and containing, rather than battling with, those feelings. She learns to recognize thoughts that are unhelpful or catastrophizing ("If I don't fix this, I will never get married or have a baby") as well as recognize the feelings underlying those thoughts. When she gives herself permission for her feelings, she can better perceive when boundaries are necessary and is encouraged to verbalize them without apology, and gain comfort with saying "no." Rather than cognitively attempt to convince the client to relax her muscles with statements such as "just relax" or "try not to contract your muscles", the client is encouraged to place the boundaries she needs and decide for herself at which point she is ready to allow the examination.

Consequently, she begins to experience feelings of control of her own body. Pain and anxiety are no longer her enemies with which she is constantly embroiled in conflict and avoidance, but valuable perceptions that she learns to recognize, accept and appreciate.

Mindfulness Based Insertion Therapy

Both standard sex therapy and physical therapy interventions include the use of vaginal inserts in the treatment of sexual pain disorders. Yet, there is little literature describing technique or protocol for insertion, including method of insertion, number of times to insert, or amount of time the insert should be inside the vagina. The advantage of working "hands on" with dilator insertion, as physical therapists and sexology physicians do, is the ability to confront and deal with anxious reactions, and to witness whether the client inserts the dilator in a disassociated manner, or, if the practitioner or her partner is assisting, experiences the insertion in a disconnected way. There is little data examining the experience of women using inserts, however, in a qualitative study that did investigate the experience of gynecological cancer patients using vaginal dilators, patients reported experiencing dilators as technical, embarrassing, invasive and aversive [15]. Mindfulness insertion allows for the act of using dilators to be combined with an awareness of the clients emotional state while using them, thus preventing feelings of resentment, obligation, lack of autonomy, or disassociation. In dilator work, clients may experience frustration and express cognitions betraying their feelings of responsibility and the need to succeed despite not really wanting to ("I was a good girl this week and made myself to do my exercises, but I hate those things and they hurt me. But I have no other choice, what is my husband supposed to do?") These cognitions may be challenged by reacting to the client without judgment or disappointment and providing the option to not work with dilators. This models differentiation and gives her permission to be autonomous about her body, without worrying about disappointing anyone. She is encouraged that she has the choice, it is her body and she can stop at any time. She is discouraged from using judgment words such as "failure" and encouraged to stay in the present moment. Dilator instruction that encourages disconnecting, such as thinking about something else, watching television, sleeping or using anesthetic agents should consider the implications of this on the client's sense of autonomy and connection.

LOOKING AT THE FUTURE

Pelvic pain affects quality of life and has a negative impact on sexuality, sexual function, and intimate relationships. Medical practitioners treating patients with CPP and their partners are confronted not only with the challenges of providing the appropriate medical diagnosis and treatment, but also with addressing their psychosexual and psychosocial concerns. Learning basic sexual history taking and counseling skills to address anxiety, depression and sexual concerns are important in effective integrative treatment.

Medical practitioners as well as physical therapists, who provide physical examination and treatment, are regularly confronted with patients who display anxiety that also perpetuates pelvic floor overactivity and painful symptoms. Addressing anxiety, with techniques such as the mindfulness approach introduced in this chapter, is likely to help decrease this overactivity and improve physical therapy outcomes. The mindfulness protocol outlined above provides a method to keep clients with CPP focused on their perceptions, emotions and thoughts during treatments, while receiving the physical component, which is the goal of the medical and physical therapy interventions. Finally, as we help our clients in achieving their treatment goals, we must be mindful that the process may reflect ups and downs rather than continual, linear improvements, and that rather than emphasize the destination, we should focus on the healing journey.

TAKE HOME MESSAGES

- The multidisciplinary model suggests that whereas medical practitioners address physiological issues and physical therapists address the pelvic floor muscles and pain, the mental health practitioners are the ones who address psycho-social and sexual aspects of CPP. However, as medical and physical therapy practitioners regularly confront clients' anxiety and distress in the clinical setting, they require basic psycho-sexual counseling skills as well.
- Addressing psychosocial and psychosexual concerns in medical and physical therapy practice includes using counseling skills such as active listening, mirroring, empathy and open discussion of sexual topics according to the PLISSIT model. The Rosenbaum Protocol, is a recently introduced intervention which provides medical and physical therapy practitioners with tools to address the clients anxious reactions, emotions, cognitions, and behaviors.

FURTHER READING

Howard HS. Sexual Adjustment Counseling for Women with Chronic Pelvic Pain. J Obstet Gynecol Neonatal Nurs. 2012 Aug 3.

Rosenbaum TY. Physiotherapy treatment of sexual pain disorders. J Sex Marital Ther. 2005 Jul-Sep;31(4):329–40.

Rosenbaum T, Owens A. The Role of Pelvic Floor Physical Therapy in the Treatment of Pelvic and Genital Pain Related Sexual Dysfunction. J Sex Med. 2008;5(3):513–23; quiz 524–5.

REFERENCES

1. Alappattu, MJ. Psychological factors in chronic pelvic pain in women: relevance and application of the fear-avoidance model of pain. Phys Ther 2011; 91:1542–50.
2. American Psychiatric Association. Diagnostic and statistical manual of mental disorders (4th ed.). Washington, DC: APA; 2000.
3. Annon J. The PLISSIT model: a proposed conceptual scheme for the behavioural treatment of sexual problems. J Sex Edu Ther 1976; 2:1–15.
4. Athanasiadis L, Papaharitou S, Salpiggidis G, et al. Educating physicians to treat erectile dysfunction patients: development and evaluation of a course on communication and management strategies. J Sex Med 2006;3:47–55.
5. Ayling, K, Ussher JM. If sex hurts, am I still a woman? The subjective experience of vulvodynia in hetero-sexual women. Arch Sex Behav 2008;37:294–304.
6. Beck JJH, Elzevier HW, Pelger RCM, et al. Multiple pelvic floor complaints are correlated with sexual abuse history. J Sex Med 2009;6:193–8.
7. Binik YM. The DSM diagnostic criteria for dyspareunia. Arch Sex Behav 2010;39:292–303.
8. Binik YM. The DSM diagnostic criteria for vaginismus. Arch Sex Behav 2010;39:278–91.
9. Borg C, de Jong,PJ, Schultz WW. Vaginismus and dyspareunia: automatic vs. deliberate disgust responsivity. J Sex Med 2010;7:2149–57.
10. Both S, van Lunsen R, Weijenborg P, Laan E. A new device for simultaneous measurement of pelvic floor muscle activity and vaginal blood flow: a test in a nonclinical sample. J Sex Med 2012;9:2888–902.
11. Boyer SC, Pukall CF. "This hurts too": pelvic examination experiences in women with dyspareunia. Poster presented at the 2011 Annual Meeting of the International Society for the Study of Women's Sexual Health (ISSWSH), Scottsdale, AZ.
12. Chung KH, Liu SP, Lin HC. Bladder pain syndrome/interstitial cystitis is associated with anxiety disorder. Neurourol Urodyn 2013;33(1):101–5.
13. Chung SD, Lin HC. Association between chronic prostatitis/chronic pelvic pain syndrome and anxiety disorder: a population-based study. PLoS One 2013;15:8.
14. Coyne KS, Margolis MK, Jumadilova Z, et al. Overactive bladder and women's sexual health: what is the impact? J Sex Med 2007;4:656–66.
15. Cullen K, Fergus K, DasGupta T, et al. From "sex toy" to intrusive imposition: a qualitative examination of women's experiences with vaginal dilator use following treatment for gynecological cancer. J Sex Med 2012;9:1162–73.
16. Desrochers G, Bergeron S, Khalifé S, et al. Fear avoidance and self-efficacy in relation to pain and sexual impairment in women with provoked vestibulodynia. Clin J Pain 2009;25:520–7.
17. Farrell J, Cacchioni T. The medicalization of women's sexual pain. J Sex Res 2012;49:328–36.
18. Ferrero S, Ragni N, Remorgida V. Deep dyspareunia: causes, treatments, and results. Curr Opin Obstet Gynecol 2008;20:394–99.
19. Gentilcore-Saulnier E, McLean L, Goldfinger C, et al. Pelvic floor muscle assessment outcomes in women with and without provoked vestibulodynia and the impact of a physical therapy program. J Sex Med 2010;7:1003–22.
20. Gil KM, Somerville AM, Cichowski S, Savitski JL. Distress and quality of life characteristics associated with seeking surgical treatment for stress urinary incontinence. Health Qual Life Outcomes 2009;7:8.
21. Harlow BL, Wise LA, Stewart BG. Prevalence and predictors of chronic lower genital tract discomfort. Am J Obstet Gynecol 2001;185:545–50.
22. Hartmann D, Strauhal MJ, Nelson CA. Treatment of women in the United States with localized, provoked vulvodynia: practice survey of women's health physical therapists. J Women's Health Phys Ther 2007;31:5.
23. Haugstad GK, Haugstad TS, Kirste UM, et al. Mensendieck somatocognitive therapy as treatment approach to chronic pelvic pain: results of a randomized controlled intervention study. Am J Obstet Gynecol 2006; 194: 1303–10.
24. Heinberg LJ, Fisher BJ, Wesselmann U, et al. Psychological factors in pelvic/urogenital pain: the influence of site of pain versus sex. Pain 2004;108:88–94.

25. Hobbins D. Survivors of childhood sexual abuse: implications for perinatal nursing care. J Obstet Gynecol Neonatal Nurs 2004;33:485–497.
26. Khandker M, Brady SS, Vitonis AF, et al. The influence of depression and anxiety on risk of adult onset vulvodynia. J Womens Health (Larchmt) 2011;20:1445–51.
27. Knoepp LR, Shippey SH, Chen CCG, et al. Sexual complaints, pelvic floor symptoms, and sexual distress in women over forty. J Sex Med 2010;7:3675–82.
28. Larsen SB, Kragstrup J. Experiences of the first pelvic examination in a random sample of Danish teenagers. Acta Obstet Gynecol Scand 1995;74:137–41.
29. Lechner ME, Vogel ME, Garcia-Shelton LM, et al. Self-reported medical problems of adult female survivors of childhood sexual abuse. J Fam Pract 1993;36:633–8.
30. Lee TT, Westrup DA, Ruzek JI, et al. Impact of clinician gender on examination anxiety among female veterans with sexual trauma: a pilot study. J Womens Health (Larchmt) 2007;16:1291–9.
31. Leeuw M, Goossens ME, Linton SJ, et al. The fear-avoidance model of musculoskeletal pain: current state of scientific evidence. J Behav Med 2007;30:77–94.
32. Lumley MA, Cohen JL, Borszcz GS, et al. Pain and emotion: a biopsychosocial review of recent research. J Clin Psychol 2011;67:942–68.
33. Melville JL, Delaney K, Newton K, Katon W. Incontinence severity and major depression in incontinent women. Obstet Gynecol 2005;106:585–92.
34. Moseley GL. Evidence for a direct relationship between cognitive and physical change during an education intervention in people with chronic low back pain. Eur J Pain 2004;8:39–45.
35. Nickel JC. Interstitial cystitis: an elusive clinical target? J Urol 2003;170:816–7.
36. Payne K, Binik Y, Amsel R, Khalifé S. When sex hurts, anxiety and fear orient attention towards pain. Eur J Pain 2004;9:427–36.
37. Reissing ED, Armstrong HL, Allen C. Pelvic floor physical therapy for women with lifelong vaginismus: A retrospective chart review and interview study. J Sex Marital Ther *2013;39*:306–20.
38. Rosenbaum TY. Addressing anxiety in vivo in physiotherapy treatment of women with severe vaginismus: a clinical approach. J Sex Marital Ther 2011;37:89–93.
39. Rosenbaum TY. An integrated mindfulness-based approach to the treatment of women with sexual pain and anxiety: promoting autonomy and mind/body connection, Sex Relat Ther 2013;28:20–8.
40. Rosenbaum TY. Physiotherapy treatment of sexual pain disorders. J Sex Marital Ther 2005;31:329–40.
41. Rosenbaum TY, Owens A. The role of pelvic floor physical therapy in the treatment of pelvic and genital pain-related sexual dysfunction (CME). J Sex Med 2008; 5:513–23; quiz 524–25.
42. Sadovsky R, Nusbaum M. Sexual health inquiry and support is a primary care priority. J Sex Med 2006;3:3–11.
43. Smith KB, Tripp D, Pukall C, Nickel JC. Predictors of sexual and relationship functioning in couples with Chronic Prostatitis/Chronic Pelvic Pain Syndrome. J Sex Med 2007;4:734–44.
44. Steege JF, Zolnoun, DA. Evaluation and treatment of dyspareunia. Obstet Gynecol 2009;113:1124–36.
45. Swahnberg K, Wijma B, Siwe K. Strong discomfort during vaginal examination: why consider a history of abuse? Eur J Obstet Gynecol Reprod Biol 2011;157:200–5.
46. Trinchieri A, Magri V, Cariani L, et al. Prevalence of sexual dysfunction in men with chronic prostatitis/chronic pelvic pain syndrome. Arch Ital Urol Androl 2007;79:67–70.
47. Tripoli TM, Sato H, Sartori MG, et al. Evaluation of quality of life and sexual satisfaction in women suffering from chronic pelvic pain with or without endometriosis. J Sex Med 2011;8:497–503.
48. van der Velde J, Laan E, Everaerd W. Vaginismus, a component of a general defensive reaction: an investigation of pelvic floor muscle activity during exposure to emotion-inducing film excerpts in women with and without vaginismus. Int Urogynecol J Pelvic Floor Dysfunct 2001;12:328–31.
49. Watts G, Nettle D. The role of anxiety in vaginismus: a case-control study. J Sex Med 2010;7:143–8.
50. Wehbe SA, Whitmore K, Kellogg-Spadt S. Urogenital complaints and female sexual dysfunction (Part 1). J Sex Med 2010;7:1704–13.
51. Weijmar Schultz W, Basson R, Binik Y, et al. Women's sexual pain and its management. J Sex Med 2005;2:301–16.
52. Weitlauf JC, Frayne SM, Finney JW, et al. Sexual violence, posttraumatic stress disorder, and the pelvic examination: how do beliefs about the safety, necessity, and utility of the examination influence patient experiences? J Womens Health (Larchmt) 2010;19:1271–80.
53. Wendt E, Fridlund B, Lidell E. Trust and confirmation in a gynecologic examination situation: a critical incident technique analysis. Acta Obstet Gynecol Scand 2004;83:1208–15.
54. Wijma B, Gullberg M, Kjessler B. Attitudes towards pelvic examination in a random sample of Swedish women. Acta Obstet Gynecol Scand 1998;77:422–8.
55. Yanikkerem E, Ozdemir M, Bingol H, et al. Women's attitudes and expectations regarding gynaecological examination. Midwifery 2009;25:500–8.

CHAPTER 12

Research, Assessment, and Treatment of Sex Related Pain

Katy Vincent

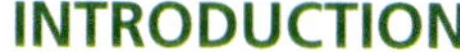

INTRODUCTION

Pain related to sexual activity is a significant and frequently under-estimated problem. Recent estimates suggest that up to 45% of women [62] and 5–8% of men [19; 50] experience sex-related pain at some time in their lives, although many never present for investigation or treatment [19; 33]. Unfortunately, for those who do present there is little data available from which to formulate evidence-based treatment strategies and therefore the treatment prescribed frequently depends on the specialty, or even the individual practitioner, that the patient is referred to.

Sex-related pain is unique amongst pain conditions by virtue of the fact that it has been considered in the context of the precipitating activity (Sex) rather than the key symptom (Pain). Clearly the intimate nature of sexual intercourse and the associations with sexual dysfunction and fertility do mean that sex-related pain may have important differences from other chronic pain conditions. However, a failure to focus on the pain means that many of the advances in other areas of chronic pain have not been considered in the context of sex-related pain [35]. In line with the IASP definition [7], the Diagnostic and Statistical Manual of Mental Disorders, 5th Edition (DSM-V) has recently revised their classification of dyspareunia, now considering it as a pain condition rather than a sexual dysfunction [6].

This chapter will firstly consider the difficulties associated with researching pain related to sex, before reviewing some of the more recent experimental findings.

In the context of a chronic pain condition, areas for assessment of the patient presenting with sex-related pain will then be considered and a multi-disciplinary approach to management presented. The chapter will conclude with a brief review of some of the more unusual sex-related pain conditions.

BASIC ASPECTS

What is Sex-Related Pain?

Traditionally a discussion of sex-related pain would focus on dyspareunia, defined as "pain associated with vaginal penetration" and limited to females. However, more recent definitions and classifications [4–7] acknowledge that this can be a problem for both males and females and do not focus specifically on penile penetration of the vagina, thereby including both anal dyspareunia and digital penetration. The DSM-V classification also allows the inclusion of pain outside of sexual activity such as with tampon insertion or gynaecological examination, both frequent correlates of dyspareunia [35].

Additionally, although not as commonly reported, both men and women can experience pain with, or immediately after, orgasm/ejaculation [2,34,37] either as a component of penetrative sexual activity or alone. Although not covered by the definitions of dyspareunia, this remains a sex-related pain and will therefore briefly be considered here. Both IASP and DSM only include sex-related pain within the pelvis/genitals in their definitions; however, headache related to sexual activity is well characterized [24,61] and thus will also briefly be discussed at the end of this chapter.

DESCRIBING THE SUBJECT

Research into Sex-Related Pain

There are a number of difficulties inherent to conducting research into sex-related pain. As already discussed, definitions of dyspareunia and sex-related pain vary and are themselves "umbrella terms" for a variety of different pain experiences and underlying pathologies, therefore it can be difficult to define and identify a homogenous population to investigate. Once the population has been identified, it can be difficult to collect accurate data, both because the questionnaires used are in the majority unvalidated and of difficulties accounting for the intimate nature of pain in laboratory based experimental paradigms. Analysis strategies for therapeutic studies also need to consider the confounder of frequency of intercourse. Thus, a partially successful treatment may lead to an increase in the frequency of intercourse with a concomitant increase in the number of painful episodes experienced, that if not properly accounted for could lead to the false assumption that the treatment was unsuccessful. Alternatively, if other psychosexual and behavioral factors are not also addressed a successful treatment may not be identified if the patient/couple are not engaging in intercourse. Despite the World Health Organization (WHO) considering that "all persons have the right to pursue a satisfying and pleasurable sexual life" [44], funding for research into sex-related pain remains difficult to secure. Even if funding is in place, it can be difficult and time-consuming to obtain ethical approval for many of the intimate procedures and questions necessary for these studies and recruitment particularly of appropriate, matched pain-free controls can be challenging.

To date, the majority of research into sex-related pain has fallen within one or more of the following themes which will briefly be considered below:

- epidemiology
- associations
- phenotyping
- pain mechanisms
- treatment

Epidemiology

Although a number of groups report on the epidemiology of dyspareunia or sex-related pain (e.g. [22,36,50,69]), these are not easy studies to undertake well. As already discussed there are issues surrounding the choice of definition and because of a reluctance to seek help for such a personal problem, if only healthcare-utilizers are considered then it is likely that the true prevalence will be under-estimated. Community studies are therefore most likely to give accurate estimates, however, although some validated questionnaires exist for assessing sexual function and sex-related pain (e.g. The Female Sexual Function Index (FSFI) [55]), these may not be accurately completed. Large-scale population studies comprising face-to-face interviews would, however, be prohibitively expensive, with the risk that some subjects may still not wish to answer accurately or may decline to be involved. The high prevalence reported in some studies (e.g. [19,50,62]), however, provides strong support for future funding applications.

Associations

Studies into the associations of sex-related pain are easier to undertake. Again, there can be difficulties in defining both the population of interest and the comparison population (e.g. pain-free controls, patients with other chronic pain conditions or patients with other sexual dysfunctions) and extrapolating from these specific cohorts to the population in general. However, the results of such studies can be of use in identifying novel therapeutic treatment and preventative targets and again to support future funding applications. Table 1 summarizes some of the associations identified in patients with dyspareunia.

Phenotyping

As discussed, sex-related pain covers a broad range of symptoms. Even if more specific definitions are used such as "deep dyspareunia in females" or "vulval pain syndrome" it is still likely that the underlying cause(s) or associations may be different. In order to optimize treatment for an individual or to design the most effective trial of a novel treatment, strategies by which these patients can be phenotyped need to be developed. Meana and colleagues proposed a phenotyping strategy including symptom descriptors, a clinical examination (including colposcopy), transvaginal ultrasound scan, microbiological investigations and psychological assessment [39]. Interestingly, they found that the levels of psychological distress and sexual impairment varied depending on the findings of the physical examination. More recently, it has been suggested that sensory testing is additionally included [31,32]. Whilst there are valid arguments that laboratory based genital sensory testing paradigms have little relevance to the experience of pain during sexual intercourse [14], these studies clearly suggest that there is more than one phenotype with the same clinical presentation. For example, in one study of women seen in a vulvar vestibulitis clinic, all of whom had experienced dyspareunia for more than six months and had severe pain in more than one location on the vestibule with the

TABLE 1 Associations of Dyspareunia

Biological	Psychological/Cognitive	Social/Sexual
Pain with first tampon use [32]	Psychological distress [49,67]	Sexual dysfunction [29,42]
Abnormal HPA axis activity [3,20]	Hypervigilance [46]	Guilt [25]
NOT related to unhealthy lifestyle [17]	Catastrophising [30,39]	Religious orthodoxy/ importance [16]
	Anxiety [26,38]	Partner behavior/ response [52,53]
	Disgust [15]	

HPA hypothalamic-pituitary-adrenal

cotton swab test, the authors were able to identify 4 subgroups on the basis of forearm pain threshold and psychological and cognitive measures [31] (Fig. 1c). In view of the relatively small sample size (n=28), 2 of these subtypes are less convincing (type 3 and 4), however, it can clearly be seen that in type 1 (representing 19% of the sample), the women had a low pain threshold and high levels of anxiety, whilst in type 2 (also 19%), pain thresholds were high and anxiety levels low. Type 3 and 4 women had less marked alterations in their pain thresholds, being only moderately low, but did have high and low levels of anxiety respectively.

Pain Mechanisms

In order to identify novel treatments for sex-related pain, it is crucial that the mechanisms underlying the generation of pain symptoms in these patients are identified. It is likely that a wide variety of mechanisms are at play and therefore accurate phenotyping of patients is necessary before these can be fully elucidated. Nonetheless, particularly in the vulval pain syndromes, significant advances are being made in this area.

As with other chronic pain conditions, women with vulval pain demonstrate altered responses to experimental noxious stimuli, both on the vulva [15,29,51] and at distant sites [29,51] (Fig. 1a-b). Furthermore, women with longstanding vulval pain show altered adaption to noxious stimuli on the hand [67] compared to those with no pain or a shorter

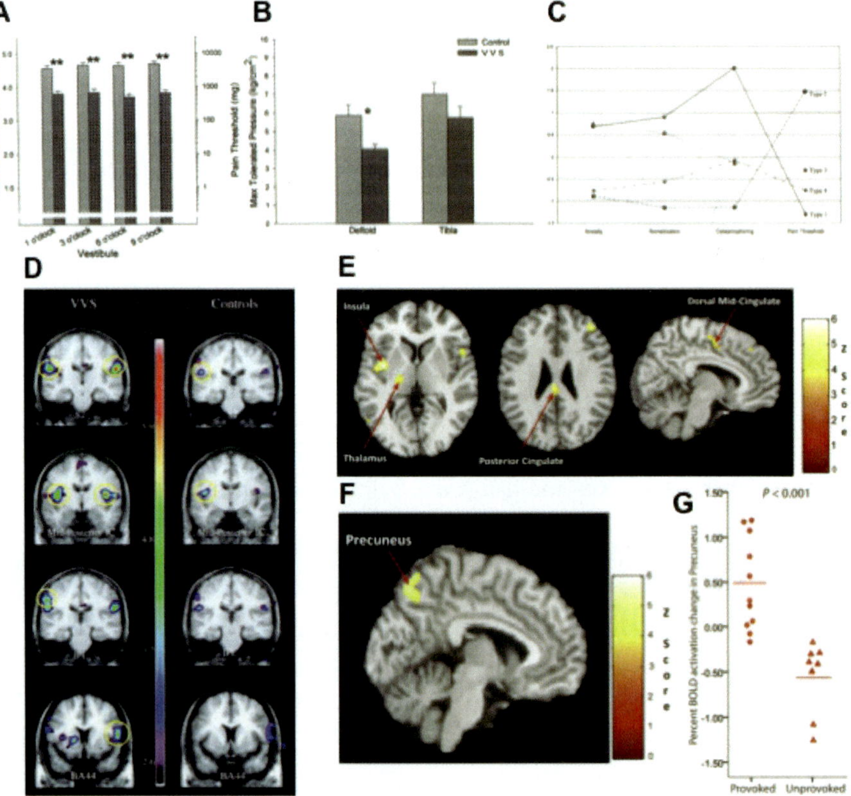

FIGURE 1 Pain mechanisms in vulval pain: Women with vulval pain show increased pain responses to noxious stimuli on the vulva (A) and at distant sites (B). Variations in pain response and anxiety may contribute to discrete phenotypes (C) [30]. Central mechanisms appear to augment pain in women with vulval pain syndromes, both in response to stimuli on the vulva (D) and the thumb (E) [51], however, phenotypes may also be identified by clinical presentation and reflect different central mechanisms (F and G) [31].

history. Similarly men with chronic pelvic pain syndrome have lower pain thresholds on their genitals/perineum/pelvis [20] and at distant sites [20,56] when compared to pain-free men and demonstrate increased sensitization to thermal stimuli on their perineum [65]. Although one study could not demonstrate a difference in either thermal or electrical thresholds on penis, perineum or distant sites [66].

Two brain imaging studies have been undertaken in women with vulval pain. In the first, the response to vulval pressure was assessed in women with vulval pain and pain-free controls and a central augmentation of pain was demonstrated [52] (Fig. 1d). The second, investigated the response to pressure pain on the thumb (e.g. a site distant from where the clinical pain is experienced) and looked for differences between subgroups of vulvodynia patients. There findings strongly support the need to carefully phenotype patients as they were able to demonstrate marked differences in the brain response to noxious stimulation between women with provoked and unprovoked vulval pain and more subtle differences between those with primary and secondary vulval pain [32] (Fig. 1f-g).

Whilst these findings support the idea that both men and women suffering from sex-related pain may have features in common with other chronic pain conditions, the relevance of these findings to the experience of pain during intercourse is harder to see. The few recent studies that have investigated the influence of sexual arousal and orgasm on sensory perception may help with our understanding. However, these studies have been relatively small and have produced contradictory results (Table 2).

Treatments

There have been few good quality randomized controlled trials investigating treatment options for sex-related pain. As with the other areas of research discussed, such studies are

TABLE 2 **Influence of Arousal and Orgasm on Sensory Perception**

	Pain-Free Women	Women with Vulval Pain	Pain-Free Men	Men with Pelvic Pain
Influence of Arousal	↓ pain sensitivity [63]	X	↔ pain sensitivity [45]	X
	↑ pain sensitivity [44,47]	↑ pain sensitivity [47]		
	↔ tactile detection [63]		↓ tactile sensitivity [45]	
	↔ pleasurable sensitivity [44]			
Influence of Orgasm	↓ pain sensitivity further [63]	X	X	X
	↑ pain sensitivity [44]			
	↔ tactile detection [63]			
	↓ pleasurable sensitivity [44]			

↑ increase
↓ decrease
↔ no effect
X not studied in this group of subjects

hampered by the heterogenous population presenting with sex-related pain or dyspareunia and the lack of a robust method of phenotyping patients. Furthermore, at present there is no gold standard treatment option to which to compare any novel treatment.

Assessment of Sex-Related Pain

The treatment of sex-related pain should ideally be individualized and multi-disciplinary. Therefore the aim of the assessment is to identify potential causative or maintaining factors or underlying pain mechanisms in order to rationalize the components of a treatment package. As always, the assessment of a patient with sex-related pain should include a detailed history, thorough examination and appropriate investigations. However, sexual dysfunction in the partners of those suffering with sex-related pain can also develop [17,35,57] and therefore an assessment of the partner may be required. It is also important to establish what the patient and potentially their partner want from treatment. Although this might appear obvious, pain-free sex may not always be the goal. For example, some may just want validation of a medical cause to their symptoms whilst others may want a pregnancy and therefore be requesting referral for consideration of assisted conception techniques.

There are a wide variety of causes of pain with intercourse, many of which are reversible or subject to modification (Table 3). It is important that any assessment undertaken of a patient presenting with sex-related pain identifies or excludes these causes. Any pathology identified should be treated appropriately, however, the patient should then be carefully reassessed at a suitable interval post-treatment to ensure the pain has resolved. Many of the pathologies associated with sex-related pain are common (e.g. endometriosis, diabetes, drug use or abuse) and may therefore be an incidental finding rather than the cause of the pain. Alternatively, although they may not have been the initial cause, secondary factors such as musculoskeletal alterations and psychosexual issues may have taken over to maintain the pain such that treatment of the initial causative factor has no or minimal benefit.

Additionally, the history should establish the frequency of painful episodes and whether the pain can also occur at times not related to sex, and if it is provoked or occurs spontaneously. Such facts are important for two reasons, firstly they may point towards specific causes or potential pain mechanisms and secondly they may influence both the treatments that are considered by the clinician and those that may be acceptable to the patient. For example, a young woman whose pain only occurs with intercourse and gynaecological examinations who does not currently have a partner may consider a daily medical treatment unnecessary, whilst a woman whose pain is additionally provoked by sports and wearing tight clothes and occurs without provocation is likely to be highly motivated to try such a treatment.

Vaginismus is a common cause and consequence of sex-related pain both in women who suffer with pain and in the partners of men with sex-related pain [17,35,57]. Without identifying and treating this component, it is unlikely that pain-free intercourse will be achieved even if any other underlying factors are treated successfully. Similarly an assessment of the psychological/cognitive state of the patient and potentially their partner may point towards the need for a psychological or behavioural component within the treatment package.

Treatment of Sex-Related Pain

As described already, as with any chronic pain condition, treatment strategies should be individualized and multidisciplinary, including treatment of: any underlying physical

TABLE 3 **Possible Causes of Sex-Related Pain in A) Women and B) Men**

A.

Vulval	Vaginal	Pelvic	Musculoskeletal	Systemic
vulval pain syndrome	vaginismus	endometriosis	pelvic floor tension	hypo-estrogenism
herpes simplex	congenital structural abnormality	IBS	pelvic floor trigger point	inadequate arousal
post-episiotomy/ tear	inadequate lubrication	BPS/IC		psychological
pudendal neuropathy	radiation vaginitis	urethral syndrome		abuse history
	post-surgery e.g. mesh, posterior repair	chronic PID		partner's sexual dysfunction
		adnexal pathology		drugs e.g. antihistamines, marijuana
				diabetes

B.

Penile	Scrotal/ perineal	Pelvic	Musculoskeletal	Systemic	Iatrogenic
ejaculatory duct stones	pudendal neuropathy	prostatitis	pelvic floor tension	diabetes	post-surgery e.g. radical prostatectomy, bowel resection, hernia repair
balantitis		IBS	pelvic floor trigger point	psychological	drugs e.g. anti-depressants
herpes simplex		BPS/IC		female sexual dysfunc- tion	radiation therapy
urethritis					circumcision
Peyronie's disease					
frenulum breve					

causes; vaginismus if present; psychological distress (in either partner). Associated issues such as fertility and contraception should be addressed and the value of support groups should not be under-estimated [35]. However, there is sparse data from which to inform an evidence-based treatment plan.

There have been small trials of gabapentin [11], lamotrigine [41], desipramine and topical lidocaine [23], and BOTOX [49] in women with vulval pain, although, the results have not been particularly convincing. However, this may represent under-powered studies with a heterogenous sample rather than poor efficacy of the medication being investigated and therefore in a patient complaining of unprovoked pain or frequent episodes of provoked pain, particularly if "neuropathic" descriptors are used it would be reasonable to consider a regular pharmacological option.

Cognitive behavioral therapy (CBT) has been shown to be effective at reducing pain both in the context of provoked vulval pain [12,38] and in vaginismus [60,63]. Even more impressive, however, are the results of studies assessing the effectiveness of an Exposure-based treatment in women with lifelong vaginismus (e.g. women who have never been able to have intercourse). This program involved a maximum of three 2 hour sessions during one week, during which the women performed vaginal penetration exercises on herself initially in the presence only of a female therapist and then subsequently with her partner. Only ten women participated in the original study, however, nine of these women had intercourse after treatment and in 5 of these this was possible within the first week of treatment [58]. Moreover, the results remained at one year follow up. The authors then went on to perform a larger waiting-list controlled trial recruiting 70 women. In this study, 89% of the treated women reported intercourse by the end of the 5 week follow up period as opposed to only 11% of the control women over the 3 month control period [59]. Women in the treatment group in this study also reported significant reduction in coital fear, coital pain and sexual distress.

Special Cases

Male Ejaculatory/Post-Orgasmic Pain

Pain with or after ejaculation/orgasm in men is surprisingly common: reported in up to 4% of otherwise healthy men and up to 58% of men with another pelvic condition [36]. Perhaps unsurprisingly, however, 88–91% of men experiencing this symptom consider it to be a serious problem [34]. The pains associated with ejaculation/orgasm are varied, being located in the abdomen, pelvis or genitals [8,9] and lasting from minutes to 24 hours [8,9]. Although the aetiology of the condition is not completely understood, there are a number of known associations, including post-radical prostatectomy, ejaculatory duct stones, use of anti-depressants and pudendal neuropathy [34]. Treatment can be medical, physiotherapy or interventional. Good responses have been demonstrated with reboxetine, tamsulosin and topiramate [34], however, only tamulosin has been subjected to a placebo controlled randomized trial [42]. Similarly good results have been shown with physiotherapy, specifically treatments targeting pelvic floor trigger points [4]. Alternatively, if ejaculatory duct obstruction is present this can be relieved by dilation or resection of the ducts or if there is any evidence of a pudendal neuropathy or pudendal entrapment the nerve can be injected or surgically released [34].

Female Orgasmic Pain

In contrast to pain associated with male orgasm/ejaculation there is little to no literature on female orgasmic pain (dysorgasmia), despite the fact that an internet search will reveal copious personal descriptions of this problem. Whilst there is no published evidence to support any aetiological theories, it is plausible that both musculoskeletal factors and neuropathic mechanisms could be involved in generating the pain. In support of this, a very small case series (n=3) found a response to amitriptyline in all the women studied [2]. Other non-peer-reviewed documents also suggest the use of NSAIDs and physiotherapy. However, the one recent study implicating the use of low dose combined oral contraceptive pills (COCPs)

[Rosenblum et al., unpublished] was flawed in a number of ways and therefore, to date there is no convincing evidence supporting a hormonal imbalance in the aetiology of dysorgasmia and thus no rationale to consider hormonal therapies.

Sexual Headache

Although not an abdominal or pelvic pain, sexual headache could be considered as a sex-related pain condition and therefore deserves a brief consideration here. As with the other types of sex-related pain discussed, the true prevalence of headaches specifically associated with sexual activity remains unknown, however, a lifetime prevalence of around 1% has been estimated [24,28], being 3–4 fold more common in men than women [61]. The International Classification of Headache Disorders recognizes two primary sexual headache disorders and one secondary, which may be associated with sexual activity:

Primary Headache Associated with Sexual Activity

Preorgasmic Headaches

- **A.** Dull ache in the head and neck associated with awareness of neck and/or jaw muscle contraction and fulfilling criterion B
- **B.** Occurs during sexual activity and increases with sexual excitement
- **C.** Not attributed to another disorder

Orgasmic Headache

- **A.** Sudden severe ("explosive") headache fulfilling criterion B
- **B.** Occurs at orgasm
- **C.** Not attributed to another disorder

Headache Attributed to Spontaneous (or Idiopathic) Low CSF Pressure [1]

However, it is important to remember that other serious secondary causes such as a subarachnoid haemorrhage (SAH), subdural haematoma or carotid/vertebral artery dissection may all present with a headache brought on by sexual activity. Thus investigation to exclude such causes is crucial on first presentation of a sexual headache [61].

Sexual headaches may well share some of their pathophysiology with other headache conditions, including vasospasm and musculoskeletal factors, and in some cases coexist, however, the exact cause remains uncertain [61]. Once underlying pathology has been excluded, it is important that both the patient and their partner are reassured as to the benign nature of these headaches and to ensure that they understand that they are usually self-limiting. No one treatment appears to be successful in all cases, but efficacy has been reported with the following taken prior to sexual activity: indomethacin, triptans, ergots, benzodiazepines; or with long-term prophylaxis using daily indomethacin, propranolol, metoprolol or diltiazem [25,61].

PRACTICAL IMPLICATIONS

It can be seen from the discussion above that more research is needed in the field of sex-related pain, in particular to identify underlying pain mechanisms, novel treatment targets and to confirm the efficacy of many of the treatments currently in use. Hopefully, the recent reclassification as a pain condition rather than a sexual dysfunction will facilitate this, in addition to supporting the concept of an individualized multidisciplinary treatment package in line with other chronic pain conditions. However, the precipitating activity should not be forgotten. Pain with sex has a number of unique associations and implications that can have a significant impact on the quality of life of both the patient and their partner. Thus, the value of support groups for these couples is enormous.

LOOKING AT THE FUTURE

Successful strategies for phenotyping patients both in terms of clinical presentation and the underlying pain mechanisms will be invaluable in the future. Without such strategies, it is unlikely that effective treatments will be identified for such a heterogeneous group of patients. Treatments that do appear effective, however, need to be subjected to rigorous randomized placebo-controlled trials wherever possible such that evidence based practice can be improved in this area.

TAKE HOME MESSAGES

- Sex-related pain should be considered as a chronic pain condition rather than a sexual dysfunction.
- The intimate nature of the precipitating activity and the impact on personal relationships, fertility and quality of life are unique and thus these should not be forgotten in any assessment and treatment strategy.
- Treatment plans need to be individualized and multi-disciplinary.
- More research is required in the field of sex-related pain.

FURTHER READING

Lahaie M, Binik Y. Dyspareunia and vaginismus. In: G Gebhart, RF Schmidt (eds). Encyclopedia of Pain. New York: Springer, 2013.

van Lankveld JJ, Granot M, Weijmar Schultz WC, et al. Women's sexual pain disorders. J Sex Med 2010;7(1 Pt 2): 615–631.

Binik YM. The DSM diagnostic criteria for vaginismus. Arch Sex Behav 2010;39(2):278–291.

Binik YM. The DSM diagnostic criteria for dyspareunia. Arch Sex Behav 2010;39(2):292–303.

DEFINITIONS

- Dyspareunia: "recurrent or persistent genital pain associated with sexual intercourse in either a male or a female" [4]
- "pain perceived within the pelvis associated with penetrative sex" [7]
- Vaginismus: "recurrent or persistent involuntary muscle spasms of the outer third of the vagina which interfere with sexual intercourse" [6,13]
- "inability to experience desired vaginal penetration during intercourse" [10]

REFERENCES

1. The International Classification of Headache Disorders: 2nd edition. Cephalalgia 2004;24 Suppl 1:9–160.
2. Ajay B, Penny J, Kurian J. Dysorgasmia or pain at orgasm: A case series. International J Gynaecol Obstet 2009;107S2:S558.

3. Anderson RU, Orenberg EK, Chan CA, et al. Psychometric profiles and hypothalamic-pituitary-adrenal axis function in men with chronic prostatitis/chronic pelvic pain syndrome. J Urol 2008;179(3):956–960.
4. Anderson RU, Wise D, Sawyer T, Chan CA. Sexual dysfunction in men with chronic prostatitis/chronic pelvic pain syndrome: Improvement after trigger point release and paradoxical relaxation training. J Urology 2006;176(4):1534–1538.
5. Association AP. Diagnostic and Statistical Manual of Mental Disorders IV. Washington, DC: American Psychiatric Publishing, 2000.
6. Association AP. Diagnostic and Statistical Manual of Mental Disorders V. Arlington, VA: American Psychiatric Publishing, 2013.
7. Baranowski A, Abrams P, Berger RE, et al. Taxonomy of Pelvic Pain. Classification of Chronic Pain: IASP, 2012.
8. Barnas J, Parker M, Guhring P, Mulhall JP. The utility of tamsulosin in the management of orgasm-associated pain: a pilot analysis. Eur Urol 2005;47(3):361–365.
9. Barnas JL, Pierpaoli S, Ladd P, et al. The prevalence and nature of orgasmic dysfunction after radical prostatectomy. BJU Int 2004;94(4):603–605.
10. Basson R, Leiblum S, Brotto L, et al. Revised definitions of women's sexual dysfunction. J Sex Med 2004; 1(1):40–48.
11. Ben-David B, Friedman M. Gabapentin therapy for vulvodynia. Anesth Analg 1999;89(6):1459–1460.
12. Bergeron S, Binik YM, Khalife S, et al. A randomized comparison of group cognitive-behavioral therapy, surface electromyographic biofeedback, and vestibulectomy in the treatment of dyspareunia resulting from vulvar vestibulitis. Pain 2001;91(3):297–306.
13. Binik YM. The DSM diagnostic criteria for vaginismus. Arch Sex Behav 2010;39(2):278–291.
14. Bohm-Starke N, Brodda-Jansen G, Linder J, Danielsson I. The result of treatment on vestibular and general pain thresholds in women with provoked vestibulodynia. Clin J Pain 2007;23(7):598–604.
15. Bohm-Starke N, Hilliges M, Brodda-Jansen G, et al. Psychophysical evidence of nociceptor sensitization in vulvar vestibulitis syndrome. Pain 2001;94(2):177–183.
16. Borg C, de Jong PJ, Schultz WW. Vaginismus and dyspareunia: automatic vs. deliberate disgust responsivity. J Sex Med 2010;7(6):2149–2157.
17. Cherner RA, Reissing ED. A Comparative Study of Sexual Function, Behavior, and Cognitions of Women with Lifelong Vaginismus. Arch Sex Behav 2013;42(8):1605–14.
18. Christensen BS, Gronbaek M, Pedersen BV, et al. Associations of unhealthy lifestyle factors with sexual inactivity and sexual dysfunctions in Denmark. J Sex Med 2011;8(7):1903–1916.
19. Clemens JQ, Meenan RT, Rosetti MCO, et al. Incidence and clinical characteristics of National Institutes of Health type III prostatitis in the community. J Urology 2005;174(6):2319–2322.
20. Davis SN, Maykut CA, Binik YM, et al. Tenderness as measured by pressure pain thresholds extends beyond the pelvis in chronic pelvic pain syndrome in men. J Sex Med 2011;8(1):232–239.
21. Ehrstrom S, Kornfeld D, Rylander E, Bohm-Starke N. Chronic stress in women with localised provoked vulvodynia. J Psychosom Obstet Gynaecol 2009;30(1):73–79.
22. Ferris JA, Pitts MK, Richters J, et al. National prevalence of urogenital pain and prostatitis-like symptoms in Australian men using the National Institutes of Health Chronic Prostatitis Symptoms Index. BJU Int 2010;105(3):373–379.
23. Foster DC, Kotok MB, Huang LS, et al. Oral desipramine and topical lidocaine for vulvodynia: a randomized controlled trial. Obstet Gynecol 2010;116(3):583–593.
24. Frese A, Eikermann A, Frese K, et al. Headache associated with sexual activity: demography, clinical features, and comorbidity. Neurology 2003;61(6):796–800.
25. Frese A, Rahmann A, Gregor N, et al. Headache associated with sexual activity: prognosis and treatment options. Cephalalgia 2007;27(11):1265–1270.
26. Fritzer N, Haas D, Oppelt P, et al. More than just bad sex: sexual dysfunction and distress in patients with endometriosis. Eur J Obstet Gynecol Reprod Biol 2013;169(2):392–396.
27. Gates EA, Galask RP. Psychological and sexual functioning in women with vulvar vestibulitis. J Psychosom Obstet Gynaecol 2001;22(4):221–228.
28. Gaul C, Visscher CM, Bhola R, et al. Team players against headache: multidisciplinary treatment of primary headaches and medication overuse headache. J Headache Pain 2011;12(5):511–519.
29. Giesecke J, Reed BD, Haefner HK, et al. Quantitative sensory testing in vulvodynia patients and increased peripheral pressure pain sensitivity. Obstet Gynecol 2004;104(1):126–133.
30. Gonen M, Kalkan M, Cenker A, Ozkardes H. Prevalence of premature ejaculation in Turkish men with chronic pelvic pain syndrome. J Androl 2005;26(5):601–603.
31. Granot M, Lavee Y. Psychological factors associated with perception of experimental pain in vulvar vestibulitis syndrome. J Sex Marital Ther 2005;31(4):285–302.

32. Hampson JP, Reed BD, Clauw DJ, et al. Augmented central pain processing in vulvodynia. J Pain 2013;14(6): 579–589.
33. Harlow BL, Wise LA, Stewart EG. Prevalence and predictors of chronic lower genital tract discomfort. Am J Obstet Gynecol 2001;185(3):545–550.
34. Ilie CP, Mischianu DL, Pemberton RJ. Painful ejaculation. BJU Int 2007;99(6):1335–1339.
35. Lahaie M, Binik Y. Dyspareunia and vaginismus. In: Gebhart G, Schmidt RF (eds). Encyclopedia of Pain: Springer, 2013: 5000.
36. Latthe P, Latthe M, Say L, et al. WHO systematic review of prevalence of chronic pelvic pain: a neglected reproductive health morbidity. BMC Public Health 2006;6:177.
37. Litwin MS, McNaughton-Collins M, Fowler FJ, et al. The National Institutes of Health chronic prostatitis symptom index: Development and validation of a new outcome measure. J Urology 1999;162(2):369–375.
38. Masheb RM, Kerns RD, Lozano C, et al. A randomized clinical trial for women with vulvodynia: Cognitive-behavioral therapy vs. supportive psychotherapy. Pain 2009;141(1):31–40.
39. Meana M, Binik YM, Khalife S, et al. Biopsychosocial profile of women with dyspareunia. Obstet Gynecol 1997;90:583–589.
40. Meana M, Lykins A. Negative affect and somatically focused anxiety in young women reporting pain with intercourse. J Sex Res 2009;46(1):80–88.
41. Meltzer-Brody SE, Zolnoun D, Steege JF, et al. Open-label trial of lamotrigine focusing on efficacy in vulvodynia. J Reprod Med 2009;54(3):171–178.
42. Nickel JC, Narayan P, McKay J, Doyle C. Treatment of chronic prostatitis/chronic pelvic pain syndrome with tamsulosin: a randomized double blind trial. J Urol 2004;171(4):1594–1597.
43. Nunns D, Mandal D. Psychological and psychosexual aspects of vulval vestibulitis. Genitourin Med 1997;73(541–544).
44. Organisation WH. Defining Sexual Health: Report of a Technical Consultation on Sexual Health, 28–31 January 2002, Geneva, 2002.
45. Paterson LQ, Amsel R, Binik YM. Pleasure and pain: the effect of (almost) having an orgasm on genital and nongenital sensitivity. J Sex Med 2013;10(6):1531–1544.
46. Payne K, Thaler L, Kukkonen T, et al. Sensation and sexual arousal in circumcised and uncircumcised men. J Sex Med 2007;4(3):667–674.
47. Payne KA, Binik YM, Amsel R, Khalifâe S. When sex hurts, anxiety and fear orient attention towards pain. Eur J Pain 2005;9(4):427–436.
48. Payne KA, Binik YM, Pukall CF, et al. Effects of sexual arousal on genital and non-genital sensation: a comparison of women with vulvar vestibulitis syndrome and healthy controls. Arch Sex Behav 2007;36(2):289–300.
49. Petersen CD, Giraldi A, Lundvall L, Kristensen E. Botulinum toxin type A-a novel treatment for provoked vestibulodynia? Results from a randomized, placebo controlled, double blinded study. J Sex Med 2009;6(9): 2523–2537.
50. Pitts M, Ferris J, Smith A, et al. Prevalence and correlates of three types of pelvic pain in a nationally representative sample of Australian men. J Sex Med 2008;5(5):1223–1229.
51. Pukall CF, Binik YM, Khalife S, et al. Vestibular tactile and pain thresholds in women with vulvar vestibulitis syndrome. Pain 2002;96(1–2):163–175.
52. Pukall CF, Strigo IA, Binik YM, et al. Neural correlates of painful genital touch in women with vulvar vestibulitis syndrome. Pain 2005;115(1–2):118–127.
53. Rosen NO, Bergeron S, Glowacka M, et al. Harmful or helpful: perceived solicitous and facilitative partner responses are differentially associated with pain and sexual satisfaction in women with provoked vestibulodynia. J Sex Med 2012;9(9):2351–2360.
54. Rosen NO, Bergeron S, Sadikaj G, et al. Impact of Male Partner Responses on Sexual Function in Women With Vulvodynia and Their Partners: A Dyadic Daily Experience Study. Health Psychol 2013 Nov 18 [Epub ahead of print].
55. Rosen R, Brown C, Heiman J, et al. The Female Sexual Function Index (FSFI): a multidimensional self-report instrument for the assessment of female sexual function. J Sex Marital Ther 2000;26(2):191–208.
56. Shoskes DA, Berger R, Elmi A, et al. Muscle tenderness in men with chronic prostatitis/chronic pelvic pain syndrome: the chronic prostatitis cohort study. J Urol 2008;179(2):556–560.
57. Smith KB, Pukall CF, Tripp DA, Nickel JC. Sexual and relationship functioning in men with chronic prostatitis/ chronic pelvic pain syndrome and their partners. Arch Sex Behav 2007;36(2):301–311.
58. ter Kuile MM, Bulte I, Weijenborg PTM, et al. Therapist-Aided Exposure for Women With Lifelong Vaginismus: A Replicated Single-Case Design. J Consult Clin Psych 2009;77(1):149–159.

59. ter Kuile MM, Melles R, de Groot HE, et al. Therapist-Aided Exposure for Women With Lifelong Vaginismus: A Randomized Waiting-List Control Trial of Efficacy. J Consult Clin Psych 2013;81(6):1127–1136.
60. ter Kuile MM, van Lankveld JJ, de Groot E, Melles R, et al. Cognitive-behavioral therapy for women with lifelong vaginismus: process and prognostic factors. Behav Res Ther 2007;45(2):359–373.
61. Turner IM, Harding TM. Headache and sexual activity: a review. Headache 2008;48(8):1254–1256.
62. van Lankveld JJ, Granot M, Weijmar Schultz WC, et al. Women's sexual pain disorders. J Sex Med 2010;7(1 Pt 2): 615–631.
63. van Lankveld JJDM, ter Kuile MM, de Groot HE, et al. Cognitive-behavioral therapy for women with lifelong vaginismus: A randomized waiting-list controlled trial of efficacy. J Consult Clin Psych 2006;74(1):168–178.
64. Whipple B, Komisaruk BR. Elevation of pain threshold by vaginal stimulation in women. Pain 1985;21(4): 357–367.
65. Yang CC, Lee JC, Kromm BG, et al. Pain sensitization in male chronic pelvic pain syndrome: why are symptoms so difficult to treat? J Urol 2003;170(3):823–826; discussion 826–827.
66. Yilmaz U, Ciol MA, Berger RE, Yang CC. Sensory perception thresholds in men with chronic pelvic pain syndrome. Urology 2010;75(1):34–37.
67. Zhang Z, Zolnoun DA, Francisco EM, et al. Altered central sensitization in subgroups of women with vulvodynia. Clin J Pain 2011;27(9):755–763.
68. Zolnoun D, Park EM, Moore CG, et al. Somatization and psychological distress among women with vulvar vestibulitis syndrome. Internatl J Gynaecol Obstet 2008;103(1):38–43.
69. Zondervan KT, Yudkin PL, Vessey MP, et al. Chronic pelvic pain in the community--symptoms, investigations, and diagnoses. Am J Obstet Gyn 2001;184(6):1149–1155.

CHAPTER 13

Bladder Pain

Ursula Wesselmann and Peter Czakanski

INTRODUCTION

Chronic nonmalignant pain syndromes in the urogenital area are well described but poorly understood pain syndromes. The primary focus of this chapter will be a specific urogenital pain syndrome: bladder pain syndrome/interstitial cystitis (BPS/IC). The intent of this chapter is to give an overview of the neurobiology of the urogenital floor, to discuss the current terminology and taxonomy of BPS/IC and then to highlight the present state of research of the pathophysiological mechanisms of BPS/IC. These research findings will be discussed in the context of clinical diagnosis and treatment approaches of BPS/IC.

While the focus of this chapter is on BPS/IC, it is important to recognize that chronic pain in the bladder area is just one of the clinical presentations of the chronic non-malignant urogenital pain syndromes. In the female patient these pain syndromes include vulval pain syndrome, clitoral pain syndrome, urethral pain syndrome, coccyx pain syndrome and generalized perineal pain. The "counterparts" in the male patient are testicular pain syndrome, prostate pain syndrome, penile pain syndrome, as well as coccyx pain syndrome and generalized perineal pain.

BPS/IC was initially regarded as bladder disease [40]. However, decades of research have failed to establish infectious etiologies or other clear etiologies related to the bladder tissue, until the clinical presentation of BPS/IC was recognized as "a chronic pain syndrome in its own right". There is significant heterogeneity in temporal characteristics and pain experiences in subgroups of patients with BPS/IC. Increasing evidence based on epidemiological studies demonstrates, that BPS/IC often occurs in the context of multiple comorbidities including other chronic pain conditions and that BPS/IC can be preceded by prodromal symptoms for many years, before the full-blown disease develops.

Patients with BPS/IC are typically evaluated and treated initially by urologists, gynecologists, family medicine practitioners, and internists. Although these patients seek medical care because they are looking for help to alleviate their urogenital discomfort and pain, in clinical practice much emphasis has been placed on finding a specific etiology and specific pathologic markers for urogenital disease. These patients typically undergo many diagnostic tests and procedures, but in many cases the examination and workup remain unrevealing and no specific cause of the pain can be identified. In these cases, it is important to recognize that pain is not only a symptom of urogenital disease, but that the patient is suffering from a chronic urogenital pain syndrome.

BASIC ASPECTS

Definitions and Taxonomy

While BPS/IC was initially regarded as a bladder disease, it is now recognized that there is a heterogeneous spectrum of still poorly defined disorders, which present with pain perceived in the bladder area and urinary symptoms. The terms painful bladder syndrome (PBS) and bladder pain syndrome (BPS) have been coined to include all patients with bladder pain [18,25]. The broader definition BPS/IC "an unpleasant sensation perceived to be related to the urinary bladder, associated with lower urinary tract symptoms of more than six weeks duration, in the absence of infection or other identifiable causes" was coined by the Society for Urodynamics and Female Urology, and has been used in both the European and American Urological Guidelines for the diagnosis and treatment of these conditions [18,25]. The International Association for the Study of Pain IASP has recently introduced an updated visceral pain taxonomy (http://www.iasp-pain.org/PublicationsNews/Content.aspx?ItemNumber=1673&navItemNumber=677). The IASP classification defines bladder pain syndrome as the occurrence of persistent or recurrent pain perceived in the urinary bladder region, accompanied by at least one other symptom, such as pain worsening with bladder filling and day-time and/or night-time urinary frequency. There is no proven infection or other obvious local pathology. The IASP definition explicitly recognizes that bladder pain syndrome is often associated with negative cognitive, behavioral, sexual, or emotional consequences as well as with symptoms suggestive of lower urinary tract and sexual dysfunction. The International Society for the Study of Bladder Pain Syndrome (ESSIC) has suggested a standardized scheme of subclassifications to acknowledge differences in this heterogeneous spectrum of disorders (http://www.essic.eu/). Pain in BPS/IC patients has been characterized to worsen with certain food or drink and/or worsen with bladder filling and/or improve with urination in 97% of cases, adding descriptors to the pain experience that might be sensitive criteria for diagnosing BPS/IC [50].

For most of the 20th century BPS/IC was diagnosed cystoscopically by Hunner's ulcers and glomerulations. However, Hunner's ulcers are uncommon and the importance of gomerulations is currently questioned [40]. Cystoscopy is not a required diagnostic test according to the latest American Urological Association guideline [24,25].

Only a minority of BPS/IC patients have evidence of an end-organ abnormality, moving away from an organ-centered understanding of chronic pain located in the bladder area to a conceptualization based on pathophysiological mechanisms of pelvic pain and integrating psychosocial and sexual dimensions has resulted in a transformation of the field that is reflected in all areas from research to clinical practice [2,17,40,61,62]. BPS/IC is recognized as a chronic visceral pain syndrome, a disease in its own right.

This concept of "chronic visceral pain as a disease" has received increased attention in the medical sub-specialties not only in urology but also in gynecology over the last 15 years. In fact visceral pain is the most frequent form of pain, felt by most people at one time or another, the number one reason for patients to seek medical attention (http://www.iasp-pain.org/Advocacy/Content.aspx?ItemNumber=1089; accessed March 1, 2014). With this statement the International Association for the Study of Pain (IASP) launched the GOBAL YEAR AGAINST VISCERAL PAIN (October 2012-October 2013), raising awareness that despite the striking prevalence of visceral pain, it is often insufficiently treated as it is considered just a symptom of an underlying disease.

Epidemiology

Based on different case definitions and populations studied estimated prevalence data of BPS/IC vary, ranging from 0.06 to 30% [16]. Estimates are difficult to compare, because BPS/IC includes a heterogeneous group of conditions and unfortunately there are no established biomarkers or tests to diagnose BPS/IC. The diagnosis is based on the presence of clinical symptoms and exclusion of other conditions, which are recognized causes of these symptoms, such as urinary tract infections or cancer. A recent population-based symptom prevalence estimate study in adult females in the USA concluded that there are 3.3 to 7.9 million women age 18 and older in the USA with BPS/IC, however, only 9.7% of these women reported being assigned a diagnosis of BPS/IC [5]. While earlier studies reported a female predominance of BPS/IC of about 5:1 or greater, a recent study showed that the prevalence of BPS/IC symptoms in men approaches that in women [45], highlighting the fact that BPS/IC may be under-diagnosed and under-treated in men.

DESCRIBING THE SUBJECT

The Urogenital Floor – Clinically Relevant Neuroanatomy

The urogenital floor is a highly specialized area of the body, and the neuroanatomy is complex. Compared with other areas of the body, there has been fairly little research on the neuroanatomy and neurophysiology of the pelvic floor. The fact that these areas of the body often are considered taboo in our society also may account for the scarcity of research on this topic. In the context of BPS/IC it is important to recognize, that the urogenital floor is responsible for executing several basic biologic functions, not only micturition (disturbances of micturition are a hallmark of BPS/IC), but also defecation, copulation, and reproduction. The coordination of these diverse functions depends on precise nervous system control, as well as endocrine and other local control mechanisms. A detailed review of the neurobiology of the urogenital floor is provided by Burnett and Wesselmann [11,12]. Briefly, the urogenital floor is innervated by both components of the autonomic nervous system (sympathetic and parasympathetic divisions), as well as the somatic nervous systems [60] (Figs. 1 and 2). Sensations from the pelvic floor are mainly conveyed via the sacral afferent parasympathetic system, and to a lesser extent via afferents traveling with the thoracolumbar sympathetics.

Within the pelvis, the inferior hypogastric plexus (pelvic plexus) is regarded as the major neuronal integrative center. It innervates multiple pelvic organs, including the urinary bladder, proximal urethra, distal ureter, rectum, internal anal sphincter, as well as genital and reproductive tract structures. The inferior hypogastric plexus receives sympathetic and parasympathetic input. Sympathetic nerves originate in the thoracolumbar segments of the spinal cord (T10-L2) and condense into the superior hypogastric plexus located just inferior to the aortic bifurcation. Preganglionic efferents originate largely in the intermediolateral cell column whereas afferents have their cell bodies located in dorsal root ganglia of these segments. Nerve fibers project from the superior hypogastric plexus as paired hypogastric plexuses and fuse distally before diverging bilaterally into branches destined for the inferior hypogastric plexuses. Additional sympathetic innervation to pelvic organs may involve preganglionic nerves, which synapse on postganglionic nerves originating in sympathetic chain ganglia. Parasympathetic preganglionic nerve efferents are thought to arise from cell

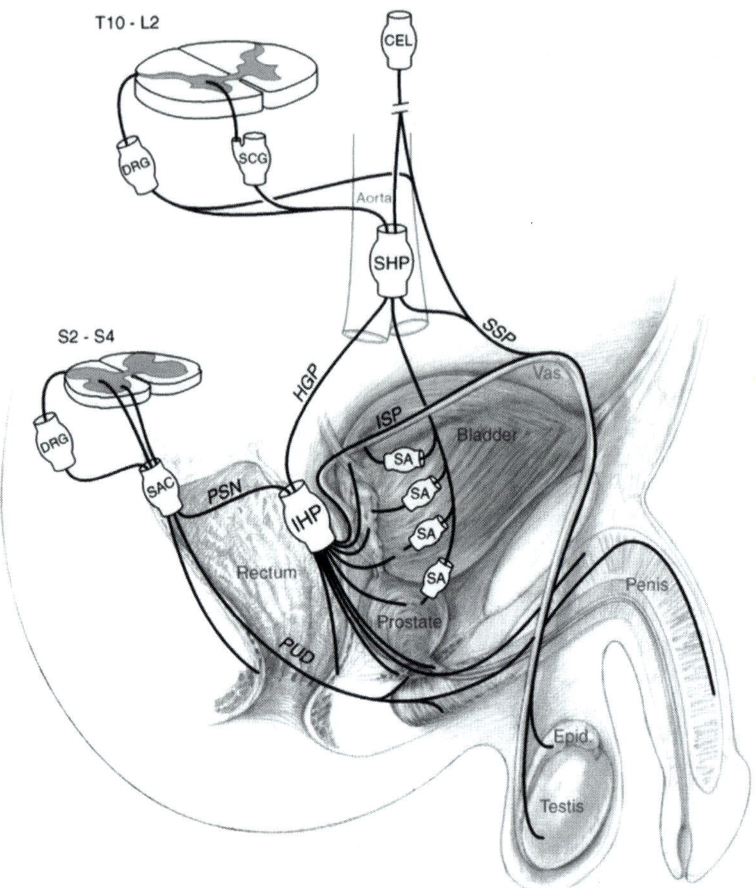

FIGURE 1 Schematic drawing showing the innervation of the pelvic floor in males. Although this diagram attempts to show the innervation in humans, much of the anatomic information is derived from animal data. CEL, celiac plexus; DRG, dorsal root ganglion; HGP, hypogastric plexus; IHP, inferior hypogastric plexus; ISP, inferior spermatic plexus; PSN, pelvic splanchnic nerve; PUD, pudendal nerve; Epid., epididymis; SA, short adrenergic projections; SAC, sacral plexus; SCG, sympathetic chain ganglion; SHP, superior hypogastric plexus; SSP, superior spermatic plexus. (From: Wesselmann U, Burnett AL, Heinberg LJ. The urogenital and rectal pain syndromes. Pain 1997; 73: 269–294 [ref. 60]. This figure has been reproduced with permission of the International Association for the Study of Pain® (IASP). This figure may not be reproduced for any other purpose without permission.)

bodies of the sacral parasympathetic nucleus located in the sacral spinal cord (S2–S4) and fuse as the pelvic splanchnic nerve before entering the inferior hypogastric plexus. Parasympathetic afferents have cell bodies located in the S2–S4 dorsal root ganglia and course also within the pelvic splanchnic nerve.

Somatic efferent and afferent innervation to the urogenital floor originates from sacral spinal cord levels S2 to S4. Sacral nerve roots emerge from the spinal cord to form the sacral plexus, and give rise to the pudendal nerve. The pudendal nerve also receives postganglionic axons from the caudal sympathetic chain ganglia. Thus the pudendal nerve carries somatic and autonomic nerve fibers. The pudendal nerve runs medial to the internal pudendal vessels along the lateral wall of the ischiorectal fossa dorsal to the sacrospinous ligament. First a branch splits off to become the dorsal nerve of the penis (or clitoris), then the remaining pudendal nerve fibers distribute a medial branch to the anal canal, dorsal branches to the urethral sphincter, and dorsolateral branches to the anterior perineal musculature. The

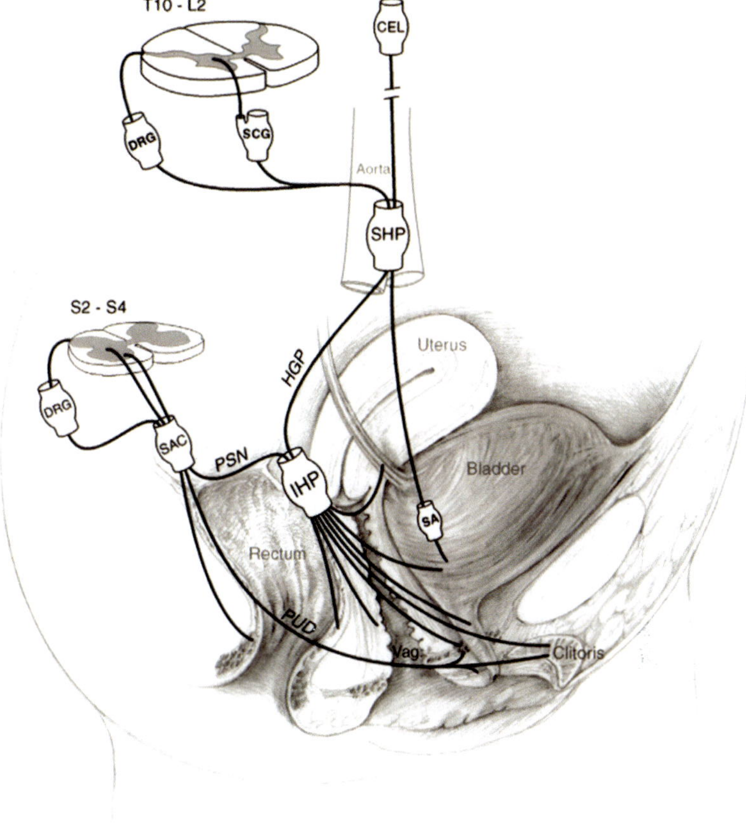

FIGURE 2 Schematic drawing showing the innervation of the pelvic floor in females. Although this diagram attempts to show the innervation in humans, much of the anatomic information is derived from animal data. CEL, celiac plexus; DRG, dorsal root ganglion; HGP, hypogastric plexus; IHP, inferior hypogastric plexus; PSN, pelvic splanchnic nerve; PUD, pudendal nerve; SA, short adrenergic projections; SAC, sacral plexus; SCG, sympathetic chain ganglion; SHP, superior hypogastric plexus; Vag., vagina (From: Wesselmann U, Burnett AL, Heinberg LJ. The urogenital and rectal pain syndromes. Pain 1997; 73: 269–294 [ref. 60]. This figure has been reproduced with permission of the International Association for the Study of Pain® (IASP). This figure may not be reproduced for any other purpose without permission.)

posterior perineal musculature is supplied by nerves originating predominantly from sacral level S4. Branches of the S4–5 nerve roots form the coccygeal plexus, distributing fibers to the perineal, perianal, and scrotal (labial) skin.

Etiologies and Pathophysiological Mechanisms

At present there is no universally accepted etiology for BPS/IC and proposed etiologies, which are not mutually exclusive include inflammation, mast cell activation, urothelial dysfunction/glycosaminoglycan defects, presence of anti-proliferative factor, autoimmune mechanisms, genetic predisposition and early-in-life experiences [47,49]. As it is increasingly being recognized that BPS/IC shares many aspects with other chronic pain syndromes, neurophysiological mechanisms including peripheral and central sensitization have been explored. These multiple etiologies reflect the heterogeneity of the patient population.

In BPS/IC multiple pain sites are common. Warren et al. [55] explored whether a careful and systematic description of pain of BPS/IC might provide insights to the pathogenesis of the disease. It has been questioned if indeed the generator of pain in BPS/IC is the bladder [55]. The suprapubic site is the usual area of normal bladder filling sensation. This site is the most common pain site in subjects with BPS/IC [20,55]. The best recognized stimulus of visceral pain is distension of a hollow organ [32]. Of patients with BPS/IC, 84% to 90% report worsening of pain with bladder filling, which suggests that the bladder is a visceral organ involved in BPS/IC [51]. These findings might imply that the bladder is in fact the generator of pain in BPS/IC. This is a hypothesis, which was tested by Warren et al. [55]. Clinical observations have documented that in BPS/IC multiple pain sites are common and consistent with these observations, BPS/IC patients in this epidemiological study reported multiple pains. Pain could be consolidated at 4 sites including, suprapubic, urethral, genital and non-genitourinary. The data demonstrated that suprapubic prominence and changes in the voiding cycle are features consistent with BPS/IC, but do not prove that the bladder is the pain generator in BPS/IC and that the pain sites described by patients are referred from it. Women, who in other contexts might have been diagnosed with urethral pain syndrome or vulval pain syndrome, did not differ in pertinent variables from women, who had BPS/IC without pain at these sites.

Early histological examinations of bladder lesions of patients diagnosed with BPS/IC revealed mucosal ulceration, pancystitis and perineural inflammatory infiltrates. However a search for a chronic viral or bacterial etiology rendered negative results [1,19], including a search for bacterial and viral DNA in bladder biopsies from patients with BPS/IC. The surface of the bladder urothelium is lined by a glycosaminoglycan layer and a defect in this protective layer has been proposed to cause the symptoms of BPS/IC, but the etiology of this breakdown in the urothelial barrier and its consequences for the clinical features of BPS/IC are still an issue for debate [47,49]. Morphological studies have demonstrated mast cell proliferation and activation in patients with BPS/IC [43]. Many symptoms such as pain, frequency, edema and ulcerations could possibly be related to mast cell release, and targeted pharmacotherapy to inhibit mast cell activation has been suggested as a therapeutic avenue [43].

Several groups have tried to identify biomarkers to identify patients with BPS/IC and to predict treatment responses. An antiproliferative factor (APF) that profoundly inhibits bladder cell proliferation has been identified in the urine of patients with BPS/IC [28]. It has been proposed that in patients with BPS/IC this peptide inhibits bladder epithelial regeneration following damage, such as that caused by bacterial cystitis [27]. A mouse model of BPS/IC based on AFP inhibition of bladder epithelial repair has been developed recently [26]. Urinary nerve growth factor (NGF) has been reported to be increased in patients with BPS/IC and a decrease in urinary NGF levels was associated with greater pain reduction after treatment, suggesting that urinary NGF levels might be a useful biomarker to detect the severity of the disease in patients with BPS/IC [31].

Numerous receptors have been shown to be increased in bladder tissue of patients with BPS/IC using immunohistochemical staining, including cannabinoid receptor-1, transient receptor potential vanilloid receptor subtype-1, and TRPM8 [33,34,35]. It has been suggested that these receptors might play a role in the pathophysiology of BPS/IC and may provide targets for pharmacological therapy [6]. Molecular studies have recently demonstrated that microRNAs may mediate the down-regulation of neurokinin-1 receptor in BPS/IC [42].

A genetic predisposition to some sub-groups of BPS/IC has been explored. Warren et al. [54] reported that adult female first relatives of patients with BPS/IC may have a prevalence of BPS/IC 17 times that found in the general population. This suggests, but does not prove, a genetic susceptibility of BPS/IC.

It has been observed that anxiety and stress may initiate and worsen urinary symptoms in BPS/IC. Life stress is associated with greater BPS/IC symptoms [41] and stress-related mechanisms can be associated with inflammatory processes within the bladder that sometimes accompany BPS/IC [43].

Psychophysical studies, using a similar approach as in patients with neuropathic pain, have confirmed hypersensitivity to somatic stimuli in patients with BPS/IC [21,30,37]. Consistent with findings in patients with fibromyalgia and IBS, conditioned pain modulation responses were significantly different in patients with BPS/IC compared to healthy controls, indicating that a deficit in endogenous pain inhibitory systems may contribute to BPS/IC [36]. f-MRI imaging studies in women with BPS/IC have demonstrated that these patients present with a sensorimotor component to their pathology involving an alteration in the intrinsic oscillations and connectivity within a cortico-cerebellar network previously associated urinary bladder function [29].

Numerous animal models have been established of bladder pain [summarized in detail in: reference 23], which have employed mechanical stimulation, chemical and infectious agents, as well as specific etiologic factors, such as stress. These models are sometimes used to explore specific etiological aspects of BPS/IC and possible therapies. Rodent models have used overdistension of the urinary bladder, inflammation with intravesical instillation of agents producing both direct signs of visceral pain perception (abnormal behavior) and referred hyperalgesia. Cyclophosphamide-induced cystitis in rats follows administration of the drug intraperitoneally, mimicking the equivalent human condition of cyclophosphamide-induced cystitis, rather than BPS/IC. However, this rodent model has also been used to understand neurophysiological aspects of bladder pain relevant to BPS/IC and to study potential treatments. The advantage of the cyclophosphamide-induced cystitis bladder pain model in mice has allowed genetic studies to be undertaken. Mice that lack the receptor for substance P (NK1) did not develop either primary hyperalgesia after bladder inflammation or referred hyperalgesia. Neonatal bladder inflammation, similar to animal studies modelling other pain syndromes, produces bladder hypersensitivity in adulthood. It is thus proposed that this model may be useful to study early-in-life experiences which might result in BPS/IC in adulthood. An animal model of stress-induced bladder mast cell activation in 1997 [44], has been used by as a model of interstitial cystitis. However, the behavioral aspects of this model, will have to be quantified with respect to pain [23]. A naturally occurring disease has been described in cats, which has many features of BPS/IC in humans [9]. This model has been proposed to study the effects of stressors on the severity of clinical signs as well as newly proposed therapies for BPS/IC patients [8,9].

Comorbid Conditions

Clinical observations suggest, that there is substantial overlap observed between BPS/IC and other pelvic/abdominal pain syndromes. These observations could be explained neurophysiologically by referred visceral pain mechanisms to other visceral and somatic areas with overlapping spinal cord projections (Figs. 1 and 2). In addition, in a report [15] for BPS/IC and fibromyalgia, there is increasing evidence of the co-occurrence of BPS/IC with chronic pain syndromes in other "non-pelvic" body areas, raising the question of systemic alterations of pain modulatory mechanisms.

Recently, these clinical observations have been confirmed by several epidemiological studies, which have demonstrated a substantial overlap between urological and non-urological unexplained clinical conditions [10]. These epidemiological studies require validated case definitions to identify comorbid conditions in large populations, and the results of these studies depend on the range of comorbidities that are screened for. For example, vulval pain syndrome in women and prostate pain syndrome in men are pain comorbidities, which have only more recently been included in such efforts, probably because these areas are considered taboo [10,38,45]. In a recent study, the overlap between men with BPS/IC and chronic prostatitis/ chronic pelvic pain syndrome was reported as 17% [45]. These findings suggested that BPS/IC may be part of a more generalized systemic disorder [10,53]. It has been proposed that BPS/IC is a functional somatic syndrome rather than a urological condition [40].

Patients with BPS/IC typically present with fibromyalgia, chronic fatigue syndrome, irritable bowel syndrome, temporomandibular disorder, migraine, chronic pelvic pain, vulval pain syndrome, low back pain, sicca syndrome, allergies, asthma, depression, and anxiety [53]. Several studies have also confirmed the coexistence of endometriosis and BPS/IC, ranging from 16% - 78% [48]. Epidemiological studies have demonstrated that the odds ratios for BPS/IC increases with increasing numbers of antecedent non-bladder syndromes [52,58]. The distribution of non-bladder syndrome types was skewed, with allergy overrepresented in those with few non-bladder syndromes and the classic functional somatic syndromes of fibromyalgia, chronic fatigue syndrome, and irritable bowel syndrome were overrepresented in those with many non-bladder syndromes [58]. BPS/IC was also significantly associated with previous female hormone use and a history of fewer pregnancies [52].

In addition, epidemiological studies have revealed that before the onset of BPS/IC, the presence of multiple non-bladder syndromes is strongly associated with a history of multiple surgeries [56]. Understanding these temporal relationships will be of utmost importance, since surgical practice in patients who present with these characteristics might need to be modified. Until the association between these non-bladder syndromes and surgeries is understood, patients presenting with ambiguous indications for surgeries should be questioned about functional somatic syndromes and other syndromes and alternatives to surgery might have to be considered.

A common theme to this group of comorbid disorders could be related to the autonomic nervous system, and indeed a recent study [4] identified a high level of autonomic dysfunction in subjects with BPS/IC including poor sleep function, Raynaud's like symptoms, and orthostatic symptoms.

Women with BPS/IC experience very high levels of sexual dysfunction [7,22]. However, most of these women do not seek medical help, and those who do seek help seldom get treatment, despite the fact that 88% of these women reported one or more general sexual dysfunction symptoms [7]. These data call for urgent changes in current clinical practice [13], since women with BPS/IC maybe unlikely to initiate discussion of sexual dysfunction due to the stigma and discomfort with discussing these issues during the medical encounter. Similar issues are likely to play a role for men who suffer from BPS/IC, but detailed studies are lacking. Treatment for sexual dysfunction will require a concerted effort of a team of clinicians experienced in urology, pain management, physical therapy and sex therapy.

The average BPS/IC onset age is in the 30s or 40s. Many female patients with BPS/IC recall having urinary symptoms decades before the onset of BPS/IC [57]. This prodrome is associated with non-bladder syndromes and predicts BPS/IC and also its poor prognosis. BPS/IC with a prodrome might have a different pathogenesis. These studies have important clinical implications and suggest that females with frequency, pelvic pain with urinary features, or bladder pain may be at risk for full-blown BPS/IC years later. From a clinical standpoint, this could have important implications, since triggers that result in full-blown BPS/IC may be preventable in this high-risk group.

PRACTICAL IMPLICATIONS

The shift in conceptualizing BPS/IC as a chronic visceral pain syndromes in its own right rather than an end-organ disease (bladder disease) has resulted in new approaches in basic science and clinical research as well as in the clinical management of BPS/IC:

Realizing the sometimes marked differences in the expression and function of receptors in visceral and somatic pathways has led to new pharmacological research explorations of both new and previously overlooked potential therapeutic targets [6,59], which might provide new avenues for treating BPS/IC in the future.

Based on the recognition that BPS/IC is a heterogeneous group of conditions, and learning from previously failed clinical trials, which showed that the discovery of a single target for the treatment of BPS/IC is unlikely, the National Institutes of Health (NIH) in the USA have launched a multi-disciplinary research network (http://www.mappnetwork.org/), embracing a systemic "whole body" approach in the study of BPS/IC focusing on 5 major areas: Epidemiology of Disease, Phenotyping of Urological and Non-Urological symptoms, Neuroimaging / Neurobiology Studies, Identification of Biomarkers of Disease, Characterizations of Organ Cross-Talk / Pain Pathways.

Clinical guidelines have been developed in several countries over the last 10 years proposing an integrated approach to urogenital pain syndromes by a multi-disciplinary team of healthcare providers [16,17,18,25].

The need for a multidisciplinary team approach to urogenital and pelvic pain syndromes, as suggested in these clinical guidelines, will require changes in the healthcare system to allow a coordinated involvement of multiple teams, beyond the historic boundaries of medical sub-specialties and of primary and secondary care. This has recently been address in the British Pain Society's Pelvic Pain Patient Pathway Map [3] and in the Pain Report of the Institute of Medicine in the USA, issued at the request of Congress as part of President Obama's Health Reform legislation [39]. Similar work at a government level has also occurred under the auspices of NHS England where specialized pain services delivering highly specialized pain management have been defined, based on the need identified in The National Pain Audit for England and Wales and the Health Survey for England.

LOOKING AT THE FUTURE

In conclusion, these events are an important step forward and highlight these chronic urogenital pain conditions (a specific one is BPS/IC), which often are under-recognized despite the high impact on the quality of life of the patient and a high societal burden [4,46]. Further research studies are urgently needed to explore the interactions of the different comorbid conditions in patients with BPS/IC and the response to treatment, specifically the effect of treating one comorbid condition on the associated comorbid conditions. Given the many comorbidities observed in this patient population, it will be important to identify which patients will be at risk to develop other chronic pain syndromes and to design strategies for early intervention.

TAKE HOME MESSAGES

- BPS/IC presents rarely as an isolated clinical problem. There is growing evidence of multiple co-morbid conditions in patients presenting with BPS/IC, and further screening for those comorbidities (beyond the bladder!) is indicated [10], so that they can be treated.
- A comprehensive multi-disciplinary treatment plan is indicated [16,25] for BPS/IC and the associated comorbid conditions.
- Such a comprehensive multi-disciplinary approach to diagnose and treat BPS/IC will require a transformation of the healthcare system to allow collaboration of different medical sub-specialties and primary and secondary healthcare providers [3].

FURTHER READING

Engeler D, Baranowski AP, Elneil S, et al. Guidelines on Chronic Pelvic Pain. European Association of Urology 2013.

Hanno PM, Burks DA, Clemens JQ, et al. AUA guideline for the diagnosis and treatment of interstitial cystitis/ bladder pain syndrome. J Urol 2011;185(6):2162–2170.

ACKNOWLEDGMENTS

Research support: NIH grants DK066641 (NIDDK), HD39699 (NICHD, Office of Research for Women's Health).

REFERENCES

1. Al-Hadithi HN, Williams H, Hart CA, et al. Absence of bacterial and viral DNA in bladder biopsies from patients with interstitial cystitis/chronic pelvic pain syndrome. J Urol 2005;174(1):151–154.
2. Baranowski AP, Abrams P, Berger RE, et al. Urogenital pain--time to accept a new approach to phenotyping and, as a consequence, management. Eur Urol 2008;53(1):33–36.
3. Baranowski AP, Lee J, Price C, Hughes J. Pelvic pain: a pathway for care developed for both men and women by the British Pain Society. Br J Anaesth 2014;112(3):452–459.
4. Beckett MK, Elliott MN, Clemens JQ, et al. Consequences of interstitial cystitis/bladder pain symptoms on women's work participation and income: results from a national household sample. J Urol 2014;191(1):83–88.
5. Berry SH, Elliott MN, Suttorp M, et al. Prevalence of symptoms of bladder pain syndrome/interstitial cystitis among adult females in the United States. J Urol 2011;186(2):540–544.
6. Blackshaw LA. TRPs in visceral sensory pathways. Br J Pharmacol 2014;171(10):2528–2536.
7. Bogart LM, Suttorp MJ, Elliott MN, et al. Prevalence and correlates of sexual dysfunction among women with bladder pain syndrome/interstitial cystitis. Urology 2011;77(3):576–580.
8. Buffington CA, Westropp JL, Chew DJ, Bolus RR. Risk factors associated with clinical signs of lower urinary tract disease in indoor-housed cats. J Am Vet Med Assoc 2006;228(5):722–725.
9. Buffington CA. Idiopathic cystitis in domestic cats--beyond the lower urinary tract. J Vet Intern Med 2011;25(4):784–796.
10. Bullones Rodriguez MA, Afari N, Buchwald DS. Evidence for overlap between urological and nonurological unexplained clinical conditions. J Urol 2013;189(1 Suppl):S66–74.
11. Burnett AL, Wesselmann U. History of the neurobiology of the pelvis. Urology 1999;53(6):1082–1089.
12. Burnett AL, Wesselmann U. Neurobiology of the pelvis and perineum: Principles for a practical approach. J Pelvic Surg 1999(5):224–232.
13. Carrico DJ, Sherer KL, Peters KM. The relationship of interstitial cystitis/painful bladder syndrome to vulvodynia. Urol Nurs 2009;29(4):233–238.
14. Chelimsky G, Heller E, Buffington CA, et al. Co-morbidities of interstitial cystitis. Front Neurosci 2012;6:114.

15. Clauw DJ, Schmidt M, Radulovic D, et al. The relationship between fibromyalgia and interstitial cystitis. J Psychiatr Res 1997;31(1):125–131.
16. Engeler D, Baranowski AP, Elneil S, et al. Guidelines on Chronic Pelvic Pain. European Association of Urology 2013.
17. Engeler DS, Baranowski AP, Dinis-Oliveira P, et al. The 2013 EAU guidelines on chronic pelvic pain: is management of chronic pelvic pain a habit, a philosophy, or a science? 10 years of development. Eur Urol 2013;64(3):431–439.
18. Fall M, Baranowski AP, Elneil S, et al. EAU guidelines on chronic pelvic pain. Eur Urol 2010;57(1):35–48.
19. Fall M, Johansson SL, Vahlne A. A clinicopathological and virological study of interstitial cystitis. J Urol 1985;133(5):771–773.
20. FitzGerald MP, Kenton KS, Brubaker L. Localization of the urge to void in patients with painful bladder syndrome. Neurourol Urodyn 2005;24(7):633–637.
21. Fitzgerald MP, Koch D, Senka J. Visceral and cutaneous sensory testing in patients with painful bladder syndrome. Neurourol Urodyn 2005;24(7):627–632.
22. Gardella B, Porru D, Nappi RE, et al. Interstitial cystitis is associated with vulvodynia and sexual dysfunction—a case-control study. J Sex Med 2011;8(6):1726–1734.
23. Giamberardino MA, Wesselmann U, Costantini R, Czakanski P. Animal Models of Urogenital Pain. In: Handwerker HO, Arendt-Nielsen L (eds). Pain Models: Translational Relevance and Applications. Washington, DC: IASP Press, 2013: 183–200.
24. Hanno P, Andersson KE, Birder L, et al. Chronic pelvic pain syndrome/bladder pain syndrome: taking stock, looking ahead: ICI-RS 2011. Neurourol Urodyn 2012;31(3):375–383.
25. Hanno PM, Burks DA, Clemens JQ, et al. AUA guideline for the diagnosis and treatment of interstitial cystitis/bladder pain syndrome. J Urol 2011;185(6):2162–2170.
26. Keay S, Leitzell S, Ochrzcin A, et al. A mouse model for interstitial cystitis/painful bladder syndrome based on APF inhibition of bladder epithelial repair: a pilot study. BMC Urol 2012;12:17.
27. Keay S, Warren JW. A hypothesis for the etiology of interstitial cystitis based upon inhibition of bladder epithelial repair. Med Hypotheses 1998;51(1):79–83.
28. Keay SK, Szekely Z, Conrads TP, et al. An antiproliferative factor from interstitial cystitis patients is a frizzled 8 protein-related sialoglycopeptide. Proc Natl Acad Sci U S A 2004;101(32):11803–11808.
29. Kilpatrick LA, Kutch JJ, Tillisch K, et al. Alterations in resting state oscillations and connectivity within sensory and motor networks in women with interstitial cystitis/painful bladder syndrome. J Urol 2014. [Epub ahead of print] doi: 10.1016/j.juro.2014.03.093
30. Lai HH, Gardner V, Ness TJ, Gereau RWt. Segmental Hyperalgesia to Mechanical Stimulus in Interstitial Cystitis/Bladder Pain Syndrome: Evidence of Central Sensitization. J Urol 2014;191(5):1294–1299.
31. Liu HT, Tyagi P, Chancellor MB, Kuo HC. Urinary nerve growth factor level is increased in patients with interstitial cystitis/bladder pain syndrome and decreased in responders to treatment. BJU Int 2009;104(10):1476–1481.
32. McMahon SB, Dmitrieva N, Koltzenburg M. Visceral pain. Br J Anaesth 1995;75(2):132–144.
33. Mukerji G, Yiangou Y, Agarwal SK, Anand P. Increased cannabinoid receptor 1-immunoreactive nerve fibers in overactive and painful bladder disorders and their correlation with symptoms. Urology 2010;75(6):1514 e1515–1520.
34. Mukerji G, Yiangou Y, Agarwal SK, Anand P. Transient receptor potential vanilloid receptor subtype 1 in painful bladder syndrome and its correlation with pain. J Urol 2006;176(2):797–801.
35. Mukerji G, Yiangou Y, Corcoran SL, et al. Cool and menthol receptor TRPM8 in human urinary bladder disorders and clinical correlations. BMC Urol 2006;6:6.
36. Ness TJ, Lloyd LK, Fillingim RB. An endogenous pain control system is altered in subjects with interstitial cystitis. J Urol 2014;191(2):364–370.
37. Ness TJ, Powell-Boone T, Cannon R, et al. Psychophysical evidence of hypersensitivity in subjects with interstitial cystitis. J Urol 2005;173(6):1983–1987.
38. Nguyen RH, Veasley C, Smolenski D. Latent class analysis of comorbidity patterns among women with generalized and localized vulvodynia: preliminary findings. J Pain Res 2013;6:303–309.
39. Pizzo PA, Clark NM, Carter-Pokras O, et al. Relieving Pain in America: A Blueprint for Transforming Prevention, Care, Education, and Research. Institute of Medicine Report (Committee on Advancing Pain Research, Care, and Education, Board on Health Sciences Policy), The National Academies Press, 364 pages. 2011
40. Potts JM, Payne CK. Urologic chronic pelvic pain. Pain 2012;153(4):755–758.

41. Rothrock NE, Lutgendorf SK, Kreder KJ, et al. Stress and symptoms in patients with interstitial cystitis: a life stress model. Urology 2001;57(3):422–427.
42. Sanchez Freire V, Burkhard FC, Kessler TM, et al. MicroRNAs may mediate the down-regulation of neurokinin-1 receptor in chronic bladder pain syndrome. Am J Pathol 2010;176(1):288–303.
43. Sant GR, Kempuraj D, Marchand JE, Theoharides TC. The mast cell in interstitial cystitis: role in pathophysiology and pathogenesis. Urology 2007;69(4 Suppl):34–40.
44. Spanos C, Pang X, Ligris K, et al. Stress-induced bladder mast cell activation: implications for interstitial cystitis. J Urol 1997;157(2):669–672.
45. Suskind AM, Berry SH, Ewing BA, et al. The prevalence and overlap of interstitial cystitis/bladder pain syndrome and chronic prostatitis/chronic pelvic pain syndrome in men: results of the RAND Interstitial Cystitis Epidemiology male study. J Urol 2013;189(1):141–145.
46. Suskind AM, Berry SH, Suttorp MJ, et al. Health-related quality of life in patients with interstitial cystitis/bladder pain syndrome and frequently associated comorbidities. Qual Life Res 2013;22(7):1537–1541.
47. Theoharides TC, Whitmore K, Stanford E, et al. Interstitial cystitis: bladder pain and beyond. Expert Opin Pharmacother 2008;9(17):2979–2994.
48. Tirlapur SA, Kuhrt K, Chaliha C, et al. The 'evil twin syndrome' in chronic pelvic pain: a systematic review of prevalence studies of bladder pain syndrome and endometriosis. Int J Surg 2013;11(3):233–237.
49. Vij M, Srikrishna S, Cardozo L. Interstitial cystitis: diagnosis and management. Eur J Obstet Gynecol Reprod Biol 2012;161(1):1–7.
50. Warren JW, Brown J, Tracy JK, et al. Evidence-based criteria for pain of interstitial cystitis/painful bladder syndrome in women. Urology 2008;71(3):444–448.
51. Warren JW, Brown V, Jacobs S, et al. Urinary tract infection and inflammation at onset of interstitial cystitis/painful bladder syndrome. Urology 2008;71(6):1085–1090.
52. Warren JW, Clauw DJ, Wesselmann U, et al. Sexuality and reproductive risk factors for interstitial cystitis/painful bladder syndrome in women. Urology 2011;77(3):570–575.
53. Warren JW, Howard FM, Cross RK, et al. Antecedent nonbladder syndromes in case-control study of interstitial cystitis/painful bladder syndrome. Urology 2009;73(1):52–57.
54. Warren JW, Jackson TL, Langenberg P, et al. Prevalence of interstitial cystitis in first-degree relatives of patients with interstitial cystitis. Urology 2004;63(1):17–21.
55. Warren JW, Langenberg P, Greenberg P, et al. Sites of pain from interstitial cystitis/painful bladder syndrome. J Urol 2008;180(4):1373–1377.
56. Warren JW, Morozov V, Howard FM, et al. Before the onset of interstitial cystitis/bladder pain syndrome, the presence of multiple non-bladder syndromes is strongly associated with a history of multiple surgeries. J Psychosom Res 2014;76(1):75–79.
57. Warren JW, Wesselmann U, Greenberg P, Clauw DJ. Urinary Symptoms as a Prodrome of Bladder Pain Syndrome/Interstitial Cystitis. Urology 2014;83(5):1035–1040.
58. Warren JW, Wesselmann U, Morozov V, Langenberg PW. Numbers and types of nonbladder syndromes as risk factors for interstitial cystitis/painful bladder syndrome. Urology 2011;77(2):313–319.
59. Wesselmann U, Baranowski AP, Borjesson M, et al. EMERGING THERAPIES AND NOVEL APPROACHES TO VISCERAL PAIN. Drug Discov Today Ther Strateg 2009;6(3):89–95.
60. Wesselmann U, Burnett AL, Heinberg LJ. The urogenital and rectal pain syndromes. Pain 1997;73: 269–294.
61. Wesselmann U. Guest Editorial: Pain - the neglected aspect of visceral disease. Eur J Pain 1999(3):189–191.
62. Wesselmann U. Interstitial Cystitis - a chronic visceral pain syndrome. Urology 2001;6A:32–39.

CHAPTER 14

Male Genital Pain

Bert Messelink

INTRODUCTION

Male genital pain can be perceived in bladder, prostate, urethra and male genital organs: penis and scrotum. Bladder pain is discussed in chapter 13. In this chapter we will use the terms that are proposed by the International Association for the Study of Pain (IASP)[1]. The definitions used are from the European Association of Urology guideline on chronic pelvic pain [2]. There is a strong relation between male genital pain and sexual activity because the genital organs are the key parts of the sexual activity. Pain perceived in those will have a strong influence on the performance of sexual tasks. Male genital pain is perceived in the penis or the scrotum. The urethra is part of the penis. It has a function in urinating and in expelling sperm during ejaculation. Scrotal pain is perceived in either the testicles, the epididymis or both. Because they are lying outside the body patients can easily palpate them and feel structures they believe are the cause of their pain. Acute pain in the genital organs is often reported and in most cases based on infection. After treating the acute illness, prevention of chronification is important

BASIC ASPECTS

Terminology

For all pain syndromes in this chapter, the definition states that there is no proven infection or other obvious local pathology. Furthermore, the pain syndrome is often associated with negative cognitive, behavioral, sexual, or emotional consequences, as well as with symptoms suggestive of lower urinary tract, sexual, or bowel dysfunction.

General

The male genital organs consist of the penis and the scrotum. Also included in this chapter is the prostate, a male organ positioned around the most proximal part of the urethra and playing an important role in the ejaculatory process, prostate fluid being the carrier for the sperm cells. The prostate is well known in urology because prostate enlargement is one of the most diagnosed problems in men with voiding symptoms.

The relation between male genital pain and sexual dysfunction is obvious. Sexual dysfunction is the most reported functional complaint in patients with genital pain. Patients with genital pain will also quite often report micturition and defecation problems. One of the central mechanisms that relate pain to dysfunction could be an overactivity of the pelvic floor muscles.

Diagnostic

When a patient presents with male genital pain, it is important to do good diagnostics, starting with a multifunctional history (Lower Urinary Tract, defecation, sexual function, myofascial function, psychological aspects.). Physical examination starts with examining the organ or region where the pain is perceived and is then broadened to every part of the whole pelvic region. Of special importance is the testing of the function of the pelvic floor muscles. The patient as a whole may also need to be examined, especially for musculoskeletal elements and possible neurological signs. Uroflowmetry is helpful in diagnosing the function of the bladder-urethra complex. It also helps in illustrating dysfunctional voiding and thereby clarifying the role of the pelvic floor muscles in voiding and in maintaining the pain.

Treatment

Almost all well known diseases in the field of male genital pain will present as acute problems. Treatment of the acute pain is important to prevent chronification. As with all other chronic pain syndromes a multidisciplinary approach is the way forward. This approach cannot be highlighted too often. Without any delay a patient should be referred for pain management if no well know disease is present. Pain then is a condition in its own right and should be treated as such. In pain management approaching the muscles attached to and surrounding the pelvis is very important. Apart from this myofascial aspect, other functional symptoms need to be addressed as well as the psychological aspects in an early phase of the process. In male genital pain there is often a role for both a sexologist as well as a pain medicine psychologist. Medication can be added to the other treatment options. Tricyclic antidepressants are of value in the first line treatment when symptoms of neuropathic pain are present. The best advice in all pain syndromes is to get a team involved, and to have the first line doctors refer patients early after well know diseases are ruled out.

DESCRIBING THE SUBJECT

Prostate Pain Syndrome

Definition

Prostate pain syndrome is the occurrence of persistent or recurrent episodic pain in the region of the prostate over at least 3 out of the past 6 months, which is convincingly reproduced by prostate palpation.

General

Prostate pain has been one of the first subjects involved in the whole new approach of chronic pelvic pain. Getting rid of the "prostatocentric approach" was a start of looking with a fresh approach into the problems formerly called chronic prostatitis [20]. The problem of these old terms is that they are organ-confined and are based on causal relations between feeling the pain at a certain place and the origin of the pain lying within that place/organ. Nowadays we know that chronic pain is a sensory process and that the central nervous system plays an important role. This is also true for prostate pain syndrome [24]. For the prostate pain patient, this is often quite hard to believe. Especially when a patient also reports LUTS and has an enlarged prostate, the conclusion seems to be inevitable. In daily practice, questionnaires are easy to use and will provide subjective measures that can be used to evaluate symptoms. Both the National Institutes of Health Chronic Prostatitis Symptom Index (NIH-CPSI) [15] and the International Prostate Symptom Score (I-PSS) [17] can be used for this purpose.

Well Known Diseases

An infection of the prostate can be present but most of the times is a clinical presentation with illness, high fever and abnormal blood tests. Culture of the semen can be done but is of limited information. Prostate cancer is important for the patient but seldom presents with pain.

Treatment

A lot of work has been done on the use of antibiotics, which is not surprising because of the idea of infection. Trying a course of antibiotics for 3–6 weeks is an option that can be used. If there is no effect after 3 weeks treatment should be terminated [4]. When LUTS are present then alpha-blockers can be used. Studies do not have a clear outcome in favor of these drugs [25] but long-term (more than 3 months) treatment can be tried [6]. Alfa blockers show the best results when used in patients with a short history of pain (<1 year), who have not been treated before with these drugs and have a high score on micturition problems in the NIH-CPSI.

Penile Pain

Definition

Penile pain syndrome is the occurrence of pain within the penis that is not primarily in the urethra.

General

The penis has two important aspects. First it is the organ needed for procreation by delivering the semen into the vagina of the female partner. Second it is the most prominent male sex-organ, indispensable for the lust experience of the man. The penis is a somato-neurovascular organ. The nervous innervation is quite unique compared to other organs [5]. The same is true for the vascular aspects. Sensory thresholds for touch and warmth are dependent on the sexual arousal state. Talking about an organ being so 'sensitive' it is easy to imagine that it may lead to painful experiences. Add to this its special role in male sexual functioning and the bio-psycho-social model is fully represented. The second aspect of the penis is the close anatomical relationship with the urethra. Penile and urethral pain can therefore be easily mixed up. Patients will talk about pain perceived in the urethra or pain perceived in the penis. Where the pain is perceived depends on the circumstances: pain during voiding will be linked to the urethra, pain during erection and intercourse to the penis.

Well Known Diseases

Looking for skin pathology (especially the foreskin) and change of sensibility are important. Penile pain can be a result from pathology in the bladder or from bladder pain.

Treatment

In cases where no well known diseases are found, no specific management for penile pain syndrome is evidenced based. Patients should than be referred to a specialised pain clinic for pain management.

Urethral Pain Syndrome

Definition

Urethral pain syndrome is the occurrence of chronic or recurrent episodic pain perceived in the urethra. Urethral pain syndrome may occur in men and women.

General

Urethral pain is a complaint seldom mentioned by men and as said before, often confused with penile pain. There are no good evidence based ideas on the mechanism of urethral pan syndrome. Two explanations are found in literature. First it is thought that urethral pain syndrome is a special form or nothing other than bladder pain perceived in the urethra [19]. Both the bladder and urethra are covered with urothelium and if the theory about epithelial damage is right this could be a good explanation for urethral pain as well. Another theory that might explain urethral pain is called hypersensitivity of the urethra, after repeated infections [13].

Well Known Diseases

To rule out well known diseases it is important to look for infection by doing a urinary culture and a swab culture from the urethral lumen. Urethroscopy can be considered but it must be realized that this procedure itself can cause urethral pain and damage to the urethral wall. Indirectly voiding dysfunctions caused by urethral pathology may lead to chronic pain in the bladder and urethra.

Treatment

Hardly any data is available on treatment of urethral pain syndrome in men.

Scrotal Pain Syndrome

Definition

Scrotal pain syndrome is the occurrence of persistent or recurrent episodic pain localized within the organs of the scrotum. Scrotal pain syndrome is a generic term and is used when the site of the pain is not clearly testicular or epididymal.

General

Not much is known about chronic scrotal pain in the sense of etiology. Most authors think that referred pain is an important phenomenon. The most reported somatic pathological findings are cysts in the epididymis and even in the testis (very rarely).

Well Known Diseases

We do know a few diseases that are found in the testis and epididymis like varicoceles and spermatoceles but they do not directly cause pain in most affected patients. Regularly patients mention that they have palpated a tumor and that this is the cause of the pain. For the physician it is important to realize that palpating a painful mass does not say anything about the origin of the scrotal pain syndrome. Often it is the other way round. Patients experience pain and start feeling if there is something wrong. At that time they do feel a cyst and the story is complete. There is some evidence that multiple cysts in the epididymis might give a painful sensation due to compression of the epididymis. Performing ultrasound of the scrotal content is often done but seldom gives information that helps in treating the pain [9]. The best result one can get is that the patient can be reassured there is no cancer inside.

Treatment

When all conservative treatment options have been used and failed, surgery can be discussed with the patient. Be aware of the fact that surgery itself always causes pain and that removal of a so called ´abnormal´ structure localized at the site of the perceived pain does not bring any guarantee of diminishing the pain. Patients should be informed that more pain afterwards is a real risk of surgery [23]. The approach that seems to be the most effective, is microsurgical denervation. No randomized trials are available but three cohort studies reported good results. All studies included patients with chronic scrotal pain who did not react on conservative treatment. All had no abnormalities on scrotal ultrasound. They also had pain relief of $> 50\%$ after a spermatic cord block. The denervation is done at the inguinal level, under magnification. The studies show effects ranging from 71–96%. Testicular atrophy is seen in 3–7% of the operated patients [22] [11]. The next surgical option is epididymectomy which showed the best results in patients with pain after vasectomy, pain on palpation of the epididymis and when ultrasound has found multiple cysts. The worst results are seen in patients with chronic inflammatory changes in the epididymis [23]. Orchiectomy is the last resort. No studies are available that can help in deciding the moment of doing the orchiectomy. When considering orchiectomy be sure to have a good talk with your patient to inform him on all aspects of this procedure, including phantom pain and subsequent pain on the other side. It seems advisable to do an orchiectomy via the inguinal route instead of via the scrotal approach [7].

Special

Post Vasectomy Pain Syndrome

This is pain that has started after a man has undergone a vasectomy. There must be a clear temporal relation between the vasectomy and the start of the pain. Be careful to not mix up post-operative pain with post vasectomy pain syndrome. The former being a normal reaction to tissue damage during surgery, the latter is a pain syndrome with all the general aspects described before. It is important to treat the acute pain because this will reduce the chance of developing a pain syndrome. Good explanation about these two types of pain before doing the vasectomy is important. Post vasectomy pain can start long after the operation, even more than a year later. It is reported in up to 20% of patients having had a vasectomy [18]. The severity of the pain is low, only 2–6% have a VAS score greater than 5, less than 1% of the patients with pain report severe pain, noticeably affecting their daily life [16]. There seems to be a reduced risk of developing post vasectomy pain when vasectomy is done using the no-scalpel technique (in which the urologist uses a special clamp with very sharp tips to puncture the scrotal skin, instead of a scalpel): 11.7% compared with 18.8% respectively [14]. The etiology of the well know diseases in post-vasectomy are not clear. The most logical explanation is that it has to do with the cutting and ligation of the vas deferens. Obstruction of the epididymal production may be a causative factor. However, the results from studies do not support this as a simple explanation.

Treatment

Special treatment option in the post vasectomy pain syndrome is doing a re-vaso-vasostomy. This theoretically will repair the epididimal outflow and stop the epididymal congestion. Results vary and are often presented as very good [12]. It is important to realize that cutting and ligating the vas yields somatic changes but also psychological ones. It is potentially the end of a man's lifetime period of reproduction. Adequate pre-operative counseling is important. Anxiety about the vasectomy procedure appears to be based on the fear of pain [21].

Post-Inguinal Hernia Repair

It is well known that inguinal hernia repair can lead to chronic pain. Unfortunately almost all study reports do not provide any more information than chronic pain. Scrotal pain is part of the chronic pain after inguinal hernia repair but we do not know how often. Asking for a history of surgery in the inguinal canal is of course mandatory in patients with scrotal pain syndrome. The most reliable explanation seems to be the fact that most of the nerves that are supplying the scrotal content enter the scrotum via the inguinal route. Any damage to the nerves or direct surrounding structures can play a role in the pain syndrome [3]. Again it is important to make a difference between post-operative pain and post hernia repair pain syndrome.

In the field of inguinal hernia surgery an international working group has produced guidelines for prevention and management of postoperative chronic pain following inguinal hernia surgery. They have stated that identifying and preserving all three inguinal nerves is the most important way of preventing pain [24]. In studies that have explicitly mentioned scrotal pain, a difference in incidence has been noted between laparoscopic and open hernia repair. The frequency of scrotal pain being significantly higher in the laparoscopic than in the open group [8,10].

PRACTICAL IMPLICATIONS

The clinician, treating male patients with genital pain, should realize that this pain syndrome is very closely related to bladder and sexual function. Be aware of the fact that we are talking about pain syndromes that need a multifactorial approach. If you are not capable of dealing with all these factors by yourself, become part of a team with colleagues from other disciplines and treat this patient in a multidisciplinary fashion. It is advisable to start at the basic cross point: is this pain a symptom or a disease at its own right. Rule out the well known diseases and start treating the pain and the patient.

The Level A recommended treatments are available in the EAU guideline on Chronic Pelvic Pain [2]. Below these recommendations are summarized.

Prostate Pain Syndrome

- Alpha-blockers are recommended for patients with a duration of PPS < 1 year.
- Single use of antimicrobial therapy (quinolones or tetracyclines) is recommended in treatment-naïve patients over a minimum of 6 weeks with a duration of PPS < 1 year.
- Consider high-dose pentosan polysulphate to improve symptoms and quality of life in PPS.
- Pregabalin is not recommended for use in PPS.

Penile and Urethral Pain Syndrome

- It is recommended to start with general treatment options for chronic pelvic pain.

Scrotal Pain Syndrome

- It is recommended to include the risk of post-vasectomy pain in the counseling of patients planned for vasectomy.
- To reduce the risk of scrotal pain, open inguinal hernia repair should be preferred over laparoscopic repair.
- It is recommended that during inguinal hernia repair all the nerves in the spermatic cord are identified.
- For patients who are treated surgically, microsurgical denervation of the spermatic cord is first choice.

LOOKING AT THE FUTURE

More research needs to be done on male urogenital pain. It would be great if researchers all use the same definitions, like we did in this chapter. Especially for the scrotal pain we need more information on how to predict which patient might benefit from surgery if all conservative measures fail.

Research should also focus on the sexological aspects of male genital pain. By doing so we will get a better view on the whole person who presents with pain. Sexology is, in its nature a bio-psycho-social discipline. That might help the somatic specialist to get more insight in this pain patient.

We need to keep working on the use of the appropriate terminology, so that we get more understanding of looking at perceived pain in a specific patient and not just look at the organ that is thought to be the cause of the pain by the patient.

Male genital pain is in most parts of the world the area of the urologist. It is important that they are aware of the fact that genital pain is not exclusively urological pain. This means that a multidisciplinary approach must be the rule in every practice dealing with male genital pain.

TAKE HOME MESSAGES

- Male urogenital pain is a compilation of pain syndromes whereby pain is perceived in male genital region.
- All general principles that are used in pain management should be applied to male urogenital pain.
- Multidisciplinary approach is mandatory in dealing with male urogenital pain.
- There is a strong relation of male urogenital pain and sexual functioning.

FURTHER READING

EAU guideline on Chronic Pelvic Pain. http://www.uroweb.org/gls/pdf/25_Chronic_Pelvic_Pain_LR.pdf

Baranowski A, Fall M, Abrams P (eds). Urogenital Pain in Clinical Practice. New York: Dekker, 2007

Flor H, Turk D. Chronic Pain. An integrated biobehavioral approach. IASP Press, 2011

Engeler DS, Baranowski AP, Dinis-Oliveira P, et al. The 2013 EAU Guidelines on Chronic Pelvic Pain: Is Management of Chronic Pelvic Pain a Habit, a Philosophy, or a Science? 10 Years of Development. Eur Urol. 2013;64(3):431–9.

REFERENCES

1. IASP. http://www.iasp-pain.org. Last accessed July 17, 2014.
2. Engeler D, Baranowski AP, Borovicka J, et al. Guidelines on Chronic Pain. European Association of Urology 2013. http://www.uroweb.org/gls/pdf/25_Chronic_Pelvic_Pain_LR.pdf Last Accessed July 17, 2014.
3. Alfieri S, Amid PK, Campanelli G, et al. International guidelines for prevention and management of post-operative chronic pain following inguinal hernia surgery. Hernia. 2011;15(3):239–49.
4. Anothaisintawee T, Attia J, Nickel JC, et al. Management of chronic prostatitis/chronic pelvic pain syndrome: A systematic review and network meta-analysis. JAMA. 2011;305(1):78–86.
5. Bleustein CB, Arezzo JC, Eckholdt H, Melman A. The neuropathy of erectile dysfunction. Int J Impot Res 2002;14(6):433–9.
6. Cheah PY, Liong ML, Yuen KH, et al. Terazosin therapy for chronic prostatitis/chronic pelvic pain syndrome: a randomized, placebo controlled trial. J Urol 2003; 169(2):592–96.
7. Davis BE, Noble MJ, Weigel JW, et al. Analysis and management of chronic testicular pain. J Urol. 1990;143(5):936–9.
8. Eklund A, Montgomery A, Bergkvist L, et al. Chronic pain 5 years after randomized comparison of laparoscopic and Lichtenstein inguinal hernia repair. Br J Surg. 2010;97(4):600–8.
9. Haarst EP van, Andel G van, Rijcken TH, et al. Value of diagnostic ultrasound in patients with chronic scrotal pain and normal findings on clinical examination. Urology 1999;54(6):1068–72.
10. Hallén M, Bergenfelz A, Westerdahl J. Laparoscopic extraperitoneal inguinal hernia repair versus open mesh repair: long-term follow-up of a randomized controlled trial. Surgery. 2008;143(3):313–7.
11. Heidenreich A, Olbert P, Engelmann UH. Management of chronic testalgia by microsurgical testicular denervation. Eur Urol 2002;41(4):392–7.
12. Horovitz D, Tjong V, Domes T, et al. Vasectomy reversal provides long-term pain relief for men with the post-vasectomy pain syndrome. J Urol. 2012;187(2):613–7.
13. Kaur H, Arunkalaivanan AS. Urethral pain syndrome and its management. Obstet Gynecol Surv 2007;62(5):348–51.
14. Leslie TA, Illing RO, Cranston DW, et al. The incidence of chronic scrotal pain after vasectomy: a prospective audit. BJU Int 2007;100(6):1330–3.
15. Litwin MS, McNaughton-Collins M, Fowler FJ Jr, et al. The National Institutes of Health chronic prostatitis symptom index: development and validation of a new outcome measure. Chronic Prostatitis Collaborative Research Network. J Urol 1999;162(2):369–75.
16. Manikandan R, Srirangam SJ, Pearson E, et al. Early and late morbidity after vasectomy: a comparison of chronic scrotal pain at 1 and 10 years. BJU Int. 2004;93(4):571–4.

17. Mebust WK, Bosch R, Donovan J, et al. Symptom evaluation, quality of life and sexuality. In: Cockett ATK, Khoury S, Aso Y, et al. Proceedings of the 2nd Consultation on Benign Prostatic Hyperplasia (BPH), Paris. Channel Islands: Scientific Communication International Ltd, 1993: 131–138.
18. Nariculam J, Minhas S, Adeniyi A, et al. A review of the efficacy of surgical treatment for and pathological changes in patients with chronic scrotal pain. BJU Int 2007;99(5):1091–3.
19. Parsons CL. The role of a leaky epithelium and potassium in the generation of bladder symptoms in interstitial cystitis/overactive bladder, urethral syndrome, prostatitis and gynaecological chronic pelvic pain. BJU Int. 2011;107(3):370–5.
20. Potts JM. Chronic pelvic pain syndrome: a non-prostatocentric perspective. World J Urol 2003; 21(2):54–56.
21. Sandlow JI, Westefeld JS, Maples MR, Scheel KR. Psychological correlates of vasectomy. Fertil Steril. 2001;75(3):544–8.
22. Strom KH, Levine LA. Microsurgical denervation of the spermatic cord for chronic orchialgia: long-term results from a single center. J Urol. 2008;180(3):949–53.
23. Sweeney CA, Oades GM, Fraser M, et al. Does surgery have a role in management of chronic intrascrotal pain? Urology. 2008;71(6):1099–102.
24. Yang CC, Lee JC, Kromme BG, et al. Pain sensitization in male chronic pelvic pain syndrome: why are symptoms so difficult to treat? J Urol 2003;170(3):823–826.
25. Yang G, Wei Q, Li H, et al. The effect of alpha-adrenergic antagonists in chronic prostatitis/chronic pelvic pain syndrome: a meta-analysis of randomized controlled trials. J Androl 2006;27(6):847–52.

CHAPTER 15

Gynaecological Aspects of Chronic Pelvic Pain

Suzy Sohier Elneil

INTRODUCTION

The main gynaecological condition that is often associated with chronic pelvic pain is endometriosis, particularly for gynaecologists [28]. Other conditions are not often considered until a diagnostic laparoscopy is done to confirm the diagnosis. If not confirmed, that is when alternative conditions should be considered. Conversely, in abdominal and pelvic pain, much focus remains on bladder pain syndromes and chronic non-organ based conditions such as complex regional pain syndromes, with little emphasis on broader gynaecological aetiology. This group of patients are predominantly looked after by urologists and pain medicine specialists, whose gynaecological knowledge may be limited. This chapter will therefore aim to establish the position of gynaecological conditions within the realm of abdominal and pelvic pain.

This chapter will cover the basics about gynaecological disorders in chronic abdominal and pelvic pain including taxonomy, terminology, making a diagnosis, and treatment.

BASIC ASPECTS

The International Association for the Study of Pain (IASP) defines chronic pelvic pain (CPP) without obvious pathology as "chronic or persistent pain perceived in structures related to the pelvis of either men or women. It is often associated with negative cognitive, behavioral, sexual and emotional consequences as well as with symptoms suggestive of lower urinary tract, sexual, bowel, pelvic floor or gynecological dysfunction." CPP in gynaecological practice is often complex and difficult to treat, as this is a heterogeneous population group. CPP becomes chronic pelvic pain syndrome (CPPS), when this pain persists or occurs in recurrent episodic episodes associated with symptoms suggestive of lower urinary tract, sexual, bowel or gynaecological dysfunction. All this must be in the absence of infection or any other obvious pathology (IASP, 2004) [12]. Thus chronic pelvic pain of gynaecological origin can be classified as shown in Table 1.

A third of patients attending gynaecology clinics complain of pelvic pain as their major or significant symptom and approximately half of all gynaecological investigative laparoscopies are for pain. It has been suggested that up to a third of patients with CPP go on to

TABLE 1 **IASP Taxonomy for Gynaecological Conditions Associated with Chronic Pelvic Pain (Adapted)**

Axis I Region		Axis II System	Axis III End organ as pain syndrome as identified from history, examination, and investigation			Axis IV Referral characteristics	Axis V Temporal Characteristics	Axis VI Character	Axis VII Associated symptoms	Axis VIII Psychological symptoms
Chronic Pelvic Pain	Pelvic Pain Syndrome	Urological	Bladder Pain Syndrome	*Discussed in Chapter 13*		• suprapubic • inguinal • urethral • clitoral • perineal • rectal • back • buttocks	ONSET • Acute • Chronic ONGOING • Sporadic • Cyclical • Continuous TIME • Filling • Emptying • Immediate post • Late post PROVOKED	Aching Burning Stabbing Electric Other	URINARY • Frequency • Nocturia • Hesitance • Poor flow • Pis en deux • Urge • Urgency • Incontinence • Other GYNAECOLOGICAL • e.g. Menstrual SEXUAL • e.g. Female dyspareunia • impotence • Anorectal • Incontinence • Constipation MUSCULAR • Hyperalgesia • Dysfunction CUTANEOUS • Allodynia	Cognitive Behavioural Emotional
			Urethral pain Syndrome	*Discussed in Chapter 14*						
		Gynaecological	Vaginal Pain Syndrome							
			Vulvar Pain Syndrome	Generalised Vulvar Pain Syndrome						
				Localised Vulvar Pain Syndrome	Vestibular Pain Syndrome					
					Clitoral Pain Syndrome					
			Other	e.g. Endometriosis Associated Pain Syndrome						
		Anorectal	Anorectal pain syndrome							
		Neurological	e.g. Pudendal Pain Syndrome							
		Muscular	Pelvic Floor Muscle Pain Syndrome							
	Non pelvic pain syndromes	e.g. Neurological	e.g. Pudendal Neuralgia							
		e.g. urological								

have a hysterectomy. Laparoscopy has become a routine investigation of CPP and studies suggest that roughly a third of CPP sufferers have endometriosis, a third have adhesions and a third have no obvious pathology [24]. However, it has been noted that the same abnormalities were found in asymptomatic patients being investigated for infertility, and therefore, laparoscopic findings must be carefully analysed before pain is attributed to a particular pathology that may be present. The relationship of pain to pathology is unclear and the amount of pathology present does not appear to relate to the degree of pain. The aim is to try and determine a remediable cause and treat it using the most effective available therapy. However, as over a third of patients have no cause determined – this presents a therapeutic challenge to the attendant physician [15,19].

The epidemiology of CPP in women is not well defined, as often the focus in the literature is on the disease process that may be associated with the pain directly, such as endometriosis. However, there are multiple prevalent studies on chronic pain from Europe and the United States of America, where the impact of reported pain on daily activities and function are reported [22]. Quite clearly, pain has a significant impact on the quality of life. It is within these publications that one has some idea of the prevalence of CPP. Some estimate it affects up to 30% of all women at any one time.

IASP were instrumental in developing a taxonomy for all chronic pain conditions. In so doing, it has brought clarity and order to a very complex world of mixed terminology often confusing diagnosis with symptoms and clinical states. Table 1 show the taxonomy adapted from IASP for gynaecological conditions.

The International Continence Society in 2011 formed a multi-disciplinary group to formulate a view on terminology used in CPP generally. This has helped start a dialogue on the global front to unify terms used and under what circumstances. This approach was applied to multiple other CPP conditions. No document has been published as yet, though the proceedings are available from the International Continence Society directly [14].

CPP is known to be a difficult condition to classify and contain, and unsurprisingly the pathological basis of the condition remains poorly understood. The basic premise remains that some sort of insult to a designated organ may have triggered an inflammatory response, which gradually led to widespread neurological sensitization in the organ and then globally spread to the rest of the pelvis. In essence, the pain is caused by an overwhelming sensory response, which clearly will have a centralized element to it. In the process the musculo-skeletal system becomes involved, as do other muscle groups resulting in a generalized 'hyper-contractile' state throughout the body, as seen in facial pain states [14], which further intensifies the pain making it difficult to control but also making it possibly amenable to non-pharmacological means of therapy, such as physiotherapy.

DESCRIBING THE SUBJECT

Aetiology of CPP in Women

The aetiology of CPP in women is multifactorial and often affects multiple systems. It is rare for only one organ system to be affected, as pain in one system such as the reproductive system often affects other systems in the pelvis, such as the lower urinary tract. The commonest well-defined causes of gynaecological pain include dysmenorrhoea, infection, endometriosis, adenomyosis, gynaecological malignancy, injuries related to childbirth and pain associated with pelvic organ prolapse and prolapse surgery, particularly where mesh is involved [22].

In cases where the pain is more diffuse, such as vaginal and vulvar pain syndromes, the origins can be many and include:

- History of sexual abuse
- History of chronic antibiotic use
- Hypersensitivity to yeast infections, allergies to chemicals or other substances
- Abnormal inflammatory response (genetic and non-genetic) to infection and trauma
- Nerve or muscle injury or irritation
- Hormonal changes

These aetiological factors can also apply to other pelvic conditions in women. Therapeutic options remain limited and require a multi-disciplinary pain management approach, with psychological and physiotherapy input.

The aetiology of CPP is shown in Table 2.

The commonest conditions encountered in gynaecology, as outlined above, tend to be recognised easily by many gynaecologists. However, the less commonly recognised conditions can be missed and patients can be told that 'nothing untoward has been found', which can be incredibly frustrating for the patient. It is important to raise awareness of these other conditions. Equally important is to recognise the gastrointestinal and urological associations, as they can be key to understanding the patient's symptoms.

Aetiological Types of CPP in Women

Common Gynaecology CPP Conditions

- Endometriosis lesions occur more frequently in CPP patients than controls. The endometriotic tissue can be found covering the entire peritoneal cavity and is often found directly on top of different abdominal and pelvic organs [28]. However, the symptoms do not correlate well with the extent of the pathology (Fig. 1). Patients may present with pain which is usually periodic and associated with menses (dysmenorrhea), intercourse (deep dyspareunia), passing urine or defecation [28], occasionally the pain is continuous and can have a huge impact on quality of life [20].

TABLE 2 **Causes of Chronic Pelvic Pain (CPP)**

Commonly recognised gynaecological causes of CPP	• Endometriosis • Dysmenorrhoea • Chronic pelvic inflammatory disease • Adhesions • Postpartum trauma • Perineal pain syndrome
Less commonly recognised gynaecological causes of CPP	• Myofascial pain • Pelvic congestion/varicosity syndrome • Urogynaecology conditions, such as descending perineum syndrome • Post-surgical pain after gynaecology oncology or urogynaecology surgery
Gastrointestinal/Urological associations	• Bladder pain syndrome (Interstitial cystitis) • Ano-rectal pain disorders • Irritable bowel syndrome

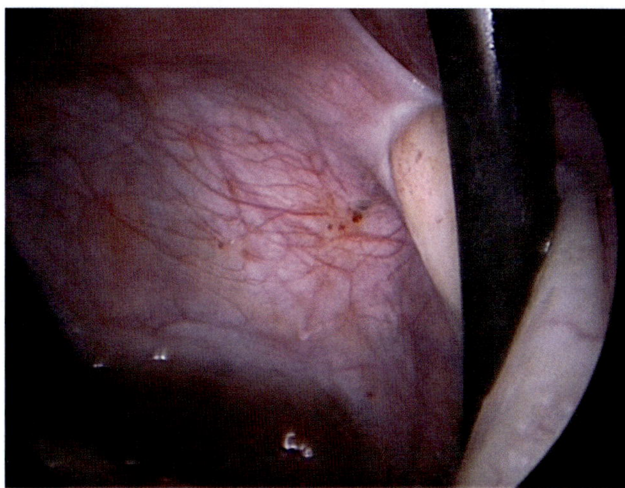

FIGURE 1 Fine spots of endometriosis seen on the peritoneal surface of the pelvis in a patient being investigated for pain.

The definitive diagnosis is best made by laparoscopy [28]. Pain associated with endometriosis may be treated medically or surgically, currently there is a great push for extensive surgery to get rid of any active disease. However, despite extensive surgery and medical treatment, it has a recurrence rate of 50% in 5 years [30] (Fig. 1).

- **Chronic Pelvic Inflammatory Disease (PID):** Acute PID usually results from ascending infection [1]. Multiple partners and previous sexually transmitted disease are known risk factors. The scarring, inflammation and adhesions from acute PID is thought to cause chronic PID. The pain is usually intermittent with episodes being precipitated by intercourse, eating, defecation, or heavy activity. Many causative organisms have been identified, including – Chlamydia, Trachomatis, Neisseria Gonorrhoeae, gram negative bacilli, Haemophlus Influenzae, streptococci, mycoplasma and various anaerobes [18]. Though the investigation and treatment of acute PID is well covered in standard gynaecological texts, the treatment of chronic PID is not well determined and often unsatisfactory. A single course of broad spectrum antibiotics (e.g. Tetracycline or Doxycycline) may be beneficial, but many patients eventually undergo radical surgery whereby the uterus, tubes and ovaries, if they are involved, are all removed. Sadly, surgical management is usually unsuccessful. No direct correlation between physical findings and pain has been found.
- **Adhesions:** Commonly occur following surgery, but they may also occur as a part of the chronic PID or in their own right [27]. Much pain in gynaecology is attributed to adhesions, though it remains to be seen whether they are truly the cause of pain [21]. A specific pain syndrome associated with adhesions is seen when the adhesions trap the ovaries following hysterectomy (residual ovarian syndrome) or the ovarian remnants following a previous oophorectomy (ovarian remnant syndrome) [33]. Both of these syndromes cause pelvic pain often with deep dyspareunia and post coital ache. There is no correlation between pain and the density of adhesions, or indeed the localisation of the ovaries. Adhesions are usually treated by laparoscopic adhesiolysis and concomitant adhesion-prevention intra-abdominal fluids, but they often recur.
- **Perineal Pain Syndrome:** Perineal pain is perhaps the most complex of the chronic pelvic pain syndromes in women. The perineum overlies the pelvic outlet and is bound posteriorly by the coccyx and buttocks and anteriorly by the external genitalia in women. The perineum derives its nerve supply primarily from various branches

of the pudendal nerve. It also receives some fibres from the anterior labial branches of the ilioinguinal, genital branch of the genitofemoral, perforating cutaneous and muscular branches of the S2,3,4 and anococcygeal nerves. The patient with CPP will often complain that clothing irritates her (possibly suggesting allodynia or allergy) or that the vulva is always moist and sensitive (infection or hyperhidrosis). The effect of the pain on micturition and sexual activity can also be reported. It is important to differentiate between pain only associated with sexual activity (dyspareunia) and pain associated with nonsexual touch, which, obviously, may affect sexual activity [2]. Previous operations, allergies, trauma, psychological issues and psychosocial circumstances must be evaluated.

A complete examination of the abdomen, female genital tract, musculo-skeletal system, and neurological system should be carefully carried out.

The causes of female perineal pain are summarised in Table 3 and discussed accordingly.

Less Common Causes of Gynaecological Pain

- **Myofascial pain:** This is the most common somatic diagnosis followed by atypical cyclic pain, gastrointestinal causes, urological causes and pelvic vascular congestion [9]. It is often caused by lower abdominal wall scars producing pelvic sensations. Nerve entrapment may also occur. Treatment includes local anaesthetic injections with or without steroid, pelvic floor physiotherapy and biofeedback [4,6]. However, as a cause of gynaecological pain it is often not recognised.
- **Pelvic congestion/varicosity syndrome:** Pelvic varicosities have been under investigation as a possible cause of CPP, but their role has never been proven [29]. The pain is said to be throbbing and burning in nature, but there is no definitive imaging or other investigative technique that has been used that has clarified what the pathognomonic anatomical findings are [3,7]. It is known to worsen on standing and with prolonged activity. Medical therapy including non-steroidal anti-inflammatory drugs, hormonal therapies such as danazol (androgen) and gonadotrophin releasing hormone analogues and extensive surgery (laparoscopic excisional surgery, injecting and/or tying off of the veins, hysterectomy and bilateral salpingo-oophrectomy, laparoscopic uterine nerve ablation and pre sacral neurectomy) have all been tried but appear to have failed [25]. Clinical psychology has also been tried (Table 3).
- **Gastrointestinal and urological associations:** Gastrointestinal problems such as constipation and irritable bowel syndrome may cause CPP and similarly there is cross reporting of patients with urological disease and CPP [12,13]. However, anorectal pain disorders are very common in women especially after traumatic childbirth and in the menopause, as outlined in Table 4.
- **Post-gynaecology oncology and urogynaecology surgical pain:** Increasingly it has become recognised that certain types of surgery lead to CPP in women. Gynaecology oncology surgery is often radical and extensive with many nerve pathways being disrupted in the pelvis resulting in pain. Many recover within six months, but in some cases the pain persists and is often difficult to treat, especially if adjuvant radiotherapy is used in the pelvis. In urogynaecology surgery, the advent of mesh kit procedures for urinary incontinence and prolapse has resulted in an increase in chronic 'obturator nerve pain' and other CPP states [10,11,16,31]. Often surgical removal of the mesh partially or in its entirety offers some relief, but in a proportion of patients CPP

TABLE 3 **Aetiology of Female Perineal Pain**

Vulval pain disorders	*Vulval Pain Syndrome*	Chronic vulvar discomfort (burning, stinging, irritation, or rawness) affecting the vulva and the vestibule.
	Generalised Vulval Pain Syndrome	Hyperaesthetic vulva, as a consequence of neuropathic pain. Management includes neuropathic analgesics, physical interventions, counselling, and psychology.
	Localised Vulval Pain Syndrome	Distinguished from generalised vulval pain syndrome as it is more focal in nature and pain is intermittent. Most likely an inflammatory condition.
	Infection and ulceration	Secondary to viral, bacterial, fungal, and protozoal agents producing painful infections secondary to tissue destruction and nerve involvement. Often presents as a 'burning' sensation. Tumours must be ruled out
	Trauma	Neuropathic pain from tissue damage and scarring (obstetric injury and traumatic sexual intercourse). May necessitate surgery.
Vulvo-vaginal and urethral pain disorders	*Vulvo-vaginal pain*	Secondary to hormonal changes (including the post-partum period), infection, injury, or allergic reaction. May lead to abscess formation and sinus tract formation. Malignancy must be ruled out.
	Acute urethritis	Acute urethritis independent of proven bacterial cystitis usually associated with sexually transmitted diseases (especially gonorrhoea) and responds to antibiotics.
	Allergies	Due to soap, clothing, perfumes, deodorants, spermicidals, latex sheaths, detergents, as well as some foods. The pain generally responds to local measures.
	Pelvic floor muscle spasm	Tension myalgia of the levator ani muscle can cause pelvic, vaginal, back, perineal, and rectal pain. Caused by poor posture, trauma infection and emotional tension. Can be continuous with exacerbation after intercourse or excercise.
Perineal pain disorders	*Descending Perineum Syndrome*	Characterised by a dull ache in the posterior part of the perineum and anal canal. Often exacerbated by defecation and standing. Surgery and neuropathic analgesics may be helpful, depending on the cause.
	Pudendal Neuralgia	Pain is well localised to the distribution of the pudendal nerve. Neuropathic analgesics should be considered, as well as pudendal nerve blocks or pulsed radio-frequency.
	Sympathetically maintained pain	Some authors suggest that some vulval pain syndromes are maintained by the sympathetic nerves - a type of complex regional pain syndrome or reflex sympathetic dystrophy. Neuropathic analgesia should be considered.
	Other neuropathic disorders	May be caused by various neuropathic disorders and it may be referred from various pelvic, gynaecological, urological, colo-rectal disorders, or diseases of the hip joint, upper thigh, or adductor tendons and pubis. All can cause pain to radiate to the perineum.

TABLE 4 **Ano-Rectal Pain Disorders in Women**

Ano-rectal pain disorders	*Coccyx pain syndrome*	Tenderness in the coccyx exacerbated by pressure over the coccyx, secondary to a fall, sitting in a poor position or obstetric trauma. Local pathology, lumbosacral disc disease and pathology within the pelvis need to be ruled out. Pain frequently radiates to the perineal, gluteal and posterior sacral regions. Diagnosis is based on clinical symptoms and signs, rectal examination, x-rays and other system examinations (e.g. genito-urinary). Treatments includes sitting supports, massage, local heat, injection of local anaesthetic with steroid, caudal block, pelvic floor relaxation techniques, and biofeedback.
	Piriformis syndrome	The Piriformis muscle arises from the inner aspect of the sacrum, runs laterally throughout the sciatic notch, passing over the sciatic nerve, inserting into the greater trochanter. Thus, spasms produce both local pain and sciatic nerve radicular pain. Onset of pain may be associated with pelvic trauma or exercise, but is often idiopathic. Pain is exacerbated by internal rotation of the hip (Freiberg's sign) or resisted external rotation (Pace's sign). Trigger point injections into the piriformis may be diagnostic. Stretching exercises may help.
	Neuropathic pain	May result from disease process at all levels within the nervous system, causing pain in the pelvis and perineum (burning and poorly localised). Associated with hyperalgesia, hyperaesthesia and paraesthesia. Peripheral neuropathies of the iliohypogastric, ilioinguinal or genitofemoral nerves (may be caused by tumour or trauma) are characterised by a burning aching pain in the distribution of the affected nerve. Relief comes from local anaesthetic infiltration to the affected nerve, which can be diagnostic and therapeutic, and thus repeatable.
	Pudendal neuralgia	Characterised by a mild to severe burning with occasional bouts of lancing pain, cutaneous hyperalgesia, hyperaesthesia, paraesthesia and numbness. It may prevent sitting or on sexual intercourse. Treatment includes tricyclic antidepressants, other neuropathic analgesics, local anaesthetic blocks and lignocaine infusions. Simple analgesics are not helpful.

persists despite removal of the mesh. Even standard urogynaecology conditions such as vaginal hysterectomy and posterior colporraphy may result in CPP [26,32]. In these situations, the pudendal nerve is often thought to become entrapped [2,17,23].

PRACTICAL IMPLICATIONS

Clinical History and Examination

Taking a detailed medical history is essential to making a diagnosis. The nature, frequency and site of the pain, its relationship to precipitating factors and the menstrual cycle, may provide vital clues to the aetiology. A detailed menstrual and sexual history, including any history of sexually transmitted diseases and vaginal discharge is mandatory. Discrete inquiry about previous sexual trauma is considered appropriate.

Abdominal and pelvic examination will exclude any gross pelvic pathology (tumours, scarring and reduced uterine mobility), as well as demonstrating the site of tenderness if present. Abnormalities in muscle function should also be sought.

Once all the above conditions have been excluded, the physician may well be left with patients with unexplained pelvic pain. It is, of course, imperative to consider pain associated with the urinary and gastrointestinal tract at the same time. For example, patients with bladder pain quite often present with dyspareunia due to bladder base tenderness.

Investigations can be limited in the chronic pain patient, but it is important to rule out any potential treatable pathology and as such specialised imaging and diagnostic procedures such as laparoscopy, cystoscopy and hysteroscopy could well have a place.

Management and Understanding the Needs of Patients

Therapy in CPP can only be improved if the physician understands pain mechanisms and their impact in the pelvis. Much research has focused on the peripheral structures and not at the spinal cord and brain, which drive the central mechanisms of pain. If that is not addressed, limiting treatment to a 'local problem' will often, not be effective for long term management. The multidisciplinary approach to CPP maintains the importance of central mechanisms and approaches the patient holistically. The best results will be obtained from this approach as it considers all possible causes and incorporates all members of the team that will help the patient. The team should include gynaecologists or urogynaecologists, urologists/gastroenterologists, pain medicine specialists, clinical psychologists, physiotherapists and specialist pain nurses, Current management of CPP in women, by gynaecologists, tends to focus of determining a 'surgical remedial cause' [5]. An ethos shift must take place so that good practice can ensue in managing these patients. As well as conventional medical and surgical treatments for CPP, psychology, physiotherapy, acupuncture, transcutaneous nerve stimulation and neuromodulation should be considered. Psychological management not only of the patient but also of the partner may be required.

More importantly, managing CPP in women is not about just focussing on the pelvis, but it is also about understanding the pain in the context of the rest of the body. The physician needs to understand that they are not 'taking over the patient', but listening to them so they can understand their needs, manage their expectations and determine a management course that can bring them to terms with their condition. It needs a 'hand-in-hand' approach. This approach needs time, patience and perseverance but it can be eminently rewarding.

LOOKING AT THE FUTURE

As in all aspects of medicine, the more a model of care is promoted and discussed the more likely it will take hold especially when it becomes apparent that it truly improves patient care. The aim would be to raise the profile of CPP in all arenas and in particular raising the profile amongst the gynaecology fraternity. The message about pain mechanisms, taxonomy and pain management strategies in a multi-disciplinary setting needs to be encouraged [8].

CPP in women is seen in daily practice, though its severity and impact on daily life is not always recognized. Thus, when women are seen in any setting they need to be questioned about pain symptoms they may have, so they can be addressed.

TAKE HOME MESSAGES

- CPP in women is a common condition, but its impact on women's quality of life is often under recognized. Women need to be encouraged to discuss pain issues freely.
- Pain mechanisms in chronic pelvic pain in women have a central sensitization basis to their pathophysiology. Thus, they must be managed holistically. The commonest gynaecological condition that affects women with CPP is endometriosis, though more recently recognized causes include urogynaecological procedures including the insertion of mesh for stress urinary incontinence and utero-vaginal prolapse.
- A good history and examination is the key to starting therapy, though there is some role for investigations such as diagnostic laparoscopy.
- All treatment for this group of patients is best managed within the realms of a multidisciplinary team which incorporates pain medicine specialists, gynaecologists, urologists, functional gastroenterologists, clinical psychologists, physiotherapists, and specialist nurses.

FURTHER READING

Engler DS, et al. EAU Guidelines on Chronic Pelvic Pain. Arnhem, Netherlands: European Association of Urology, 2013.

Baranowski AP, Abrams P, Fall M. Urogenital Pain in Clinical Practice. New York: Informa Healthcare Publications, 2008.

Jacobson TZ, Duffy JM, Barlow D, et al. Laparoscopic surgery for pelvic pain associated with endometriosis. Cochrane Database Syst Rev. 2009;(4):CD001300. http://www.ncbi.nlm.nih.gov/pubmed/19821276.

REFERENCES

1. Armed Forces Health Surveillance C. Acute pelvic inflammatory disease, active component, U.S. Armed Forces, 2002–2011. Msmr 2012;19(7):11–13.
2. Beco J, Climov D, Bex M. Pudendal nerve decompression in perineology: a case series. BMC Surg 2004;4:15.
3. Cheong YC, Smotra G, Williams AC. Non-surgical interventions for the management of chronic pelvic pain. Cochr Database Syst Rev 2014;3:CD008797.
4. Clinton SC, George SE, Mehnert M, et al. Pelvic floor pain: physical therapy versus injections. PM & R 2011;3(8):762–770.
5. Deguara CS, Pepas L, Davis C. Does minimally invasive surgery for endometriosis improve pelvic symptoms and quality of life? Curr Opin Obstet Gynecol 2012;24(4):241–244.
6. Diaz-Mohedo E, Baron-Lopez FJ, Pineda-Galan C. [Etiological, diagnostic and therapeutic consideration of the myofascial component in chronic pelvic pain]. Actas urologicas espanolas 2011;35(10):610–614.
7. Edo Prades MA, Ferrer Puchol MD, Esteban Hernandez E, Ferrero Asensi M. Pelvic congestion syndrome: outcome after embolization with coils. Radiologia 2012.
8. Engeler DS, Baranowski AP, Dinis-Oliveira P, et al. The 2013 EAU guidelines on chronic pelvic pain: is management of chronic pelvic pain a habit, a philosophy, or a science? 10 years of development. Eur Urol 2013;64(3):431–439.
9. Gyang A, Hartman M, Lamvu G. Musculoskeletal causes of chronic pelvic pain: what a gynecologist should know. Obstet Gynecol 2013;121(3):645–650.
10. Gyang AN, Feranec JB, Patel RC, Lamvu GM. Managing chronic pelvic pain following reconstructive pelvic surgery with transvaginal mesh. Internatl Urogynecol J 2014;25(3):313–318.

11. Hansen BL, Dunn GE, Norton P, et al. Long-Term Follow-up of Treatment for Synthetic Mesh Complications. Female Pelvic Med Reconstr Surg 2014;20(3):126–130.
12. Hauser W, Turp JC, Lempa M, et al. [Functional somatic pain syndromes-nomenclature]. Schmerz 2004;18(2):98–103.
13. Jelovsek JE, Barber MD, Paraiso MF, Walters MD. Functional bowel and anorectal disorders in patients with pelvic organ prolapse and incontinence. Am J Obstet Gynecol 2005;193(6):2105–2111.
14. Kerstein RB. Reducing chronic masseter and temporalis muscular hyperactivity with computer-guided occlusal adjustments. Compend Contin Educ Dent 2010;31(7):530–534, 536, 538 passim.
15. Lal AK, Weaver AL, Hopkins MR, Famuyide AO. Laparoscopic appendectomy in women without identifiable pathology undergoing laparoscopy for chronic pelvic pain. J Soc Laparoendosc Surg 2013;17(1):82–87.
16. Lee D, Dillon B, Lemack G, et al. Transvaginal mesh kits--how "serious" are the complications and are they reversible? Urology 2013;81(1):43–48.
17. Lee JC, Yang CC, Kromm BG, Berger RE. Neurophysiologic testing in chronic pelvic pain syndrome: a pilot study. Urology 2001;58(2):246–250.
18. Mylonas I. Female genital Chlamydia trachomatis infection: where are we heading? Arch Gynecol Obstet 2012;285(5):1271–1285.
19. Newham AP, van der Spuy ZM, Nugent F. Laparoscopic findings in women with chronic pelvic pain. S Afr Med J 1996;86(9 Suppl):1200–1203.
20. Nnoaham KE, Hummelshoj L, Webster P, et al, World Endometriosis Research Foundation Global Study of Women's Health. Impact of endometriosis on quality of life and work productivity: a multicenter study across ten countries. Fertil Steril 2011;96(2):366–373 e368.
21. Robertson D, Lefebvre G, Leyland N, et al. Adhesion prevention in gynaecological surgery. J Obstet Gynaecol Canada 2010;32(6):598–608.
22. Santosh A, Liaquat HB, Fatima N, et al. Chronic pelvic pain: a dilemma. J Pakistan Med Assoc 2010;60(4):257–260.
23. Shafik A. Pudendal canal syndrome as a cause of vulvodynia and its treatment by pudendal nerve decompression. Eur J Obstet Gynecol Reprod Biol 1998;80(2):215–220.
24. Singh N, Rashid M, Herath RP. How can we reduce negative laparoscopies for pelvic pain? J Obstet Gynaecol 2011;31(1):62–68.
25. Smith PC. The outcome of treatment for pelvic congestion syndrome. Phlebology 2012;27 Suppl 1:74–77.
26. Stav K, Dwyer PL, Roberts L. Pudendal neuralgia. Fact or fiction? Obstet Gynecol Surv 2009;64(3):190–199.
27. ten Broek RP, Issa Y, van Santbrink EJ, et al. Burden of adhesions in abdominal and pelvic surgery: systematic review and met-analysis. Bmj 2013;347:f5588.
28. Triolo O, Lagana AS, Sturlese E. Chronic pelvic pain in endometriosis: an overview. J Clin Med Res 2013;5(3):153–163.
29. Tu FF, Hahn D, Steege JF. Pelvic congestion syndrome-associated pelvic pain: a systematic review of diagnosis and management. Obstet Gynecol Survey 2010;65(5):332–340.
30. Vercellini P, Somigliana E, Consonni D, et al. Surgical versus medical treatment for endometriosis-associated severe deep dyspareunia: I. Effect on pain during intercourse and patient satisfaction. Human Reprod 2012;27(12):3450–3459.
31. Wagenlehner FM, Del Amo E, Santoro GA, Petros P. Perineal body repair in patients with third degree rectocele: a critical analysis of the tissue fixation system. Colorectal Dis 2013;15(12):e760–765.
32. Young SB, Schaffer JI, Lucero ML, Howard AE. Society of gynecologic surgeons' survey: mesh use in vaginal prolapse surgery. Female Pelvic Medicine Reconstr Surg 2010;16(6):336–339.
33. Zapardiel I, Zanagnolo V, Kho RM, et al. Ovarian remnant syndrome: comparison of laparotomy, laparoscopy and robotic surgery. Acta Obstet Gynecol Scand 2012;91(8):965–969.

CHAPTER 16

Mechanisms and Treatment of Endometriosis Associated Pain

Rukset Attar and Erkut Attar

INTRODUCTION

Endometriosis is a common, benign gynecologic disease which is characterized by the presence of uterine endometrial tissue outside of the uterus [63]. The prevalence of pelvic endometriosis is 6–10% in the general female population, up to 70% in women with pelvic pain and more than 80% if they have both pelvic pain and subfertility [45,71,81,130].

The pain symptoms most commonly attributed to endometriosis are dysmenorrhoea, dyspareunia, dysuria, dyschesia, painful gastrointestinal symptoms (such as colicky pains and irritable bowel-type symptoms), and chronic pelvic pain [56,104]. Nerve entrapment pain is a relatively rare type of endometriosis associated pain. It occurs as a result of anatomical nerve distortion by active, fibrotic lesions, especially around the sciatic and obturator nerves [93,117]. It is also postulated that nerve entrapment occurs in the complex fibrous and hypertrophic deep invasive endometriotic lesions in the recto-vaginal septum, where distortion of nerve trunks appears to occur [7], moreover adhesions can play a role in painful symptoms [69,82].

BASIC ASPECTS

Endometriosis associated pain is pelvic pain that occurs in the presence of laparoscopically confirmed endometriosis. Although the association of pain and endometriosis is widely accepted by gynecologists, the mechanisms involved in endometriosis associated pain remains unclear. The cause of pain in endometriosis is likely multifactorial, however, critical, common pathways or mechanisms may exist [55].

The most commonly suggested mechanisms for pain production in endometriosis are; production of substances such as growth factors and cytokines, the effects of active bleeding from endometriotic implants, and irritation or direct invasion of pelvic floor nerves by infiltrating endometriotic implants, especially in the cul-de-sac [111,112,119]. There is evidence that more elusive mechanisms such as neuroangiogenesis, nociceptive, or neuropathic mechanisms contribute to endometriosis associated pain [9,69,70].

These mechanisms may explain why pain relief for more than 6 months occures in only 40% to 70% of affected women treated with conventional medical or surgical therapies [9]. They may also explain the poor correlation between the extent or morphological characteristics of endometriosis and the intensity and character of the pain symptoms [15, 64,78,82,88,91,100,101,116,138]. This chapter discusses these mechanisms as well as current and future treatment modalities.

DESCRIBING THE SUBJECT

Cyclical Bleeding Within Lesions

Ectopic endometriotic lesions retain their endocrine responsiveness and undergo episodes of intraperitoneal bleeding during menstruation. This is supported by the observation of visible intraperitoneal bleeding when laparoscopy is performed during menses and by the presence of localized hemorrhage and hemosiderin-laden macrophages in lesions examined microscopically [9].

Cyclic recurrent micro-bleeding occurs as a common feature in all macroscopic entities of endometriosis [31]. It may explain the reason for severe dysmenorrhoea related to endometriosis and the fact that women with deeply infiltrating endometriosis (DIE) have the most severe dysmenorrhoea [41].

Cyclical bleeding within the implants is believed to result in a chronic inflammatory nidus that causes pelvic pain, such bleeding may explain why medical therapies such as progestins, danazol, and GnRHa that induce amenorrhea are partially effective in the relief of this symptom [9].

Immune and Inflammatory Factors

Endometriosis is described as a pelvic inflammatory process with altered immune cells function and increased number of activated macrophages in the peritoneal environment that secrete various mediators including, growth factors and cytokines [1,128]. Endometriotic lesions themselves secrete pro-inflammatory cytokines such as interleukin-8 (IL-8), which recruit macrophages and T cells to the peritoneum mediating inflammatory responses. The concentration of some chemokines such as monocyte chemoattractant protein 1(MCP-1) is increased in the peritoneal fluid of patients [63].

The evidence for IL-6 is inconsistent. Increased concentrations of IL-6 have been found in peritoneal fluid of women with endometriosis in some studies but not in others [113,115].

Concentrations of tumor necrosis factor (TNF) in peritoneal fluid are higher in women with endometriosis than those with normal pelvic anatomy [52]. It has been suggested that TNF is one of the essential factors for the pathogenesis and maintenance of endometriosis and its role in chronic pain is well documented [34,134]. The concentrations of cytokines in peritoneal fluid however, do not correlate with pain symptoms or severity of endometriosis [107].

There is little doubt that immune cells play important roles in pain generation in endometriosis. It was shown that macrophage numbers and function are greatly modified in, ectopic lesions, peritoneal fluid and eutopic endometrium of women with endometriosis [20,65]. Macrophages cause symptoms by releasing inflammatory substances such as ILs and transforming growth factors (TGFs) [153]. There is also a direct relationship between the numbers of macrophages and the density of nerve fibers in ectopic lesions [153] and in peritoneal endometriotic lesions is much higher than in normal peritoneum [148].

The nerve endings of these fibres can be stimulated by many inflammatory substances, such as histamine, serotonin, bradykinin, prostaglandins (PGs), leukotrienes, ILs, vascular endothelial growth factor (VEGF), tumor necrosis factor- alpha (TNF-alpha), epidermal growth factors, TGF-beta, platelet-derived growth factor (PDGF) and nerve growth factor (NGF) which are secreted from macrophages and endometriotic lesions [7,22] and are proposed to contribute to the generation of pain in endometriosis [148].

Moreover, there is substantial disturbance in the numbers of immature and mature dendritic cells in eutopic endometrium and in the ectopic lesions in women with endometriosis [120,121]. It was stated that macrophages and their products may play important roles in the growth and repair of nerve fibres rather than only stimulating nerve fibre endings to induce pain. Nerve fibre growth is regulated by many substances, including NGF, brain derived neurotropic factor (BDNF) and VEGF [7]. Their synthesis is also affected by macrophage activities. NGF is released from endometriotic lesions and many other cell types including macrophages. It is important in the development of the peripheral and central nervous systems (CNS). The synthesis of NGF can be up-regulated by IL-1 and basic fibroblast growth factor (FGF), both of which can increase the content of NGF mRNA up to 6-fold in astrocytes [16,87,137,158]. BDNF, another neurotrophin has a crucial role for the growth and differentiation of the peripheral system and is secreted from activated macrophage also the synthesis of BDNF, NGF and NGF receptors were up-regulated by estrogens [29,44,60,83,90,125].

Recent studies have demonstrated that VEGF produced by macrophages can act as a neurotrophic factor stimulating the growth of nerve fibres and the peritoneal fluid from women with endometriosis contains a greater concentration of VEGF than that of controls [61,114]. These studies suggest that VEGF may also play a role in increased nerve fibre density of peritoneal endometriotic lesions.

Other studies show that macrophages are essential during nerve fibre regeneration in the peripheral nervous system. It has been demonstrated that when peripheral nerve fibres are injured, macrophages invade the distal stump of damaged nerve fibres within 1 day, secrete growth factors with neurotropic properties to regenerate nerve fibres and induced Schwann cell proliferation [67]. Sensory nerve fibre regeneration is impaired when macrophage invasion is delayed [32].

Increased numbers of activated and degranulating mast cells have been found near endometriotic lesions, often close to nerve fibres [8]. In endometriosis patients activated mast cells were also shown to be abundant on the myometrial side, but in very low density in the endometrium [3]. Also mast cells produce a variety of degranulation products such as NGF that may activate and/or sensitize primary nociceptive neurons [30,53,127–129,146,163]. NGF functions as a chemoattractant for mast cells, but it can also trigger mast cell degranulation [8,139].

NGF interacts with two specific receptors: TRK-A (a high affinity receptor) and p75 (a low affinity receptor). These receptors are barely detectable in normal endometrium, but are both intensely expressed in nerve fibers and stroma in eutopic endometrium and in the stroma of ectopic lesions. This up-regulation of neurotrophin and its receptors can be a potent stimulus to branching and ingrowth of new nerve fibers [56].

Irritation and Invasion of Pelvic Nerves

Currently the most popular thesis explaining endometriosis associated pain is irritation or direct invasion of pelvic floor nerves by infiltrating implants, particularly in the cul-de-sac via secretion of matrix-degrading enzymes and acquired migratory behaviour of endometriotic cells [7,123]. Patients with the highest preoperative pain scores displayed the highest density of nerve encapsulation within endometriotic lesions and more frequent perineurial and endoneurial invasion by endometriotic cells than patients with lower preoperative pain scores [6].

Visceral Nociceptors

Pain is defined as an unpleasant sensory and emotional experience associated with actual or potential tissue damage [97]. Pain signals in sensory nerve fibers are generated through receptors called nociceptors [37]. These receptors are responsive to 'noxious' stimuli that have the potential to do harm and the potential to trigger a reflex response. They respond to excessive pressure, excessive stretch, inflammatory processes and a range of injurious chemical substances. They send signals which initiate the sensation of pain. These signals are processed in the dorsal root ganglia and the lower spinal cord, before onward transmission of a modified signal to the thalamus, limbic system and higher centres, where pain is perceived and the emotional response developed [56].

Nociceptors are found in most tissues, including the viscera including the uterus and cervix [23,24,36,54,151]. They are present in high densities in both the functional and basal layers of the endometrium of women with endometriosis, virtually none are found in the endometrium of women without endometriosis [25,26,28,147] and are also noted in ectopic endometriotic lesions [27,91,147]. It was shown that ectopic endometriotic implants developed a sensory and sympathetic nerve supply both in rats and in women [26,27]. There is a correlation between nerve fibre density in endometriotic lesions and pain severity [95]. It was demonstrated that nociceptors invaded peritoneal endometriotic lesions in women and also found invading endometriotic cysts in experiments on rats [26,27,148].

Pelvic nociceptors in adjacent organs are strongly stimulated by NGF and prostaglandin E2 [18,110]. Expression of NGF in endometriotic tissue is reported to be higher than in eutopic endometrium [7,148]. NGF plays a key role in the occurrence of pain, hyperalgesia, and neuropathic pain. NGF is strongly expressed in deep infiltrating endometriosis and its specific receptor (Trk-A) is expressed in nerves lying within deep lesions or in the vicinity of deep endometriotic lesions [7]. They are significantly sensitized by estrogen and can be regulated by molecules secreted from immune competent cells, such as mast cells, macrophages, dendritic cells, neutrophils, natural killer cells and plasma cells [56].

Neuropathic Pain

Neuropathic pain is increasingly recognized as a significant component of persistent endometriosis pain [62]. Neuropathic pain arises from damage to peripheral or central nerve fibers, resulting in erratic or persistent axonal discharges. These persistent stimuli can set up abnormal neural circuits at a spinal cord or central level resulting in persistent, prolonged or intermittent signals to the central processing and perception centres. This may lead to persistent perception of pain long after the original stimulus has been removed [56].

Neuropathic pain is usually accompanied by a nerve injury such as invasion of the brachial plexus in Pancoast's syndrome. This phenomenon occurs in deep infiltrating endometriosis where nerve invasion by endometriotic stromal cells is frequently observed [6]. Repeated surgery may cause damage to nerve fibers and especially repeated damage may trigger persistent, abnormal discharges from these damaged and regenerating pelvic and endometriotic nerve fibers, leading to the development of neuropathic pain [56].

Neuropathic pain symptoms can also be induced by inflammatory stimuli in the absence of nerve injury [38,53]. Macrophages and neutrophils release algesic mediators such as prostaglandin E2, eicosanoids, and reactive oxygen intermediates, which can sensitize nociceptors and induce hyperalgesia [85,89,109,143,152]. Histamine is a key mediator released by activated mast cells which can sensitize nociceptors [66,99]. Neuronal histamine receptors are upregulated or modulated by nerve injury [17,74]. Histamine also plays a critical role in leukocyte recruitment after mast cell activation [162]. Activated mast cells contribute directly to neuropathic hyperalgesia by releasing other mediators such as tryptase, TNF-alpha, PGs, serotonin, and IL-1 [72,127,128,131–133,141,152,154].

There is cumulative evidence that mast cells play an important role in the pathogenesis of chronic pain and neuropathic pain in many pathological conditions [49,66,89,99,109,146]. Mast cells release mediators that increase excitability of neurons, and neurotransmitters such as substance P or NGF can trigger mast cell degranulation [76].

Women with deep infiltrating endometriosis experience exacerbation of pain when pressure is exerted on deep nodular or indurated lesions at physical examination. This phenomenon of exquisite pain from a non-painful stimulus is called hyperalgesia, which is a major characteristic of neuropathic pain. It is a pain sensation that is out of proportion with the intensity of nociceptors stimulation [30]. Sympathetic and classical sensory nerve fibers contribute to hyperalgesia [164]. It was shown that the peritoneum of women with endometriosis are rich in sympathetic nerve fibers. Increased excitability of viscero-visceral convergent neurons to the spinal cord are associated with persistent neuropathic pain and hyperalgesia [14].

Generalized hypersensitivity has been demonstrated earlier in women with fibromyalgia, primary dysmenorrhea and pelvic pain during pregnancy [12,13,84]. Central hyperexcitability of the nociceptive system has been demonstrated in patients with chronic pain [11,14,79,135]. The nociceptive barrage from endometriotic tissue might also cause central hyperexcitability of dorsal horn neurons [25,59]. This central hyperexcitability might cause pelvic pain aggravated during menstruation and persist after medical or surgical ablation of the endometriotic tissue. Bajaj et al demonstrated an increased muscle nociceptor input in the form of increased post-saline pain intensity. They also showed that there are pain areas at the first dorsal interosseous muscle (FDI) of the hand, and hypersensitivity to pressure in women with endometriosis central sensitization was increased [14].

It is not yet clear how the central hyperexcitability is maintained. Evidences suggest that noxious stimuli from peripheral tissue damage sensitize central mechanisms involved in pain perception which causes alterations in central nervous system function and subsequent pain experience [42]. Muscle hyperalgesia and hyperexcitability of dorsal horn neurons might be induced by a decrease in the efficacy of the descending antinociceptive system, central sensitization due to long-lasting activation of receptive fields, or heterotopic facilitation caused by active nociceptive fibers outside the receptive fields [156].

NEUROANGIOGENESIS

The endometrium has intrinsic angiogenic potential, and endometriotic lesions tend to grow in areas with rich vascularization, suggesting that angiogenesis is a prerequisite for endometriosis development [103]. Angiogenesis is important not only for implant establishment but also for supporting ongoing lesion growth and progression [47,72,103]. In several rodent models of endometriosis, it was noted that treatment with antiangiogenic drugs reduced the surface area or volume of the endometriotic lesions. These findings indicate that a continuous angiogenic process is required for survival of the lesion after implantation [4,72,103].

Peripheral nerves track alongside blood vessels in discrete neurovascular bundles. Recent elucidation of developmental mechanisms of embryonic neurovascular patterning provides evidence for a direct link between neurogenesis and angiogenesis [80,160]. It was hypothesized that neuroangiogenesis provided innervation and engraftment of refluxed endometrial fragments [9,145]. The patterning and branching of vessels and nerves are shown to be molecularly linked with signals from each influencing the migration of the other. Ligand-receptor pairs implicated in axonal and vessel guidance include ephrins and their Eph receptors, slit ligands and their roundabout (Robo) receptors, semaphorins and their plexin and neuropilin receptors, and netrins and their DCC/ neogenin and Unc5 receptors [9].

Ephrin A1 mRNA transcripts were reduced in endometrium of women with endometriosis compared to women without endometriosis [73]. In a recent study higher expression of Slit and Robo1 proteins and increased microvascular density were observed in cases of endometrioma recurrence [124]. SemaphorinE (also referred as semaphorin 3c) is upregulated in the endometrium of women with endometriosis [73]. Class 3 semaphorins bind to neuropilinplexin receptor complexes on the axonal surface membranes of neurons and endothelial cells and stimulate cell migration [98]. The neuropilins, also described as semaphorin receptors have nanomolar affinities for vascular endothelial growth factor (VEGF) isoforms and can mediate angiogenesis [9].

Other factors may coordinate the close physical association between larger nerves and vessels. Nerve-derived VEGF is essential for the formation of arteries in skin [102]. Secretoneurin, a neuropeptide expressed in nerve fibers that are found in close apposition to blood vessels, stimulates endothelial cell migration and angiogenesis in vitro and in vivo assays [77]. This protein has been identified in capsaicin-sensitive C-afferent nerve fibers in rat endometrium, although loss-of-function studies are not yet available to definitively assign its role [43].

Vessels also provide cues for the growth and alignment of adjacent nerves. The blood vessel–derived artemin protein, a member of the glial cell–derived neurotrophic factor (GDNF) family of ligands, acts as a guidance factor for the growth of sympathetic nerve fibers along blood vessels in a variety of mouse tissues, including the gastrointestinal tract [9,68]. Knockouts of artemin or its preferred receptor GFRα cause severe defects in the migration and axonal projection of sympathetic neurons but not other types of neurons. Artemin expression in endometriosis is unknown; but artemin appears to increase cancer cell migration and invasiveness in the endometrium [108].

NGF, FGF, BDNF and neurotrophin-3 are all expressed by endometrial cells. However, only the latter two proteins appear to be quantitatively upregulated in women with endometriosis [33]. Growth-associated protein 43, a marker of neural outgrowth and regeneration, is expressed in endometriosis-associated nerve fibers but not in existing peritoneal nerves. The fibers appear to sprout from para- and perivascular nerve fibers that accompany the blood vessels [95].

It is stated that estrogen plays role in neuroangiogenesis. Estrogen exacerbates pain sensitivity by stimulating the growth of a nerve supply in parallel with the growth of new blood vessels into the ectopic endometrial tissue [9].

Treatment of Endometriosis-Associated Pain

Medical and surgical treatments can be used for endometriosis associated pain. However, the optimal treatment still remains unknown. Current therapies aim to reduce the pain and delay recurrence as disease recurs after cessation of treatment.

Surgical options for treating endometriosis include the use of unipolar or bipolar cautery, laser ablation and excision techniques [19,35,39,46,48,51,118,140,141,161]. Relief of pain following surgical treatment of endometriosis at one-year follow-up is 50–95% [112]. Laparotomy or hysterectomy are rarely necessary except for cases of severe, advanced stages of disease or cases involving coexisting malignancy [112].

Ovarian endometriomas respond very poorly to medical therapy. Therefore surgery is the primary approach for symptomatic or large endometriomas [40]. Cyst excision achieves greater improvements in symptoms of dysmenorrhea, deep dyspareunia, and nonmenstrual pain, compared with fenestration and coagulation [21]. Simple drainage of endometriomas is associated with a high risk of cyst recurrence within six months and, therefore, is not recommended as definitive therapy [50,94,154].

Laparoscopic uterosacral nerve ablation (LUNA) is a technique designed to disrupt the efferent nerve fibers in the uterosacral ligaments to decrease uterine pain for women with intractable dysmenorrhea [86,142]. However, it does not offer any added benefits beyond those that can be achieved with conservative surgery alone [112,155].

Presacral neurectomy involves interrupting the sympathetic innervation to the uterus at the level of the superior hypogastric plexus. It is proposed for treatment of midline pain associated with menses. However, it is a technically challenging procedure associated with significant risk of bleeding from the adjacent venous plexus[112].

Surgical resection of endometriotic lesions provides temporary relief in terms of reduced chronic pelvic pain and severe dysmenorrhea but the recurrence at 2 years after surgery is high [58]. Thus, medical treatment is employed at any stage of disease in many patients worldwide. Current treatment modalities are designed to induce a hypoestrogenic state, which leads to a reduction in disease progression and symptoms. Oral contraceptives (OCs), progestogens, danazol, GnRH agonists, and anti-progestogens have all been employed for the treatment of endometriosis [57].

Hormonal contraceptives are used in both a cyclic and a continuous fashion in the treatment of symptoms associated with endometriosis. Decidualization, followed by atrophy of the endometrial tissue is the proposed mechanism of action [106]. Also oral contraceptives and progestogens have been demonstrated to significantly decrease nerve fiber density [96,149,150].

Oral progestogens have been used for the treatment of endometriosis and endometriosis-associated complaints [4]. Progestogens most commonly used for this include medroxyprogesterone acetate and 19-nortestosterone derivatives. Their proposed mechanism of action is the same as OCs. A more recent proposed mechanism is progestogen-induced suppression of matrix metalloproteinases (MMP) [103].

Dienogest is a synthetic steroid that has been used as a progestogen in contraceptive pills and has been shown to be effective in endometriosis related pain [4]. The levonorgestrel-releasing intrauterine system (Lng- IUS) represents another novel approach to the medical treatment of endometriosis, however, the device is not approved for this indication by the FDA[109].

Etonogestrel subdermal implants (Implanon) are an additional treatment option and used in combination with Lng- IUS in cases of persistent pelvic pain due to endometriosis not responding to conventional treatments [4].

Danazol is a derivative of 17a-ethinyltestosterone and acts primarily by inhibiting the LH surge and steroidogenesis[103]. It produces a high androgen and low estrogen environment resulting in atrophy of the endometriotic implants and thus improvement in painful symptoms. However, its use is limited by the occurrence of androgenic side effects [4].

GnRH agonists (GnRH-a) are modified forms of GnRH that bind to pituitary receptors, but have a longer half life than native GnRH and thereby result in down-regulation of the pituitaryovarian axis and hypoestrogenism. The likely mechanism of action involves induction of amenorrhea and progressive endometrial atrophy[103]. Because of hypoestrogenic adverse effects, their use is limited to 6-months duration. "Add-back" therapy with a progestogen or a combination of estrogen and progestogen has been advocated for reducing the severity of hypoestrogenic side effects associated with GnRH agonist treatment [109].

Gestrinone (ethylnorgestrienone, R2323) is an anti-progestational steroid used in Europe for the treatment of endometriosis, the mechanism of action includes a progestational withdrawal effect at the endometrial cellular level and inhibition of ovarian steroidogenesis [103].

Aromatase inhibitors (AIs) are shown to be effective for the treatment of endometriosis and pelvic pain in pilot studies [2,10,139]. Aromatase is the key enzyme in the synthesis of estrogens and mediates the conversion of androstenedione and testesterone to estrone and estradiol (E2), the last step in steroid biosynthesis. Therefore aromatase is an excellent target for inhibition of E2 synthesis without affecting important downstream enzymes and has unique features for the aromatizing reaction, making it amenable to selective inhibition [10]. In non-randomized trials, the combination of an AI with a progestin was shown to be successful in significantly decreasing pain and reducing the amount of visible endometriosis in patients who did not tolerate or respond to medical or surgical treatments [2,126]. AI plus a combination OC was also used to treat endometriosis associated pain [5]. A significant reduction in pain was noted at the end of the study. GnRH-a with AI regimen was also investigated in the treatment of endometriosis associated pain. The efficacy of anastrozole in conjunction with goserelin was compared with goserelin alone [136]. Both treatment protocols were effective in reducing total pain scores. However, the GnRH-a with AI regimen showed a more profound, stable, and long lasting effect. The investigators stated that a novel treatment regimen with an AI with a after conservative surgery is effective to control recurrence and pain in patients with severe endometriosis. However, treatment of endometriosis associated pain with AIs is still considered investigational and is not approved by the FDA for this indication [2,144].

Other medical treatment options for endometriosis currently under investigation include RU486 (mefipristone), selective progesterone receptor modulators (SPRMs), selective estrogen receptor modulators (SERMs), GnRH antagonists, pentoxifylline, melatonin, MMP inhibitors, and agents that inhibit angiogenesis [105,106,112,122].

Therapeutic manipulation of the immune system has been promising in rodent and baboon models of endometriosis using agents such as rosiglitazone, imiquimod (a Toll-like receptor agonist), recombinant human interferon-α-2b, leflunomide, levamisole, recombinant TNF binding protein-1, or anti-TNF-α monoclonal antibodies. Tricyclic antidepressants, serotonin and norepinephrine reuptake inhibitors, calcium channel α(2)-δ ligands (gabapentin and pregabalin), 5-fluorouracil and NMDA receptor antagonists that have been designed to target neurotransmission are proposed and may prove useful in treating endometriosis pain[4,9]. Another strategy is to target neurotrophic factors or those that guide neuroangiogenesis [9].

PRACTICAL IMPLICATIONS

Pelvic pain together with infertility constitutes a major clinical problem for women with endometriosis; however, the mechanisms involved in endometriosis associated pain syndrome remain unclear. Understanding the mechanisms of pain associated with endometriosis is important since it can aid researchers in finding new treatment modalities as current therapies are expensive, carry perioperative risks, or have unpleasant side effects of hypoestrogenism with a high recurrence rate on cessation of therapy.

LOOKING AT THE FUTURE

Recent advances in molecular and clinical sciences offer a range of modalities for treatment. However, currently there is no single very successful option for the ultimate treatment. Researchers are studying new treatment modalities including: AI, RU486 (mefipristone), SPRMs, SERMs, GnRH antagonists, pentoxifylline, immunmodulator agents, 5-fluorouracil, melatonin and agents that inhibit the effect of TNF-alpha, MMP, and angiogenesis. Rigorous clinical trials have yet to be done to test if they are superior to the current standard medical treatments for endometriosis pain.

Identification of specific targets that influence the activity of neurons can be studied to develop drugs that inhibit endometriosis associated neural hyperexcitability. Also, drugs that target neurotransmission, neurotrophic factors, or neuroangiogenesis can be explored and new treatment modalities can be developed.

TAKE HOME MESSAGES

- Endometriosis is a common gynecologic disease which can be associated with pelvic pain, but there is not a direct correlation.
- The most commonly suggested mechanisms for pain production in endometriosis are; production of substances such as growth factors and cytokines, effects of active bleeding from endometriotic implants and irritation or direct invasion of pelvic floor nerves or direct invasion of those nerves by infiltrating endometriotic implants.
- Neuroangiogenesis, nociceptive, or neuropathic mechanisms also contribute to endometriosis associated pain.
- The current therapies are expensive, carry perioperative risks, or have unpleasant side effects of hypoestrogenism. Recurrence is high after the cessation of therapy.
- There is urgent need for new treatment modalities.
- Understanding the mechanisms of pain associated with endometriosis can help researchers in finding novel treatment modalities with fewer side effects and lower or no recurrences.

FURTHER READING

Baranowski AP, Fall M, Abrams P (eds). Urogenital Pain in Clinical Practice. Taylor and Francis, 2007.
Chaitow L, Jones RL (eds). Chronic Pelvic Pain & Dysfunction. UK. Elsevier Health Sciences, 2012.

DEFINITIONS

- Dysmenorrhoea is painful menstruation
- Dyspareunia is pain during intercourse
- Dysuria is pain during urination
- Dyschesia is pain during defecation
- Neuroangiogenesis is a process of coordinated neural and vascular mitogen action

REFERENCES

1. Agic A, Xu H, Finas D, et al. Is endometriosis associated with systemic subclinical inflammation? Gynecol Obstet Invest 2006;62:139–47.
2. Ailawadi RK, Jobanputra S, Kataria M, et al. Treatment of endometriosis and chronic pelvic pain with letrozole and norethindrone acetate: a pilot study. Fertil Steril 2004;81:290–6.
3. Al-Jefout M, Black K, Schulke L, et al. Novel finding of high density of activated mast cells in endometrial polyps. Fertil Steril. 2009;92(3):1104–6.
4. Al-Jefout M. Brief update on endometriosis treatment. Middle East Fertility Society Journal 2011;16:167–174
5. Amsterdam LL, Gentry W, Jobanputra S, et al. Anastrazole and oral contraceptives: a novel treatment for endometriosis. Fertil Steril 2005;84(2):300–4.
6. Anaf V, Simon P, El Nakadi I, et al. Relationship between endometriotic foci and nerves in rectovaginal endometriotic nodules. Hum Reprod 2000;15:1744–50.
7. Anaf V, Simon P, El Nakadi I, et al. Hyperalgesia, nerve infiltration and nerve growth factor expression in deep adenomyotic nodules, peritoneal and ovarian endometriosis. Hum Reprod 2002;17:1895–1900.
8. Anaf V, Chapron C, El Nakadi I, et al. Pain, mast cells, and nerves in peritoneal, ovarian, and deep infiltrating endometriosis. Fertil Steril. 2006;86(5):1336–43.
9. Asante A, Taylor RN. Endometriosis: The Role of Neuroangiogenesis. Annu Rev Physiol 2011;73:163–82.
10. Attar E, Bulun SE. Aromatase inhibitors: the next generation of therapeutics for endometriosis? Fertil Steril. 2006;85(5):1307–18.
11. Bajaj P, Bajaj P, Graven-Nielsen T, Arendt-Nielsen L. Osteoarthritis and its association with muscle hyperalgesia: An experimental controlled study. Pain 2001;93:107–114.
12. Bajaj P, Bajaj P, Madsen H, et al: Antenatal women with or without pelvic pain can be characterized by generalized or segmental hypoalgesia in late pregnancy. J Pain 2002;3(6):451–460.
13. Bajaj P, Bajaj P, Madsen H, Arendt-Nielsen L: A comparison of modality-specific somatosensory changes during menstruation in dysmenorrheic and nondysmenorrheic women. Clin J Pain 2002;18:180–190.
14. Bajaj P, Madsen H, Arendt-Nielsen L. Endometriosis is associated with central sensitization: a psychophysical controlled study. J Pain 2003:4(7):372–80.
15. Balasch J, Creus M, Fabregues F, et al. Visible and non-visible endometriosis at laparoscopy in fertile and infertile women and in patients with chronic pelvic pain: a prospective study. Hum Reprod 1996;11:387 391.
16. Bandtlow CE, Meyer M, Lindholm D, et al. Regional and cellular codistribution of interleukin 1 beta and nerve growth factor mRNA in the adult rat brain: possible relationship to the regulation of nerve growth factor synthesis. J Cell Biol 1990;111:1701–1711.
17. Baron R, Schwarz K, Kleinert A, et al. Histamine induced itch converts into pain in neuropathic hyperalgesia. Neuro Rep 2001;12:3475–8.
18. Basbaum AI, Bautista DM, Scherrer G, Julius D. Cellular and molecular mechanisms of pain. Cell. 2009;16;139(2):267–84.
19. Bateman BG, Kolp LA, Mills S. Endoscopic versus laparotomy management of endometriomas. Fertil Steril 1994;62:690–5.
20. Berbic ML, Schulke L, Markham R, et al. Macrophage expression in endometrium of women with and without endometriosis. Hum Reprod 2009;24:325–332.
21. Beretta P, Franchi M, Ghezzi F, et al. Randomized clinical trial of two laparoscopic treatments of endometriomas: cystectomy versus drainage and coagulation. Fertil Steril 1998;70:1176–80.
22. Bergqvist A, Bruse C, Carlberg M, Carlstrom K. Interleukin 1beta, interleukin-6, and tumor necrosis factor-alpha in endometriotic tissue and in endometrium. Fertil Steril 2001;75:489–495.
23. Berkley KJ, Robbins A, Sato Y. Afferent fibers supplying the uterus in the rat. J Neurophysiol 1988;59:142–63.
24. Berkley KJ, Hotta H, Robbins A, Sato Y. Functional properties of afferent fibers supplying reproductive and other pelvic organs in pelvic nerve of female rat. J Neurophysiol 1990;63:256–72.

25. Berkley KJ, Cason A, Jacobs H, et al. Vaginal hyperalgesia in a rat model of endometriosis. Neurosci. Lett. 2001;306:185–88.
26. Berkley KJ, Dmitrieva N, Curtis KS, Papka RE. Innervation of ectopic endometrium in a rat model of endometriosis. Proc. Natl. Acad. Sci. USA 2004;101:11094–98.
27. Berkley KJ, Rapkin AJ, Papka RE. The pains of endometriosis. Science 2005;308:1587–89.
28. Berkley KJ, McAllister SL, Accius BE, Winnard KP. Endometriosis-induced vaginal hyperalgesia in the rat: effect of estropause, ovariectomy, and estradiol replacement. Pain 2007;132(1):150–59.
29. Bjorling DE, Beckman M, Clayton MK, Wang ZY. Modulation of nerve growth factor in peripheral organs by estrogen and progesterone. Neuroscience 2002;110:155–167.
30. Bouaziz H, Lombard MC. La Douleur en gynécologie. Paris: Arnette Blackwell, 1997:23–40.
31. Brosens IA. Endometriosis – a disease because it is characterized by bleeding. Am J Obstet Gynecol 1997;76:263–267.
32. Brown MC, Perry VH, Lunn ER, et al. Macrophage dependence of peripheral sensory nerve regeneration: possible involvement of nerve growth factor. Neuron 1991;6:359–370.
33. Browne AS, Yu J, Sidell N, et al. Proteomic identification of neurotropic proteins in eutopic endometrium. Reprod. Sci. 2010;17(3):350A.
34. Bullimore DW. Endometriosis is sustained by tumour necrosis factor-alpha. Med Hypotheses 2003;60:84–8.
35. Busacca M, Fedele L, Bianchi S, et al. Surgical treatment of recurrent endometriosis: laparotomy versus laparoscopy. Hum Reprod 1998;13:2271–4.
36. Cervero F, Laird JM. Visceral pain. Lancet 1999;353:2145–8.
37. Cervero F, Laird JM. Understanding the signalling and transmission of visceral nociceptive events. J Neurobiol 2004;61:45–54.
38. Chacur M, Milligan ED, Gazda LS, et al. A new model of sciatic inflammatory neuritis (SIN): induction of unilateral and bilateral mechanical allodynia following acute unilateral peri-sciatic immune activation in rats. Pain 2001;94:231–44.
39. Chapron C, Dubuisson JB, Fritel X, et al. Operative management of deep endometriosis infiltrating the uterosacral ligaments. J Am Assoc Gynecol Laparosc 1999;6:31–7.
40. Chapron C, Vercellini P, Barakat H, et al. Management of ovarian endometriomas. Hum Reprod Update 2002;8:591–7.
41. Chapron C, Fauconnier A, Dubuisson JB, et al. Deep infiltrating endometriosis: relation between severity of dysmenorrhoea and extent of disease. Hum Reprod 2003;18:760–766.
42. Coderre TJ, Katz J, Vaccarino AL, Melzack R: Contribution of central neuroplasticity to pathological pain: Review of clinical and experimental evidence. Pain 1993;52:259 285.
43. Collins JJ, Wilson K, Fischer-Colbrie R, Papka RE. Distribution and origin of secretoneurinimmunoreactive nerves in the female rat uterus. Neuroscience 2000;95:255–64.
44. Conover JC, Yancopoulos GD. Neurotrophin regulation of the developing nervous system: analyses of knockout mice. Rev Neurosci 1997;8: 13–27.
45. Cramer DW. Epidemiology of endometriosis in adolescents. In: Wilson EA (ed). Endometriosis. New York: Alan Liss, 1987:5–8.
46. Crosignani PG, Vercellini P, Biffignandi F, et al. Laparoscopy versus laparotomy in conservative surgical treatment for severe endometriosis. Fertil Steril 1996;66:706–11.
47. Dabrosin C, Gyorffy S, Margetts P, et al. Therapeutic effect of angiostatin gene transfer in a murine model of endometriosis. Am. J. Pathol. 2002;161:909–18.
48. Davis GD. Management of endometriosis and its associated adhesions with the CO2 laser laparoscope. Obstet Gynecol 1986;68:422–5.
49. Dines KC, Powell HC. Mast cell interactions with the nervous system: relationship to mechanisms of disease. J Neuropathol Exp Neurol 1997;56:627– 40.
50. Donnez J, Nisolle M, Gillerot S, et al. Ovarian endometrial cysts: the role of gonadotropin-releasing hormone agonist and/or drainage. Fertil Steril 1994;62:63–6.
51. Donnez J, Nisolle M, Gillerot S, et al. Rectovaginal septum adenomyotic nodules: a series of 500 cases. Br J Obstet Gynaecol 1997;104:1014–8.
52. Eisermann J, Gast MJ, Pineda J, et al. Tumor necrosis factor in peritoneal fluid of women undergoing laparoscopic surgery. Fertil Steril 1988;50:573–9.
53. Eliav E, Herzberg U, Ruda MA, Bennett GJ. Neuropathic pain from an experimental neuritis in the rat sciatic nerve. Pain 1999;83:169–82.
54. Evans S, Moalem-Taylor G, Tracey DJ. Pain and endometriosis. PAIN 2007; 132[1): S22-S25.
55. Fauconnier A, Chapron C. Endometriosis and pelvic pain: epidemiological evidence of the relationship and implications. Hum Reprod Update 2005;11(6):595–606.

56. Fraser IS. Mysteries of endometriosis pain: Chien-Tien Hsu Memorial Lecture 2009. J Obstet Gynaecol Res. 2010;36(1):1–10.
57. Gambone JC, Mittman BS, Munro MG, et al, Chronic Pelvic Pain/Endometriosis Working Group. Consensus statement for the management of chronic pelvic pain and endometriosis: proceedings of an expert-panel consensus process. Fertil Steril 2002;78:961–72.
58. Garry R. The effectiveness of laparoscopic excision of endometriosis. Curr Opin Obstet Gynecol 2004; 16:299–303.
59. Giamberardino MA, Berkley KJ, Affaitati G, et al. Influence of endometriosis on pain behaviors and muscle hyperalgesia induced by a ureteral calculosis in female rats. Pain 2002;95:247–257.
60. Gibbs RB. Treatment with estrogen and progesterone affects relative levels of brain-derived neurotrophic factor mRNA and protein in different regions of the adult rat brain. Brain Res 1999;844:20–27.
61. Gilabert-Estelles J, Ramon LA, Espana F, et al. Expression of angiogenic factors in endometriosis: relationship to fibrinolytic and metalloproteinase systems. Hum Reprod 2007;22:2120 2127.
62. Gillett WR, Jones D. Chronic pelvic pain in women: Role of the nervous system. Exp Rev Obstet Gynecol 2009;4:149–163.
63. Giudice LC, Kao LC. Endometriosis. Lancet. 2004;364(9447):1789–99.
64. 25. Gruppo Italiano per lo Studio dell'Endometriosi: Relationship between stage, site and morphological characteristics of pelvic endometriosis and pain. Hum Reprod 2001;16:2668- 2671.
65. Halme J, Becker S, Haskill S. Altered maturation and function of peritoneal macrophages: Possible role in pathogenesis of endometriosis. Am J Obstet Gynecol 1987;156:783–789.
66. Herbert MK, Just H, Schmidt RF. Histamine excites group III and IV afferents from the cat knee joint depending on their resting activity. Neurosci Lett 2001;305:95– 8.
67. Heumann R. Regulation of the synthesis of nerve growth factor. J Exp Biol 1987;132:133–150.
68. Honma Y, Araki T, Gianino S, et al. Artemin is a vascular-derived neurotropic factor for developing sympathetic neurons. Neuron 2002;35:267–82.
69. Howard FM. An evidence-based medicine approach to the treatment of endometriosis-associated chronic pelvic pain: placebo-controlled studies. J. Am. Assoc. Gynecol. Laparosc. 2000;7:477–88.
70. Howard FM. Endometriosis and Mechanisms of Pelvic Pain. J Minim Invasive Gynecol 2009;16(5): 540–550
71. Houston DE. Evidence for the risk of pelvic endometriosis by age, race, and socioeconomic status. Epidemiol Rev 1984;6:167–91.
72. Hull ML, Charnock-Jones DS, Chan CL, et al. Antiangiogenic agents are effective inhibitors of endometriosis. J. Clin. Endocrinol. Metab. 2003;88:2889–99.
73. Kao LC, Germeyer A, Tulac S, et al. Expression profiling of endometrium from women with endometriosis reveals candidate genes for disease-based implantation failure and infertility. Endocrinology 2003;144:2870–81
74. Kashiba H, Fukui H, Morikawa Y, Senba E. Gene expression of histamine H1 receptor in guinea pig sensory neurons: a relationship between H1 receptor mRNE expressing neurons and peptidergic neurons. Mol Brain Res 1999;66:24–34.
75. Kawabata A, Kawao N, Kuroda R, et al. Peripheral PAR 2 triggers thermal hyperalgesia and nociceptive responses in rats. NeuroReport 2001;12:715–9.
76. Kessler JA, Black IB. Nerve growth factor stimulates the development of substance P in sensory ganglia. Proc Nat Acad Sci USA 1980;77:649–52.
77. Kirchmair R, Egger M, Walter DH, et al. Secretoneurin, an angiogenic neuropeptide, induces postnatal vasculogenesis. Circulation 2004;110:1121–27.
78. Kirshon B, Poindexter AN 3rd and Fast J. Endometriosis in multiparous women. J Reprod Med 1989;34:215–217.
79. Koelbaek Johansen M, Graven-Nielsen T, Schou Olesen A, Arendt-Nielsen L: Generalised muscular hyperalgesia in chronic whiplash syndrome. Pain 1999;83:229 234.
80. Kokaia Z, Lindvall O. Neurogenesis after ischaemic brain insults. Curr. Opin. Neurobiol.2003;13:127–32.
81. Koninckx PR, Meuleman C, Demeyere S, et al. Suggestive evidence that pelvic endometriosis is a progressive disease, whereas deeply infiltrating endometriosis is associated with pelvic pain. Fertil Steril 1991;55:759–65.
82. Kresch AJ, Seifer DB, Sachs LB, Barrese I. Laparoscopy in 100 women with chronic pelvic pain. Obstet Gynecol 1984;64:672–674.
83. Krizsan-Agbas D, Pedchenko T, Hasan W, Smith PG. Oestrogen regulates sympathetic neurite outgrowth by modulating brain derived neurotrophic factor synthesis and release by the rodent uterus. Eur J Neurosci 2003;18:2760–2768.
84. Lautenbacher S, Rollman GB, McCain GA: Multi-method assessment of experimental and clinical pain in patients with fibromyalgia. Pain 1994;59:45–53.

85. Levine JD, Lam D, Taiwo YO, et al. Hyperalgesic properties of 15-lipoxygenase products of arachidonic acid. Proc Nat Acad Sci USA 1996;83:5331– 4.
86. Lichten EM, Bombard J. Surgical treatment of primary dysmenorrhea with laparoscopic uterine nerve ablation. J Reprod Med 1987;32:37–41.
87. Lindholm D, Heumann R, Hengerer B, Thoenen H. Interleukin 1 increases stability and transcription of mRNA encoding nerve growth factor in cultured rat fibroblasts. J Biol Chem 1988;263:16348–16351
88. Liu DT, Hitchcock A. Endometriosis: its association with retrograde menstruation, dysmenorrhoea and tubal pathology. Br J Obstet Gynaecol 1986; 93:859–862.
89. Liu T, Van Rooijen N, Tracey DJ. Depletion of macrophages reduces axonal degeneration and hyperalgesia following nerve injury. Pain 2000;86:25–32.
90. Lu B, Figurov A. Role of neurotrophins in synapse development and plasticity. Rev Neurosci 1997;8:1–12.
91. Lundeberg T, Lund I. Is there a role for acupuncture in endometriosis pain, or "endometrialgia"? Acupunct. Med. 2008;26:94–110
92. Mahmood TA, Templeton AA, Thomson L, Fraser C. Menstrual symptoms in women with pelvic endometriosis. Br J Obstet Gynaecol 1991; 98:558–563.
93. Mannan K, Altaf F, Maniar S, et al. Cyclical sciatica: Endometriosis of the sciatic nerve. J Bone Joint Surg 2008; 90: 98–101.
94. Marana R, Caruana P, Muzii L, et al. Operative laparoscopy for ovarian cysts: Excision vs. aspiration. J Reprod Med 1996;41:435–8.
95. Mechsner S, Schwarz J, Thode J, et al. Growth-associated protein 43-positive sensory nerve fibers accompanied by immature vessels are located in or near peritoneal endometriotic lesions. Fertil. Steril. 2007;88:581–87
96. Medina MG, Lebovic DI. Endometriosis-associated nerve fibers and pain. Acta Obstet. Gynecol. Scand. 2009;:968–75
97. Merskey H, Lindblom U, Mumford JM, et al. Pain terms: A current list with definitions and notes on usage. In: Merskey H, Bogduk N (eds). Classification of Chronic Pain. Seattle: IASP Press, 1994: 207–213.
98. Miao HQ, Klagsbrun M. Neuropilin is a mediator of angiogenesis. Cancer Metastasis Rev. 2000;19:29–37
99. Mizumura K, Koda H, Kamazawa T. Possible contribution of protein kinase C in the effects of histamine on the visceral nociceptor activities in vitro. Neurosci Res 2000;37:183–90.
100. Moen MH. Endometriosis in women at interval sterilization. Acta Obstet Gynecol Scand 1987;66: 451–454.
101. Moen MH, Stokstad T. A long-term follow-up study of women with asymptomatic endometriosis diagnosed incidentally at sterilization. Fertil Steril 2002;78:773–776.
102. Mukouyama YS, Shin D, Britsch S, et al. Sensory nerves determine the pattern of arterial differentiation and blood vessel branching in the skin. Cell 2002;109:693–705
103. Nap AW, Griffioen AW, Dunselman GA, et al. Antiangiogenesis therapy for endometriosis. J. Clin. Endocrinol. Metab. 2004;89:1089–95
104. Nassif J, Trompoukis P, Barata S, et al. Management of deep endometriosis. Reprod Biomed Online. 2011;23(1):25–33.
105. Novella-Maestre E, Herraiz S, Vila-Vives JM, et al. Effect of antiangiogenic treatment on peritoneal endometriosis-associated nerve fibers . Fertil Steril 2012;98(5):1209–1217
106. Olive DL. Medical therapy of endometriosis. Semin Reprod Med 2003;21:209–22.
107. Overton C, Fernandez-Shaw S, Hicks B, et al. Peritoneal fluid cytokines and the relationship with endometriosis and pain. Hum Reprod 1996;11:380 6.
108. Pandey V, Qian PX, Kang J, et al. Artemin stimulates oncogenicity and invasiveness of human endometrial carcinoma cells. Endocrinology 2010;151:909–20
109. Perkins NM, Tracey DG. Hyperalgesia due to nerve injury: role of neutrophils. Neuroscience 2000; 101:745–57.
110. Pezet S, McMahon SB. Neutrophins: Mediators and modulators of pain. Annu Rev Neurosci 2006; 29: 507–538.
111. Porpora MG, Koninckx PR, Piazze J, et al. Correlation between endometriosis and pelvic pain. J Am Assoc Gynecol Laparosc 1999;6:429–34.
112. Practice Committee of the American Society for Reproductive Medicine. Treatment of pelvic pain associated with Endometriosis. Fertil Steril. 2008;90(5):S260–9
113. Punnonen J, Teisala K, Ranta H, et al. Increased levels of interleukin-6 and interleukin-10 in the peritoneal fluid of patients with endometriosis. Am J Obstet Gynecol 1996;174:1522–6.
114. Pupo-Nogueira A, de Oliveira RM, Petta CA, et al. Vascular endothelial growth factor concentrations in the serum and peritoneal fluid of women with endometriosis. Int J Gynaecol Obstet 2007;99:33–37.

115. Rapkin A, Morgan M, Bonpane C, Martinez-Maza O. Peritoneal fluid interleukin-6 in women with chronic pelvic pain. Fertil Steril 2000;74:325–8.
116. Rawson JM. Prevalence of endometriosis in infertile women. J Reprod Med 1991;36:513–515.
117. Redwine DB, Sharpe DR. Endometriosis of the obturator nerve. J Reprod Med 1990; 35: 434–435.
118. Redwine DB. Conservative laparoscopic excision of endometriosis by sharp dissection: life table analysis of reoperation and persistent or recurrent disease. Fertil Steril 1991;56:628–34.
119. Riley JL, Robinson ME, Wise EA, Price DD. A meta-analytic review of pain perception across the menstrual cycle. Pain 1999;81:225–35.
120. Schulke LM, Markham R, Luscombe G, et al. Endometrial dendritic cell populations during the normal menstrual cycle. Hum Reprod 2008; 23: 1574–1580.
121. Schulke L, Berbic M, Manconi F, et al. Dendritic cell populations in the eutopic and ectopic endometrium of women with endometriosis. Hum Reprod. 2009;24(7):1695–703.
122. Schwertner A, Conceição Dos Santos CC, Costa GD, et al. Efficacy of melatonin in the treatment of endometriosis: A phase II, randomized, double-blind, placebo-controlled trial. PAIN 2013;154(6):874–881
123. Sharpe-Timms KL, Cox KE. Paracrine regulation of matrix metalloproteinase expression in endometriosis. Ann. NY Acad. Sci. 2002;955:147–56
124. Shen F, Liu X, Geng JG, Guo SW. Increased immunoreactivity to SLIT/ROBO1 in ovarian endometriomas: a likely constituent biomarker for recurrence. Am. J. Pathol. 2009; 175:479–88
125. Shibata A, Zelivyanskaya M, Limoges J, et al. Peripheral nerve induces macrophage neurotrophic activities: regulation of neuronal process outgrowth, intracellular signaling and synaptic function. J Neuroimmunol 2003;142:112–129.
126. Shippen ER, West WJ Jr. Successful treatment of severe endometriosis in two premenopausal women with an aromatase inhibitor. Fertil Steril 2004;81:1395– 8.
127. Shu XQ, Mendell LM. Neurotrophins and hyperalgesia. Proc Natl Acad Sci USA 1999;96:7693– 6.
128. Siristatidis C, Nissotakis C, Chrelias C, et al. Immunological factors and their role in the genesis and development of endometriosis. J Obstetr Gynaecol Res 2006;32:162–70
129. Skaper SD, Pollock M, Facci L. Mast cells differentially express and release active high molecular weight neurotrophins. Mol Brain Res 2001;972:177– 85.
130. Snesky TE, Liu DT. Endometriosis: associations with menorrhagia, infertility, and oral contraceptives. Int J Gynaecol Obstet 1980; 17: 573–76.
131. Sommer C, Schmidt C, George A. Hyperalgesia in experimental neuropathy is dependent on the TNF receptor 1. Exp Neurol 1997;151:138–42.
132. Sommer C, Petrausch S, Lindenlaub T, Toyka K. Neutralizing antibodies to interleukin-1 receptor reduce pain associated behavior in mice with experimental neuropathy. Neurosci Lett 1999;270:25– 8.
133. Sommer C, Kress M. Recent findings on how proinflammatory cytokines cause pain: peripheral mechanisms in inflammatory and neuropathic hyperalgesia. Neurosci Lett 2004;361:184–7.
134. Sorensen J, Graven-Nielsen T, Henriksson KG, et al: Hyperexcitability in fibromyalgia. J Rheumatol 1998;25:152–155
135. Sorkin LS, Xiao WH, Wagner R, Myers RR. Tumor necrosis factor alpha induces ectopic activity in nociceptive primary afferent fibers. Neuroscience 1997;81:255– 62.
136. Soysal S, Soysal M, Ozer S, et al. The effects of postsurgical administration of goserelin plus anastrozole compared to goserelin alone in patients with severe endometriosis: a prospective randomized trial. Hum Reprod 2004;19:160–7.
137. Spranger M, Lindholm D, Bandtlow C, et al. Regulation of nerve growth factor (NGF) synthesis in the rat central nervous system: comparison between the effects of interleukin-1 and various growth factors in astrocyte cultures and in vivo. Eur J Neurosci 1990;2:69–76.
138. Strathy JH, Molgaard CA, Coulam CB, Melton LJ 3rd. Endometriosis and infertility: a laparoscopic study of endometriosis among fertile and infertile women. Fertil Steril. 1982;38(6):667–72.
139. Sugamata M, Ihara T, Uchiide I. Increase of activated mast cells in human endometriosis. Am J Reprod Immunol 2005;53:120–5.
140. Sutton C, Hill D. Laser laparoscopy in the treatment of endometriosis. Br J Obstet Gynaecol 1990;97:181–5.
141. Sutton CJ, Ewen SP, Whitelaw N, Haines P. Prospective randomized double-blind controlled trial of laser laparoscopy in the treatment of pelvic pain associated with minimal, mild, and moderate endometriosis. Fertil Steril 1994;62:696–700.
142. Sutton C, Pooley AS, Jones KD, et al. A prospective randomized, double-blind controlled trial of laparoscopic uterine nerve ablation in the treatment of pelvic pain associated with endometriosis. Gynecol Endosc 2001;10:217–22.

143. Syriatowicz JP, Hu D, Walker JS, Tracey DJ. Hyperalgesia due to nerve injury: the role of prostaglandins. Neuroscience 1999;94:587–94.

144. Takayama K, Zeitoun K, Gunby RT, et al. Treatment of severe postmenopausal endometriosis with an aromatase inhibitor. Fertil Steril 1998;69:709–13.

145. Taylor RB, Hummelshoj L, Stratton P, Vercellini P. Pain and endometriosis: Etiology, impact, and therapeutics Middle East Fertil Soc J. 2012;17(4):221–225.

146. Theodosiou M, Rush RA, Zhou XF, et al. Hyperalgesia due to nerve damage: role of nerve growth factor. Pain 1999;81:245–55.

147. Tokushige N, Markham R, Russell P, Fraser IS. High density of small nerve fibres in the functional layer of the endometrium in women with endometriosis. Hum Reprod 2006;21:782–7.

148. Tokushige N, Markham R, Russell P, Fraser IS. Nerve fibres in peritoneal endometriosis. Hum Reprod 2006;21:3001–7.

149. Tokushige N, Markham R, Russell P, Fraser IS. Effect of progestogens and combined oral contraceptives on nerve fibers in peritoneal endometriosis. Fertil. Steril. 2009;92:1234–39

150. Tokushige N, Markham R, Russell P, Fraser IS. Effects of hormonal treatment on nerve fibers in endometrium and myometrium in women with endometriosis. Fertil Steril 2008;90:1589–98.

151. Tong C, Conklin D, Clyne BB, et al. Uterine cervical afferents in thoracolumbar dorsal root ganglia express transient receptor potential vanilloid type 1 channel and calcitonin gene-related peptide, but not P2X3 receptor and somatostatin. Anesthesiology 2006;104:651–7.

152. Tracey DJ, Walker JS. Pain due to nerve damage: are inflammatory mediators involved? Inflamm Res 1995;44:407–11.

153. Tran LV, Tokushige N, Berbic M, et al. Macrophages and nerve fibres in peritoneal endometriosis. Hum Reprod. 2009 Apr;24(4):835–41

154. Vercellini P, Vendola N, Bocciolone L, et al. Laparoscopic aspiration of ovarian endometriomas: Effect with postoperative gonadotropin releasing hormone agonist treatment. J Reprod Med 1992;37:577–80.

155. Vercellini P, Aimi G, Busacca M, et al. Laparoscopic uterosacral ligament resection for dysmenorrhea associated with endometriosis: results of a randomized, controlled trial. Fertil Steril 2003;80:310–9.

156. Vercellini P, Crosignani PG, Abbiati A, et al. The effect of surgery for symptomatic endometriosis: The other side of the story. Hum Reprod Update 2009; 15: 177–188.

157. Vergnolle N, Wallace JL, Bunnett NW, Hollenberg MD. Protease activated receptors in inflammation, neural signalling and pain. Trends Pharmacol Sci 2001;22:146–52.

158. Vige X, Costa E, Wise BC. Mechanism of nerve growth factor mRNA regulation by interleukin-1 and basic fibroblast growth factor in primary cultures of rat astrocytes. Mol Pharmacol 1991;40:186–192.

159. Wagner R, Myers RR. Endoneurial injection of TNF-alpha produces neuropathic pain behaviors. NeuroReport 1996;7:2897–901.

160. Weinstein BM. Vessels and nerves: marching to the same tune. Cell 2005;120:299–302

161. Wheeler JM, Malinak LR. Recurrent endometriosis: incidence, management, and prognosis. Am J Obstet Gynecol 1983;146:247–53.

162. Yamaki K, Thorlacius H, Xie X, et al. Characteristics of histamine-induced leukocyte rolling in the undisturbed microcirculation of the rat mesentery. Br J Pharmacol 1998;123:390–9.

163. Zhang YH, Nicol GD. NGF-mediated sensitization of the excitability of rat sensory neurons is prevented by a blocking antibody to the p75 neurotrophin receptor. Neurosci Lett 2004;366:187–92.

164. Zhang G, Dmitrieva N, Liu Y, et al. Endometriosis as a neurovascular condition: estrous variations in innervation, vascularization, and growth factor content of ectopic endometrial cysts in the rat. Am. J. Physiol. Regul. Integr. Comp. Physiol. 2008;294:162–71

The ISSVD classification system divides aetiology of VP into four categories: infectious, inflammatory, neoplastic, and neurologic [32]. With inflammatory conditions, pain may result from fissures, tears, irritation of sensitized and inflamed nerve fibers, friction, and damage to irritated tissues. Since it is beyond the scope of this chapter to review in detail all vulvovaginal diseases, only the most common disorders are described.

Yeast Infection

Yeast Infection is a common cause of vulvovaginitis and in 80–90% Candida albicans is the causative agent [28]. Symptoms vary from slight discharge and discomfort to severe inflammation including itching, pain, burning, and dyspareunia. In such cases swelling, fissures and erythema are commonly seen. As signs and symptoms are often nonspecific, a laboratory diagnosis is essential. Microscopic examination may aid, but a culture is required for confirmation and identification of the specific pathogen.

Single episodes of yeast vulvovaginitis cause short-term pain. However, 5–8% of adult women suffer from recurrent or intractable candida vulvovaginitis (RVVC), defined as 4 or more symptomatic infections in a year. Evaluation of patients for RVVC usually fails to reveal precipitating causes, such as excess of estrogen, antibiotic use, and uncontrolled diabetes [40]. It is thought that recurrence results from reinfection or relapse, implying incomplete clearance with therapy. Therefore, the treatment is directed at control, rather than cure, thus requiring long term maintenance therapy [41].

Vulvovaginal Atrophy

Vulvovaginal atrophy results from inadequate estrogen levels in the vagina, most commonly occurring with menopause, but can also be secondary to lactation and medications [35]. As estrogen plays a major role in maintaining the normal vaginal environment, with its withdrawal significant changes occur causing the vagina to become pale, thin, short, narrow, and less elastic [34]. Other changes, such as diminished blood flow, decreased secretions, changes in flora and increased pH are noted as well, thus increasing the likelihood of trauma, infection, pain, and slower healing after injury [20]. Patients with vaginal atrophy may complain of dryness, dyspareunia, itching, discharge, pain, and irritative urinary symptoms [34]. Diagnosis is made by identifying characteristic changes on physical examination, noting an elevated vaginal pH, and finding parabasal cells on microscopy [29] (Fig. 1).

Desquamative inflammatory Vaginitis

Desquamative inflammatory vaginitis [29] (DIV) is a rare cause of noninfectious vaginitis, characterized by an exudative inflammation of the vagina, with erythema and purulent discharge. It can also involve the vestibule and the cervix. Typical microscopic findings include an increased number of WBCs and parabasal cells (Fig. 1).

Little is known regarding aetiology, treatment options and long term follow up. DIV tends to be chronic, with symptoms lasting months. It may accompany erosive lichen planus and blistering disorders.

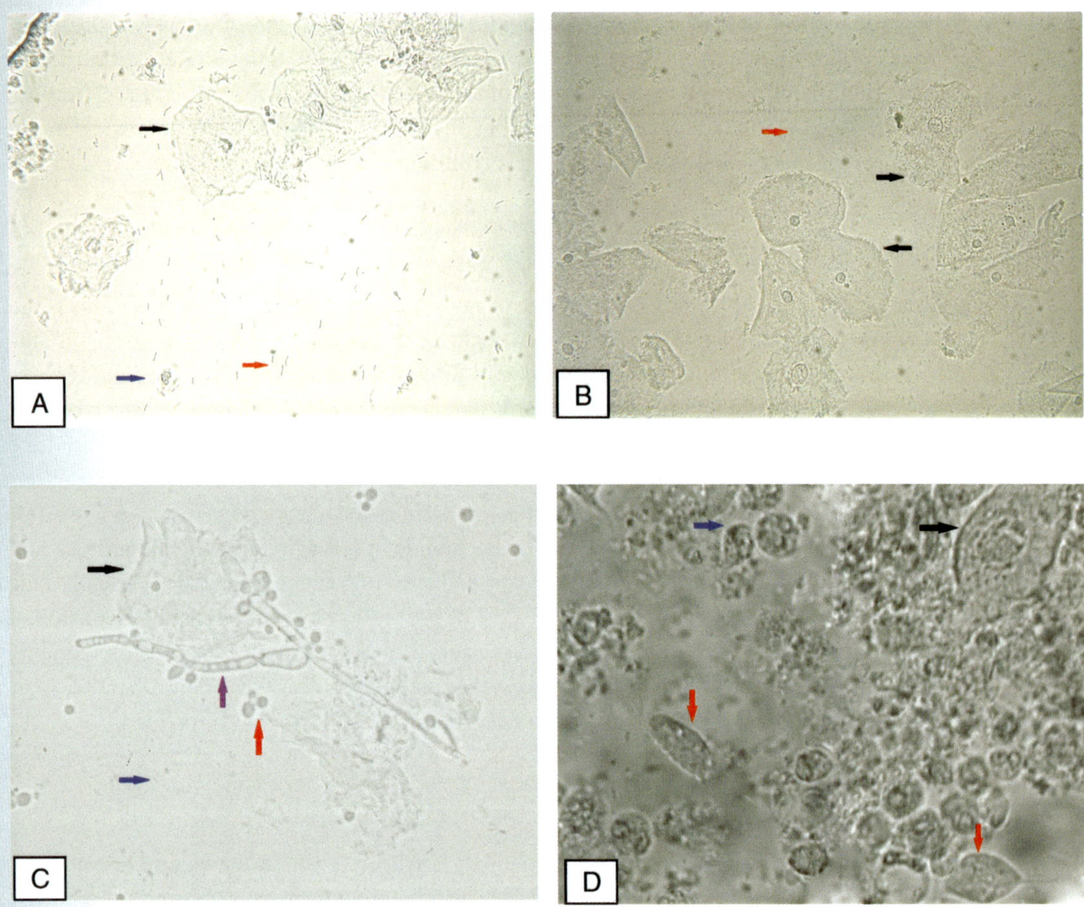

FIGURE 1 Microscopic findings of vaginal conditions

A-Normal wet mount: Mature squamous epithelial cells (black arrow), appear as large, polygonal cells. There is one or no white blood cell (blue arrow) per epithelial cell, and gram-positive rods (lactobacillus morphotypes) (red arrow) are present. This wet mount represents normal discharge, and is accompanied with normal pH (≤4.5).

B-Bacterial vaginosis (BV): clue cells (black arrow) are mature squamous epithelial cells, with adherence of abnormal bacteria to the cell. The flora is comprised of abnormal coccid bacteria (red arrow), without elevation of inflammatory cells.

C-Yeast Infection: Mature squamous epithelial cells (black arrow), rod bacteria suggestive of lactobacilli (blue arrow), hyphae (purple arrow) and budding yeast (red arrow). The specific species cannot be recognized from the smear, and a culture is required for identification.

D- Trichomoniasis: wet mount reveals an increase of inflammatory cells (blue arrow) and parabasal cells (black arrow). The parasites *Trichomonas vaginalis* are ovoid-shaped and slightly larger than inflammatory cells (red arrow), and they are best recognized by their motility.

E-Vaginal atrophy: characteristic findings are the presence of parabasal cells (black arrow), which are smaller, rounder, and have a large nucleus compared to mature squamous epithelial cells, with scanty vaginal flora as well as an elevated pH (>4.5).

F-Desquamative inflammatory vaginitis (DIV): microscopic findings show high number of white blood cells (black arrow), an increase of immature, parabasal epithelial cells and intermediate epithelial cells (blue arrow), an absence of lactobacilli and a coccoid flora (red arrow). The pH is>4.5.

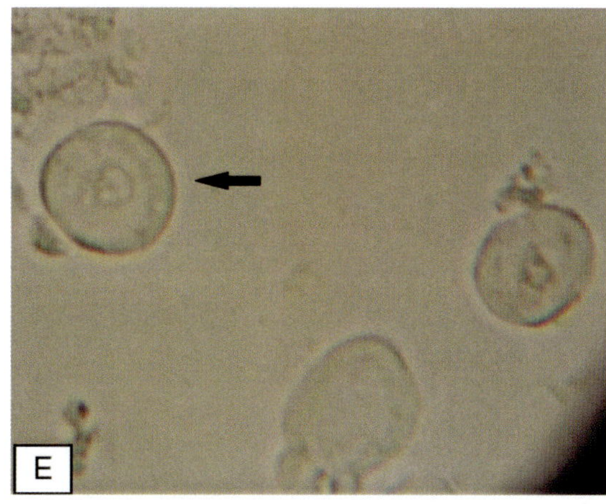

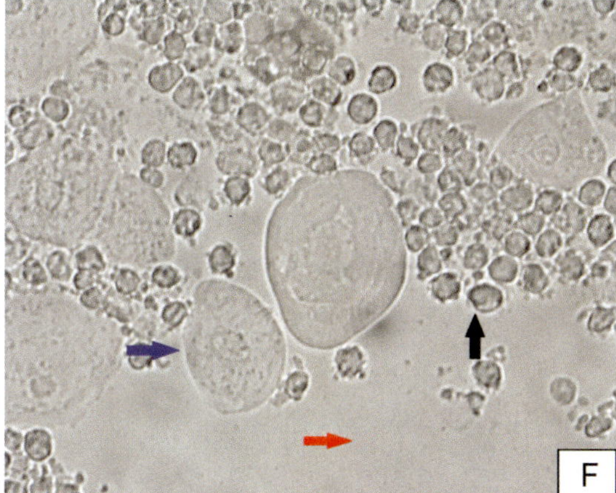

FIGURE 1 Continued

Contact Dermatitis

Contact dermatitis (CD) is an inflammation of the skin due to exposure to an exogenous agent acting as a primary irritant or an allergen. As vulvar tissue is susceptible to irritants, CD is common and can complicate all other vulvovaginal conditions. As symptoms are of nonspecific inflammation, diagnosis is based on detailed history, exclusion of infectious causes, and a high level of suspicion.

Lichen Sclerosus

Lichen sclerosus (LS) is a chronic, inflammatory skin disorder affecting 0.1–1.7% of women [12]. Classic findings include hypopigmentation, epithelial thinning or thickening, and hemorrhages. LS causes scarring of vulvar tissue, loss of normal architecture, including disappearance of labia minora, clitoral adhesions and narrowing of the introital opening. It may affect vulvar and perianal areas with the classic “figure 8” appearance or only small areas of skin. Typically, there is no vaginal involvement.

Lichen Planus

Lichen planus (LP) [31] is a systemic inflammatory mucocutaneous disorder which can involve the vagina, vulva, and vestibule. The most common variant is erosive LP, causing painful vestibular erosion that appears as deep glazed erythema. It can cause vaginitis or localized erosive lesions in the vagina. The inflammatory process can cause adhesions, fibrosis, and even complete vaginal obliteration. Introital stenosis and destruction of normal vulvar architecture can occur.

Classic LP presents with white, reticulate, lacy striae. Diagnosis is based on either physical examination findings or biopsy.

Genital Pain Syndromes: Provoked Vulvar Pain Syndrome /ProvokedVestibulodynia (PVPS/PVD) and Generalized Vulvar Pain Syndrome/ Generalized Unprovoked Vulvodynia (GVPS/GVD)

Patients with VP, in whom there is not another recognized disorder, are diagnosed with vulvar pain syndrome (VPS)/vulvodynia. The IASP and ISSVD terminology for classification of VPS/vulvodynia distinguishes between generalized and localized pain, and each of these two subgroups is further subdivided into provoked, unprovoked, or mixed (continuous pain, exacerbated by touch) [32]. The majority of presentations are either provoked VPS/ provoked vestibulodynia, formerly known as vulvar vestibulitis syndrome, or generalized VPS/generalized unprovoked vulvodynia.

PVPS/PVD

PVPS/PVD is a syndrome of provoked, localized allodynia of the vulvar vestibule, not explained by another condition, which lasts more than 3 months. PVPS/PVD was first described as a syndrome in 1987 by Dr. Friedrich [14] and was termed vulvar vestibulitis syndrome. Friedrich's criteria were: (1) severe pain in the vulvar vestibule upon touch or attempted vaginal entry; (2) tenderness to pressure localized within the vestibule; and (3) erythema of various degrees.

As inflammation is often not found, the term vestibulitis was dropped in 2003 by the ISSVD and the name was changed to PVD [32]. The diagnostic criteria remain similar to those suggested by Friedrich and include typical history of pain upon vestibular touch, such as attempted intercourse, gynecological examination, tampon insertion or other direct contact, and a suitable Q tip test which elicits severe pain or discomfort. Most patients with PVPS/PVD present with dyspareunia or a complete inability to have intercourse.

GVPS/GVD

GVPS/GVD replaced the older terminology, dysesthetic vulvodynia, essential vulvodynia, and burning vulva syndrome [32]. Patients report a continuous unpleasant pain sensation, usually burning, stinging, irritating, itching, or a feeling of rawness. Most often pain is diffuse, without clear borders. Any stimulus which results in pressure on the vulva can exacerbate the pain, including intercourse, tight fitting clothing, sitting, walking, or exercising.

DESCRIBING THE SUBJECT

Causes of Provoked Vulvar Pain Syndrome/Provoked Vestibulodynia (PVPS/PVD)

There is a belief that PVPS/PVD represents a group of distinct disorders that have been classified together simply because they produce pain in the same anatomic location [23]. Causes of these disorders include hormonal imbalance, caused mainly by hormonal contraception [7,18,21,27], nerve fiber proliferation in the vestibular mucosa, [5,6,43,44] and hyperactive pelvic floor (PF) dysfunction [37,45]. PVPS/PVD may appear with first attempts of sexual intercourse or tampon insertion (primary PVPS/PVD) or can be a new onset of pain with activities that did not illicit pain in the past (secondary PVPS/PVD) [46].

Studies found that various factors such as genetic, inflammatory mediators, recurrent vaginitis, allergy, and trauma may be involved in the development of PVPS/PVD.

A high percentage of VP patients report an antecedent history of recurrent or intractable candida vulvovaginitis, although it is unknown if this represents a true increase in incidence or an original misdiagnosis. It has been suggested that repeated vulvovaginitis is a triggering event for some women leading to chronic VP. This observation has led to hypothesis that in a patient with neurogenic vulnerability, an initiating event or series of events may lead to chronic VP [11,19,47].

Several studies point to a possible genetic involvement with polymorphisms in genes responsible for regulating inflammatory response: allele 2 of the IL-1b gene[16], mannose-binding lectin (MBL)[2], melanocortin-1 receptor (MC1R) gene[13], and the gene coding for the inflammasome component NALP3 [30]. The theory suggests that some women with PVPS/PVD have defective regulation of proinflammatory immune responses, due to genetic variations that predispose them to exaggerated inflammatory responses [15,16,30,47]. Chronic inflammation may induce changes to peripheral nociceptors or may represent an increased exaggerated neurogenic inflammation, facilitating central sensitization.

Because the diagnosis of VPS/vulvodynia is nonspecific, treatment is not evidence based and proceeds on a trial and error basis. At least 30 different therapeutic interventions have been suggested for the management of VPS/vulvodynia, yet evidence from clinical trials remains largely inconclusive [1]. Recommendations are in favor for a multi-disciplinary approach focusing on pain management and re-establishing the PF function [4].

A different approach is suggested by Goldstein[17]. He classifies PVPS/PVD groups, based on history and exam findings:

Hormonally mediated PVPS/PVD - The pain began while taking hormonal contraceptives. Typically, patients have a low calculated free testosterone and complain of dryness, decreased libido and arousal. The entire vestibule is tender and vestibular mucosa is often dry and thin. Treatment includes stopping hormonal contraception and application of topical estradiol (± testosterone) to the vestibule [9].

Hyperactive pelvic muscle dysfunction - PF muscles become tight and tender. Patients often have other symptoms suggesting hyperactivity (see below) and predisposing factors, such as musculoskeletal disorders or anxiety, may coexist. Typically, the pain is much worse at 4–8 o'clock position of the vestibule with minimal or no pain in the upper vestibule. Treatment includes PF physiotherapy, with an optional addition of muscle relaxants (diazepam suppositories), Botulinum toxin injections and cognitive behavioral therapy.

Neuroproliferative PVPS/PVD - Women have an increased number of nociceptors in the vestibular mucosa. This group is further subdivided into congenital and acquired forms.

In the congenital subgroup, vestibular pain has always been present, and there may be sensitivity to palpation of the belly button, due to common embryologic origin (the primitive urogenital sinus)[10]. With acquired neuroproliferative PVPS/PVD, the pain began after a severe allergic reaction or vaginitis. There is tenderness of the entire vestibule. Treatments include topical anaesthetics, antidepressants, antiseizure drugs, capsaicin cream and vestibulectomy.

As with PVPS/PVD, the term generalized VPS/generalized unprovoked vulvodynia describes a symptom, the question is whether we can diagnose a specific cause instead of calling it simply "vulvar pain". It is possible that some cases of GVPS/GVD may represent a pudendal nerve disorder, PF hyperactive disorder, or can be classified as an entity within the spectrum of neuropathic pain syndromes, while in other patients it represents functional pain syndrome.

PRACTICAL IMPLICATIONS

Assessment of Patients with Genital Pain

Vulvovaginitis causes itching, irritation, discharge, pain, and dyspareunia. On physical exam, erythema, edema, discharge, and tenderness may be noted. These signs and symptoms are nonspecific and represent an inflammatory response to various causes. Most disorders can be diagnosed by combining history, physical examination, and microscopic evaluation of vaginal discharge. In addition, cultures and PCR (polymerase chain reaction) assays are required to diagnose specific pathogens, while a biopsy is needed when vulvar skin is involved or when a neoplasm is suspected.

History Taking: Which Questions are Important to Ask?

History taking provides the data required to make an accurate diagnosis. Many providers use questionnaires specifically designed for evaluation of vulvovaginal complaints (see references below).

A detailed symptom history is important. This should include the nature of symptom, location, severity, duration, whether it is continuous, intermittent or cyclical, if it is provoked by touch or unprovoked, and what aggravates or relieves it. It is important to clarify whether the discomfort is localized to the external genitalia, vestibule, or deep in the vagina. Assess the effects on daily life and functioning. Inquire about prior treatments, how they were used, and what their effect was. If a woman reports painful intercourse, determine whether the pain is superficial, on penetration (likely related to a vulvar or vestibular problem), or deep (deep dyspareunia). Ask about tightening of the PF muscles: this may present as painful penetration (vaginismus), urinary frequency, urgency and hesitancy, constipation, hemorrhoids, and anal fissures. Take a brief gynecological history and inquire about menstruation, fertility, and contraception. Include in your history questions regarding skin conditions and exposure to potential irritants and allergens.

While obtaining the history, be familiar with potential diagnoses but open to various possibilities. Don't be distracted as many patients will provide speculated diagnoses they heard elsewhere or have self diagnosed using the internet. Finally, look for coexisting conditions.

Examination: What Should be Examined?

Keep in mind that VPS/vulvodynia is a diagnosis of exclusion. Many inflammatory, infectious, and dermatologic disorders present with provoked vestibular pain or unprovoked pain, and are ruled out by thorough physical examination.

The exam should always include observation, evaluation of vestibular tenderness, assessment of discharge using microscopy, pH measurement, cultures, PF muscles and adjacent organ palpation.

A bright light is recommended to examine the vulva, vagina, and cervix. To evaluate the vulva, separate the labia to assess for lesions, fissures, redness, or swelling. Gently retract the clitoral hood, exposing the clitoris. Examine the vestibule for epithelial thinning associated with estrogen deficiency or skin disorders.

Vestibular tenderness should be evaluated using the Q tip test (Fig. 2).

Examination of the vagina with a speculum can range from normal appearance of vaginal walls to diffuse redness, erosions, and petechiae suggestive of vaginitis. Note the presence of discharge, its characteristics and origin (vaginal walls or cervix). As findings on examination can be nonspecific, a microscopic examination (wet mount) should be performed. Vaginal secretions should be placed on microscopic slides and a drop of saline (0.9% NaCl) and 10% KOH should be added separately to each sample. Microscopy can allow the identification of fungal infection, trichomoniasis, parabasal cells (characterizing vaginal atrophy and estrogen deficiency) and diagnosis of DIV (Fig. 1). Cultures and PCR studies identify fungal organisms, relevant bacteria such as Group A streptococci, and sexually transmitted organisms.

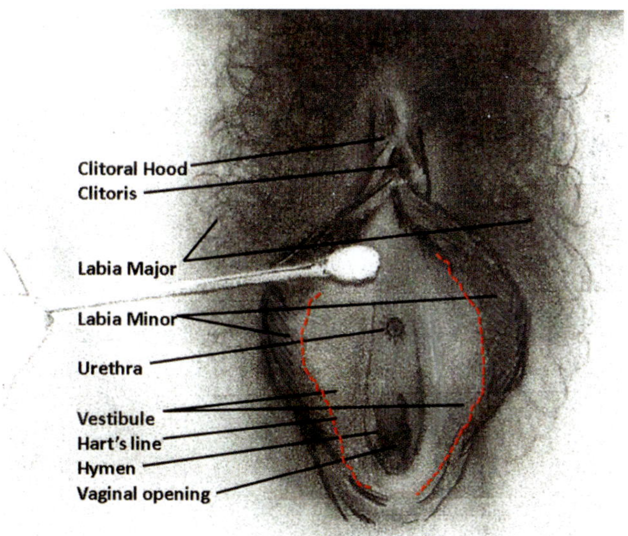

FIGURE 2 The Q-tip test

The goal of the Q-tip test is to determine if there are areas that exhibit an abnormal pain response in the genital area. Use a cotton-tipped applicator to determine whether pain is provoked by pressure at one or more points. Apply gentle pressure to the following areas: inner thighs, labia major and labia minor, interlabial sulci, clitoris, clitoral hood and perineum. Sites to be tested within the vestibule can be visualized using a clock face (1–12 o'clock). The anterior vestibular sites (2, 10, and 12) are typically assessed first, followed by the posterior sites (5, 6, and 7). Apply gentle pressure to each of these sites and ask the patient to rate the pain severity (VAS score) and describe the pain character (burning, raw etc.).

The physical exam includes digital palpation of the levator ani muscles for hyperactivity, tenderness and trigger points, palpation of the urethra, bladder trigone, pudendal nerve, uterus, and adnexa.

Additional studies, including biopsy, patch tests, or imaging should be performed, as needed.

After completion of the history and examination, the provider should be able to diagnose the causative factor such as infectious and noninfectious vaginitis, skin disorders, estrogen deficiency, etc. If all known causes are ruled out, VPS/vulvodynia can be diagnosed.

Treatment of PVD and GVD

The current VPS/vulvodynia management is described in "The Vulvodynia Guideline" (VG) published in 2005 [25], developed by an expert panel, organized by the ISSVD. The guideline is largely based on expert opinion and has several disadvantages, including the absence of differentiation between treatments for GVPS/GVD and PVPS/PVD, lack of the most up to date research and the absence of the quality of the supportive evidence utilized. Because the pathogenesis is not defined, treatment of VPS/vulvodynia is generally predicated on a trial and error basis. The result is that many therapeutic interventions are used, yet the evidence remains largely inconclusive. Modalities of treatment include vulvar care measures, topical, oral, and injectable medications, physical therapy, surgery (vestibulectomy), and complementary medicine [25].

In a review published recently, [1] Andrews evaluated all published studies regarding VPS/vulvodynia and PVPS/PVD. He sought to include only placebo-controlled randomized trials (PCRT), but not surprisingly, found only a few, so he included studies without a comparator. In most of these studies, the data analyzed was a pre-treatment assessment versus a post-treatment assessment and the primary outcome was the reported reduction in pain.

Andrews found 447 treatment articles of PVPS/PVD and GVPS/GVD, of these, 71 were eligible for review. 55 studies reported 28 different treatments for PVPS/PVD. The majority of the published studies were case series, with success rates varying from no effect to 100% improvement. There were eleven RT, five were placebo-controlled. Most studies had several methodological weaknesses, including lack of control or placebo group, non double-blind evaluation, no pre-treatment pain and functional status evaluation, non validated outcome measures of pain and sexual functioning, and no long-term outcomes.

Of the 71 eligible articles, 16 reported an evaluation of a therapy for VPS/vulvodynia, predominantly GVPS/GVD. Twelve different interventions for GVPS/GVD were evaluated. All of the VPS/vulvodynia studies had the methodological weaknesses cited above. There were no analytic studies, no RCTs, and all the studies reported a beneficial effect. Andrew's review found that there is insufficient evidence to conclude that any of the nonsurgical therapies confer a net benefit for patients with PVPS/PVD, and insufficient evidence for efficacy of any of the treatments studied for GVPS/GVD.

Furthermore, single PCRT have demonstrated evidence for a lack of benefit of topical 5% lidocaine, oral desipramine and botulinum-toxin injections. The body of evidence for other interventions was poor, and there was insufficient evidence regarding the efficacy of numerous other interventions, including steroid and anesthetics injections, multilevel nerve blocks, interferon, capsaicin, topical gabapentin, cognitive behavioral therapy, and PF physiotherapy.

Surgical therapy was also evaluated: case series of 1138 patients reported an effect of 31% to 100%, for patients who reported at least some improvement. For 12 studies reporting complete relief as an outcome, the median effect size was 67%. Therefore, there is fair evidence that vestibulectomy provides a benefit for patients with PVPS/PVD, but the size of this effect cannot be determined with confidence.

In addition, outcomes show a wide range of response to different therapies for VP syndromes, with 35% to 79% of women reporting improvement in pain scores at 6 months [19,25,38]. Nevertheless, long-term outcomes are disappointing with up to 66% of women reporting some improvement, but only 57% reporting greater than 50% improvement in pain since diagnosis [26,36], and more than half still describe severe pain and functional impairment in daily activities [26,38].

It is suggested that several parameters may be responsible for these discouraging results. First, the expression, presentation, and response to therapy result in a unique pain experience for each patient. There are also other psychological factors that adversely affect outcome, such as depression, stress, somatization, anxiety, phobic symptoms, and catastrophizing. Failure to identify and address these factors in the clinical and research settings, may affect outcome [23].

Some women have evidence of CNS dysregulation, such as enhanced systemic pain responses and more than one pain syndrome. The failure to address this central component may account for treatment failures [23].

Finally, VP syndromes may represent a diverse group of disorders with several possible pain mechanisms and the appropriate treatment for each may be different. The unfavorable outcomes to therapy can be explained by grouping patients with different conditions, and then studying an intervention that might only help one subset of the conditions. This can lead to an apparent lack of effect, secondary to dilution of the patient subpopulation [1].

VP syndromes are complex conditions with a variety of factors contributing to etiology, symptoms, and response to therapy. Most studies involve monotherapy and demonstrate disappointing results. However, an integrated approach addressing a variety of contributing factors offers the best therapeutic result [22] and in fact, several studies found that multidisciplinary approach leads to substantial improvements in VP and the resumption of intercourse [33,39,42].

LOOKING AT THE FUTURE

Management of vulvar pain syndromes can be improved if the etiology of the pain is identified or classified better. More research on epidemiology, the natural history and etiology of PVPS/PVD and GVPS/GVD is required. Given the high placebo response rate of around 50%, the only data that will give confidence about a beneficial therapeutic effect will come from PCRT. Centers should consider collaborating in large multicenter trials, and the standardization of research tools, definitions, and outcome measures is needed.

TAKE HOME MESSAGES

VPS/Vulvodynia is a diagnosis of exclusion. Many inflammatory, infectious, and dermatologic disorders present with VP and dyspareunia need to be ruled out through history, physical examination, microscopy, pH measurement, and biopsy prior to diagnosing a patient with VPS/vulvodynia.

As VP has an effect on diverse aspects of life, accurate diagnosis accompanied by rapid and suitable treatment is of major importance. It may provide immediate cure or control of chronic disorders, and therefore prevent sequelae such as PF dysfunction and emotional stress that may develop if VP is left untreated. In addition, due to the possibility that intractable vaginitis is a triggering event leading to chronic VP in vulnerable patients, a quick and accurate diagnosis is important.

Multidisciplinary approach leads to substantial improvements in VP and the resumption of intercourse, and is therefore recommended.

FURTHER READING

Books

Goldstein A, Pukall C, Goldstein I (eds). Female Sexual Pain Disorders: Evaluation and Management. Wiley-Blackwell Publishing Ltd, 2008.

Goldstein A, Pukall C, Goldstein I. When Sex Hurts: A Woman's Guide to Banishing Sexual Pain. First Da Capo Press Edition, 2011.

Stewart EG, Spencer P. The V Book: A Doctor's Guide to Complete Vulvovaginal Health. Bantam Books, 2002.

Questionnaires

International Pelvic Pain Society
http://www.pelvicpain.org/pdf/History_and_Physical_Form/IPPS-H&PformR-MSW.pdf
ISSVD
https://netforum.avectra.com/temp/ClientImages/ISSVD/3ef9c6ea-aac7-4d2b-a37f-058ef9f11a67.pdf

REFERENCES

1. Andrews JC. Vulvodynia interventions-Systemic Review and Evidence Grading. Obstet Gynecol Surv 2011;66:299–315.
2. Babula O, Danielsson I, Sjoberg I, et al. Altered distribution of mannose-binding lectin alleles at exon I codon 54 in women with vulvar vestibulitis syndrome. Am J Obstet Gynecol 2004;191:762–6.
3. Bachmann GA, Rosen R, Pinn VW, et al. Vulvodynia: a state-of-the-art consensus on definitions, diagnosis and management. J Reprod Med 2006;51: 447–456.
4. Bohm-Starke N. Medical and physical predictors of localized provoked vulvodynia. Acta Obstet Gynecol Scand 2010;89:1504–10.
5. Bohm-Starke N, Hilliges M, Falconer C, Rylander E. Increased intraepithelial innervation in women with vulvar vestibulitis syndrome. Gynecol Obstet Invest 1998;46:256–60.
6. Bornstein J, Goldschmid N, Sabo E. Hyperinnervation and mast cell activation may be used as histopathologic diagnostic criteria for vulvar vestibulitis. Gynecol Obstet Invest 2004;58:171–8.
7. Bouchard C. Use of Oral Contraceptive Pills and Vulvar Vestibulitis: A Case-Control Study. Am J Epidemiol 2002;156:254–261.
8. Buchan A, Munday P, Ravenhill G, et al. A qualitative study of women with vulvodynia: I. The journey into treatment. J Reprod Med 2007;52:15–8.
9. Burrows LJ, Goldstein AT. The Treatment of Vestibulodynia with Topical Estradiol and Testosterone. Sex Med 2013;1:30–33.
10. Burrows LJ, Klingman D, Pukall CF, Goldstein AT. Umbilical hypersensitivity in women with primary vestibulodynia. J Reprod Med 2008;53:413–416.
11. Edwards L. New concepts in vulvodynia. Am J Obstet Gynecol 2003;189:S24–30.
12. Fistarol SK, Itin PH. Diagnosis and treatment of lichen sclerosus: an update. Am J Clin Dermatol 2013;14: 27–47.
13. Foster DC, Sazenski TM, Stodgell CJ. Impact of genetic variation in interleukin-1 receptor antagonist and melanocortin-1 receptor genes on vulvar vestibulitis syndrome. J Reprod Med 2004;49:503–9.
14. Friedrich EG. Vulvar vestibulitis syndrome. J Reprod Med 1987;32:110–4.
15. Gerber S, Bongiovanni AM, Ledger WJ, Witkin SS. A deficiency in interferon-alpha production in women with vulvar vestibulitis. Am J Obstet Gynecol 2002;186:361–4.
16. Gerber S, Bongiovanni AM, Ledger WJ, Witkin SS. Interleukin-1beta gene polymorphism in women with vulvar vestibulitis syndrome. Eur J Obstet Gynecol Reprod Biol 2003;107:74–7.
17. Goldstein AT. Moving beyond the diagnosis of vestibulodynia" A holiday wish list. J Sex Med 2009;6(12): 3227–3229.
18. Goldstein A, Burrows L, Goldstein I. Can oral contraceptives cause vestibulodynia? J Sex Med 2010;7:1585–7.
19. Goldstein AT, Marinoff SC, Haefner HK. Vulvodynia: strategies for treatment. Clin Obstet Gynecol 2005;48:769–85.
20. Graziottin A, Leiblum SR. Biological and psychosocial pathophysiology of female sexual dysfunction during the menopausal transition. J Sex Med 2005;2 Suppl 3:133–145.

21. Greenstein A, Ben-Aroya Z, Fass O, et al. Vulvar vestibulitis syndrome and estrogen dose of oral contraceptive pills. J Sex Med 2007;4:1679–83.
22. Gunter J. Chronic pelvic pain: an integrated approach to diagnosis and treatment. Obstet Gynecol Surv 2003;58:615–23.
23. Gunter J. Vulvodynia: new thoughts on a devastating condition. Obstet Gynecol Surv 2007;62:812–9.
24. Haefner HK. Report of the International Society for the Study of Vulvovaginal Disease terminology and classification of vulvodynia. J Lower Genital Tract Dis 2007;11:48–9.
25. Haefner HK, Collins ME, Davis GD, et al. The Vulvodynia Guideline. 2005;9(1):40–51.
26. Jensen JT, Wilder K, Carr K, et al. Quality of life and sexual function after evaluation and treatment at a referral center for vulvovaginal disorders. Am J Obstet Gynecol 2003;188:1629–35.
27. Johannesson U, Blomgren B, Hilliges M, et al. The vulval vestibular mucosa-morphological effects of oral contraceptives and menstrual cycle. Br J Dermatol 2007;157:487–93.
28. Kennedy MA, Sobel JD. Vulvovaginal Candidiasis Caused by Non-albicans Candida Species: New Insights. Curr Infect Dis Rep 2010;12:465–470.
29. Lev-Sagie A, Nyirjesy P. Noninfectious Vaginitis. In: Goldstein A, Pukall C, Goldstein I (eds). Female Sexual Pain Disorders: Evaluation and Management. Wiley-Blackwell Publishing Ltd, 2008:105–111.
30. Lev-Sagie A, Prus D, Linhares IM, et al. Polymorphism in a gene coding for the inflammasome component NALP3 and recurrent vulvovaginal candidiasis in women with vulvar vestibulitis syndrome. Am J Obstet Gynecol 2009;200:303.e1–6.
31. Moyal-Barracco M, Edwards L. Diagnosis and therapy of anogenital lichen planus. Dermatol Ther 2004;17:38–46.
32. Moyal-Barracco M, Lynch PJ. 2003 ISSVD terminology and classification of vulvodynia: a historical perspective. J Reprod Med 2004;49:772–777.
33. Munday P, Buchan A, Ravenhill G, et al. A qualitative study of women with vulvodynia: II. Response to a multidisciplinary approach to management. J Reprod Med 2007;52:19–22.
34. North American Menopause Society. The role of local vaginal estrogen for treatment of vaginal atrophy. Menopause 2007;14:355–356.
35. Nyirjesy P. Postmenopausal vaginitis. Curr Infect Dis Rep 2007;9:480–484.
36. Reed BD, Haefner HK, Cantor L. Vulvar dysesthesia (vulvodynia). A follow-up study. J Reprod Med 2003;48:409–16.
37. Reissing ED, Brown C, Lord MJ, et al. Pelvic floor muscle functioning in women with vulvar vestibulitis syndrome. J Psychosom Obstet Gynaecol 2005;26:107–13.
38. Sadownik L. Clinical profile of vulvodynia patients. A prospective study of 300 patients. J Reprod Med 2000;45:679–84.
39. Sadownik LA, Seal BN, Brotto LA. Provoked vestibulodynia-women's experience of participating in a multidisciplinary vulvodynia program. J Sex Med 2012;9:1086–93.
40. Sobel JD. Pathogenesis of recurrent vulvovaginal candidiasis. Curr Infect Dis Rep 2002;162:332–519.
41. Sobel JD, Wiesenfeld HC, Martens M, et al. Maintenance fluconazole therapy for recurrent vulvovaginal candidiasis. N Engl J Med 2004;351(9): 876–883.
42. Spoelstra SK, Dijkstra JR, van Driel MF, Weijmar Schultz WCM. Long-term results of an individualized, multifaceted, and multidisciplinary therapeutic approach to provoked vestibulodynia. J Sex Med 2011;8:489–96.
43. Tympanidis P, Terenghi G, Dowd P. Increased innervation of the vulval vestibule in patients with vulvodynia. Br J Dermatol 2003;148:1021–7.
44. Weström L V, Willén R. Vestibular nerve fiber proliferation in vulvar vestibulitis syndrome. Obstet Gynecol 1998;91:572–576.
45. White G, Jantos M, Glazer H. Establishing the diagnosis of vulvar vestibulitis. J Reprod Med 1997;42:157–60..
46. Witkin SS, Gerber S, Ledger WJ. Differential characterization of women with vulvar vestibulitis syndrome. Am J Obstet Gynecol 2002;187:589–94.
47. Zolnoun D, Hartmann K, Lamvu G, et al. A conceptual model for the pathophysiology of vulvar vestibulitis syndrome. Obstet Gynecol Surv 2006;61:395–401;

CHAPTER 18

Functional Disorders of the Gastro-Intestinal Tract

Lalit Kumar and Anton Emmanuel

INTRODUCTION

Descriptions of gut dysfunction and its association to specific causal factors date as far back as the Papyrus records of ancient Egyptians. This traditional approach of associating identifiable factors to disease has been the basis of medical teaching for thousands of years [2]. Hence it comes as no surprise that functional disorders, comprising of a symptom cluster of unknown organic cause, did not gain recognition until recently. The paradigm shift away from conceptualizing disease in addition to recent advances in the medical technology have undoubtedly facilitated the recognition of functional gastro-intestinal disorders (FGID) as distinct clinical entities [15].

In recent years, this field has witnessed an exponential increase in the number of studies as more and more researchers and clinicians get involved with these disorders. The newly found interest seems to be justified by the fact that FGIDs affect at least one third of the population[34]. Moreover, half of all the patients seen in primary care and up to half of all referrals to specialist gastroenterologists with gastrointestinal complaints are for FGIDs [17,27].

BASIC ASPECTS

Terminology

FGID is characterized by gastro-intestinal symptoms for which no pathophysiological explanation is established, despite extensive investigations. There is no structural cause identifiable on endoscopic, radiological or histopathological investigations, nor is there any presence of infectious or neoplastic pathology. The symptomatology usually contains physiologic aberrations such as altered GI motility and secretion, visceral hypersensitivity and brain-gut deregulation.

Although the term FGID encompasses a group of prevalent syndromes categorized under six anatomical regions: oesophageal, gastro duodenal, bowel, functional abdominal pain syndrome, biliary and anorectal, it is the IBS which stands out as being the commonest and is almost synonymous with the term "functional bowel disorder". While FGIDs have been described in the medical literature since early 19th century, it wasn't until 1950 that the term irritable bowel syndrome (IBS) was first coined [8].

Taxonomy

Functional disorders comprise of cluster of symptoms rather than one individual symptom. Absence of a specific biomarker coupled with the mediocre accuracy of diagnosing FGIDs based on individual symptoms led to the development of diagnostic criteria's, which combined several symptoms together. Manning, in 1978 proposed the Manning criteria comprising of four symptoms [45] whereas Kruis and colleagues endorsed a statistical model in 1984 [36] to help diagnose IBS. Colin-Jones and his group postulated diagnostic criteria in a meeting of gastroenterologists in 1988 [13]. However, all these attempts failed to gain wide acceptances due to their modest performance and their unwieldy nature. Advent of Rome criteria changed the scene and by helping evolve our understanding of these disorders, have gained a worldwide acceptance. The Rome criteria have been revised twice since their inception, with Rome III being the current diagnostic nomenclature system. The FGIDs are classified into six major categories for adults, as shown in Table 1. Each category contains further subgroups of several disorders, each of which has its own relatively specific clinical features.

Mechanisms

The aetiologies of this heterogeneous group of disorders are still not well understood. It is plausible that FGIDs do not have a single unifying explanation and are rather multifactorial. With help of numerous research studies and advancement in medical technology, several mechanisms by which FGIDs may develop have come to light. While most of these mechanisms may vary between patients, visceral hypersensitivity and abnormal motility have often been found to be a common factor. Other elements such as dysfunction of brain-gut axis, genetic factors, infection, altered gut bacteria and intestinal inflammation, have also been found to play a role in development of FGIDs.

Visceral hypersensitivity: Two-thirds of patients with functional GI disorders have increased sensitivity to gut stimuli. In other words, these patients experience pain or discomfort, even with simple physiological activities such as gut contractions. In patients suffering from FD postprandial sensitivity to balloon distention has been reported to be significantly greater than in controls[18]. IBS patients have a higher intensity of perception and report more gastrointestinal symptoms as compared to non IBS sufferers [63].

Abnormal motility: The human gut is known to be affected by psychological and physiological stressors. These stressors have an even greater effect on FGID patients. Highly specialised mechanisms of GI tract to propulse food, absorb nutrients, and eliminate waste are often altered in functional disorders. This dysmotility causes symptoms particularly of vomiting, bloating or constipation if movement of food is too slow and diarrhoea or incontinence if it's too fast. Abnormal transit times have been reported in several studies looking at functional GI disorders [7,28,44].

Brain-gut axis: Dysfunction of the bi-directional pathways between the gastrointestinal and the central nervous system (the 'brain-gut axis') have been reported to be associated with FGIDs [33,59,71]. In simple terms, the bidirectional relationship means that the GI symptoms can not only lead to psychological distress but may themselves result as an effect of psychosocial factors. A population based study looking at this bidirectional relation found a significantly increased likelihood of developing IBS in subjects having higher levels of anxiety as compared to those without. It also reported higher levels of anxiety and depression at follow-up after diagnosis of FGID in subjects who did not have clinically elevated levels of psychological distress at baseline.

TABLE 1 Rome III Functional Gastrointestinal Disorders In Adults

- A. Functional esophageal disorders
  - A1. Functional heartburn
  - A2. Functional chest pain of presumed esophageal origin
  - A3. Functional dysphagia
  - A4. Globus
- B. Functional gastroduodenal disorders
  - B1. Functional dyspepsia
    - B1a. Postprandial distress syndrome
    - B1b. Epigastric pain syndrome
  - B2. Belching disorders
    - B2a. Aerophagia
    - B2b. Unspecified excessive belching
  - B3. Nausea and vomiting disorders
    - B3a. Chronic idiopathic nausea
    - B3b. Functional vomiting
    - B3c. Cyclic vomiting syndrome
  - B4. Rumination syndrome in adults
- C. Functional bowel disorders
  - C1. Irritable bowel syndrome
  - C2. Functional bloating
  - C3. Functional constipation
  - C4. Functional diarrhea
  - C5. Unspecified functional bowel disorder
- D. Functional abdominal pain syndrome
- E. Functional gallbladder and Sphincter of Oddi (SO) disorders
  - E1. Functional gallbladder disorder
  - E2. Functional biliary SO disorder
  - E3. Functional pancreatic SO disorder
- F. Functional anorectal disorders
  - F1. Functional fecal incontinence
  - F2. Functional anorectal pain
    - F2a. Chronic proctalgia
      - F2a1. Levator ani syndrome
      - F2a2. Unspecified functional anorectal pain
    - F2b. Proctalgia fugax
  - F3. Functional defecation disorders
    - F3a. Dyssynergic defecation
    - F3b. Inadequate defecatory propulsion

Genetic factors: Genetic predisposition has been linked to FGIDs due to several studies which have looked at over 100 genetic variants in over 60 genes and discovered few positive associations [61]. For instance, high prevalence of GNβ3 CC genotype has been reported in patients with dyspepsia [9], lower levels of IL-10, an anti-inflammatory cytokine and serotonin reuptake transporter polymorphism have been linked to IBS [23,61]. Apart from genetic predisposition a familial association has also been reported in FD and IBS [40]. A twin study demonstrated that genetic build as well as social learning adds to the risk of developing FGIDs [37]. These effects of modelling were also reported in children, of IBS suffering parents, who required more consultations as compared to children with non IBS suffering parents [38].

Inflammation and infections: Inflammation in enteric mucosa or the neural plexus has been postulated as a contributory factor to development of FGIDs for quite some time [14] but it was only in the last decade that a study revealed half of the IBS patients to have increased activated mucosal inflammatory cells [10]. Moreover, this seems to corroborate with the results from two meta-analysis looking at FD and IBS, both of which reported an increased incidence of these disorders after a bout of infection [25,54].

Altered bacterial flora: Studies looking at the role of gut flora in FGID have discovered possible associations. H. Pylori eradication in FD patients was reported to have a small but statistically significant effect in a meta-analysis [48]. Altered microbiota has been found in IBS patients [31] and is possibly related to increased abdominal symptoms after antibiotic use in these patients [46]. Further substance for the role of gut flora is imparted by improvement of symptoms in IBS patients with use of probiotic bacterial preparations [51] and eradication of small bowel bacterial overgrowth [56]. There is a need for further studies to support this newly emerging area of research in FGIDs.

DESCRIBING THE SUBJECT

Functional gastrointestinal disorders pose a significant challenge to health care professionals worldwide. They take a huge toll on health and are associated with high personal and economic costs. Over the last two decades of studying FGIDs a substantial number of scientific studies have focused on IBS due to its high prevalence. As such, IBS serves as an effective prototype for other functional GI conditions. The Rome foundation has unequivocally been the major force behind increasingly meticulous and accurate definitions of this syndrome.

Epidemiology

Functional gastrointestinal disorders are highly prevalent in the population but their global mapping is far from complete. This is primarily due to only a subset of symptomatic subjects seeking care, and the fact that this varies across cultures and countries. Moreover, the incidence rates are difficult to obtain as they require complex longitudinal population-based studies with repeated surveys as well as because of the fluctuating nature of these disorders. The few studies looking at incidence have reported unusually varying rates ranging from 0.05–4.3% for gastro esophageal reflux, from 0.8 to 5.6% for dyspepsia and from 3 to 32% for IBS. The challenges to have accurate epidemiological studies are outlined below.

Lack of common diagnostic criteria has been suggested to be one such factor. It has been known that the prevalence of IBS decreases as more Manning criteria are required to be fulfilled. While applying only two of the Manning criteria an obvious increase in IBS prevalence was reported [45]. However, no such correlation has been detected with use of any of the Rome criteria (I, II or III) [42,69].

Moreover, accuracy of these diagnostic criteria's varies in diagnosing different FGIDs. Certain symptoms such as chest pain and chronic diarrhea are likely to have a full work up done before being labeled as a functional disorder but others such as heartburn or IBS symptom cluster usually get classed as functional without much further investigation. This clearly leads to an overestimation of the occurrence of FGID since some of these symptoms may actually be due to structural or biochemical alterations which haven't been picked up due to lack of appropriate investigations.

Time span assessed by epidemiological studies is another cause of variability. Studies conducted in the recent past and of shorter time duration provide more reliable information than those conducted over a long period. However, they tend to miss subjects in long periods of remission and also those whose symptom profile has changed recently.

Difference in study population with regard to sex difference and number of people seeking medical attention, have also been ascribed to be behind this variation in epidemiological data. Whereas a female preponderance of 2:1 is seen in Western countries for chronic abdominal pain, globus and bowel disorders including constipation and incontinence, male predominance is evident in aerophagia and abdominal bloating. Females are three to four times more likely to seek health care for symptoms of all FGIDs as compared to men for IBS and constipation-like symptoms [4,6,16,47,66,68].

DIAGNOSIS OF FGIDS

Diagnosing functional disorders is often a frustrating and difficult process both for the patient and the physician. While the physicians, in ensuring that an underlying pathology is not missed, subject patients to a barrage of diagnostic tests, patients often develop a negative attitude to physician's inability in finding a defect. This extensive testing is certainly more prevalent at primary care level as compared to the specialists dealing with FGIDs [65]. There is little doubt that increasing awareness at primary care level and a persuasive communication of disease to patients will lead to a decrease in socioeconomic impact of these disorders.

Thankfully, with the advent of the Rome Criteria there has been a big transformation in the methodology of diagnosing FGIDs. The Rome criteria were developed in consensus meetings (via Delphi Approach) and have gone through three versions with the fourth version expected to be released in 2016. Over the years, they have seen a move away from consensus to evidence based knowledge [15].

The development of these criteria's has eased the diagnostic process, especially for IBS, the commonest type of functional bowel disorder. IBS has now become a positive diagnosis rather than being a 'diagnosis of exclusion'. Rome criteria to diagnose IBS are shown in Figure 1.

Apart from IBS, Rome criteria define the other FGIDs shown in Table 1. Although these criteria are increasingly becoming the diagnostic pillars, clinicians are still required to consider various other important aspects to complete the much bigger picture. It is imperative to have a thorough and a systematic approach while diagnosing FGIDs which lacks anatomic and physiologic markers.

Pre Clinic Work Up

An overview of patient's previous illnesses and co-morbidities along with history of previous specialist consultations especially for 'medically unexplained' symptoms, is generally a helpful starting point when dealing with FGIDs. There is often a pattern of patients seeking

Recurrent abdominal pain or discomfort, at least three days per month in the past three months, with symptom onset at least six months prior to diagnosis associated with two or more of the following:

1. Improvement of symptoms with defecation
2. Onset associated with a change in frequency of stool
3. Onset associated with a change in stool consistency and appearance

FIGURE 1 Rome III Criteria

numerous previous consultations and nonexistence of such a pattern would (possibly counterintuitively) indicate the possibility of organic underlying pathology. This process helps getting insight into patient's psyche and how they have responded to treatment so far. Demographic details are also quite useful in these disorders, for instance IBS is commonly seen in young to middle aged females whereas new abdominal symptoms above age of 50 raise concerns of colonic cancer and prompt further investigations. It has also been shown to be less prevalent in Asian countries than in the west [30,43].

First Consultation

In a clinical scenario, the key to diagnosing FGID is careful history taking. The clinic consultation offers a good opportunity to discern not only the main symptoms but also the psychological issues associated with FGIDs. A good consultation using open-ended questionnaires will put patients at ease and allow them to describe their symptoms clearly. Portraying a positive body language and appearing 'unhurried' is essential to make patients feel empathized with. It is important to ensure that the consultation allows sufficient time for psychosocial history to come to light as psychological distress has been associated with FGIDs [29,39]. Another reason to discuss this aspect is the fact that it has been proven to reduce return visits to the clinic by making the patient feel that they have been listened to [53]. As well as eliciting the psychological aspects, the clinic appointment should also be used to exclude any red flag symptoms that may warrant further investigations. Dietary precipitants should also be enquired about as should be any infectious precursors to the start of symptoms.

Somatization and Co-Morbidities

One of the most challenging facets of managing functional disorder patients is the high incidence of multiple co-morbidities. These include psychological disorders such as somatization disorder as well as involvement of other bodily systems. Non-cardiac chest pain has been associated with IBS [62]and functional dyspepsia(FD) has been associated with general pain, sleep disorders and osteoarthritis [72]. Due to somatization these patients are subjected to numerous unnecessary investigations and treatments [12,21,57]. Accurate documentation of co-morbidities and previous hospital attendances is vital to identify patients with somatization disorder. These patients have been reported to be more challenging to manage and having a poorer response to conventional treatments [26,52]. The Patient Health Questionnaire 15 (PHQ-15) has been shown to be a useful tool in identifying this group of patients which may warrant specific treatment [35].

Precipitating Events

A relation between FGIDs and precipitating event such as severe adverse life events and chronic stressors, infection and dietary factors, has been reported in several studies. Importance of psychosocial history has already been discussed in the chapter. Recognition of chronic stressors has been shown to be significant in predicting success of treatment [5]. Infectious pathology has been reported to be associated with IBS [60], functional dyspepsia [54] and other functional bowel disorders [67]. A documented history of an infectious episode is quintessential in avoiding needless investigations, in absence of any red flag symptoms. Dietary elements should also be routinely investigated as they are known to be associated with certain FGIDs. For instance, bran seems to worsen symptoms in IBS [22], lactose intolerance can cause IBS-like symptoms [41] and symptoms of functional dyspepsia improve by consuming smaller meals with reduced fat content [55].

Drugs

A complete drug history is important since many drugs, including over the counter medications, can mimic IBS symptoms. Particular attention should be paid to opiates, which cause constipation [49], antibiotics which cause diarrhoea and proton pump inhibitors (PPIs) which can also cause diarrhoea due to microscopic colitis [11,32,50,58,70]. Probiotics are widely used and some have a laxative effect [3] so it is always worth specifically enquiring if they are being taken since many patients do not regard them as drugs. Other rare causes of diarrhoea due to medications are cardiac medications: angiotensin converting enzyme inhibitors [64], beta-blockers, drugs affecting the central nervous system, lithium and carbamazepine [20,24], weight control medication, and lipase inhibitors[1,19].

PRACTICAL IMPLICATIONS

In patients presenting with abdominal and pelvic pain with no alarming symptoms and where no organic cause can be established, FGIDs should be considered as an alternative diagnosis. The clinician should make all efforts to develop an empathetic relationship with their patients. Patient's trust should be won by discussing the challenging nature of these disorders in a positive manner and by agreeing to the legitimacy of patient's symptoms. The psychosocial aspect constitutes an important part of these disorders and should be properly explored to manage the patient appropriately. Moreover, patients should be informed of the biopsychosocial model of these disorders, e.g. a stress or vicious-circle model.

Setting up realistic goals for treatment so that the patient aims for improvement rather than cure is essential for success of the treatment. In general, pharmacotherapy and psychotherapy have not been found to be the most effective treatments for functional disorders, yet they do produce impressive results in a few individuals. The therapeutic options should be chosen based on severity of patient's symptoms, patient's preferences and psyche, physician's own expertise, and the availability of different treatment options.

LOOKING AT THE FUTURE

FGIDs are challenging disorders mainly due to the traditional practice of conceptualizing a disease by associating it to identifiable defects. Further research is vital to develop a better understanding of these disorders and their treatment. Increasing awareness amongst clinicians and educating the general public on this rapidly growing knowledge is one of the key areas for development. While the diagnostic modality needs further development, the management of these disorders requiring different specialties needs an even more radical change in order to reduce the socioeconomic burden of these disorders.

The traditional delineation of "functional" versus "organic" is very likely to fade away in the future as the pathophysiology of these diseases is discovered.

TAKE HOME MESSAGES

- Functional bowel disorders are distinct clinical entities having a chronic and benign nature.
- Their development is most likely due to an interaction of somatic and psychosocial disease factors.
- There is a need for creating more awareness of these disorders amongst the primary care physicians in order to reduce their socioeconomic burden on the society
- It is important to communicate the diagnosis to patients in a positive and persuasive communication so as to maintain the legitimacy of the patient's complaints and uproot their efforts to find an organic cause
- The diagnosis and treatment should be according to current guidelines

FURTHER READING

Rome III Diagnostic Criteria for Functional Gastrointestinal Disorders http://www.romecriteria.org/assets/pdf/19_RomeIII_apA_885-898.pdf

REFERENCES

1. Acharya NV, Wilton LV, Shakir SA. Safety profile of orlistat: results of a prescription-event monitoring study. Int J Obes (Lond) 2006;30(11):1645–1652.
2. Ackerknecht EH. A Short history of medicine Baltimore, Johns Hopkins UP, 1982.
3. Agrawal A, Houghton LA, Morris J, et al. Clinical trial: the effects of a fermented milk product containing Bifidobacterium lactis DN-173 010 on abdominal distension and gastrointestinal transit in irritable bowel syndrome with constipation. Aliment Pharmacol Therapeut 2009;29(1):104–114.
4. Barbezat G, Poulton R, Milne B, et al. Prevalence and correlates of irritable bowel symptoms in a New Zealand birth cohort. N Z Med J 2002;115(1164):U220.
5. Bennett EJ, Tennant CC, Piesse C, et al. Level of chronic life stress predicts clinical outcome in irritable bowel syndrome. Gut 1998;43(2):256–261.
6. Bommelaer G, Dorval E, Denis P, et al. Prevalence of irritable bowel syndrome in the French population according to the Rome I criteria. Gastroenterol Clin Biol 2002;26(12):1118–1123.
7. Bouchoucha M, Devroede G, Dorval E, et al. Different segmental transit times in patients with irritable bowel syndrome and "normal" colonic transit time: is there a correlation with symptoms? Tech Coloproctol 2006;10(4):287–296.
8. Brown PW. The irritable bowel syndrome. Rocky Mountain Med J 1950;47(5):343–346.
9. Camilleri CE, Carlson PJ, Camilleri M, et al. A study of candidate genotypes associated with dyspepsia in a U.S. community. Am J Gastroenterol 2006;101(3):581–592.
10. Chadwick VS, Chen W, Shu D, et al. Activation of the mucosal immune system in irritable bowel syndrome. Gastroenterology 2002;122(7):1778–1783.
11. Chande N, Driman DK. Microscopic colitis associated with lansoprazole: report of two cases and a review of the literature. Scand J Gastroenterol 2007;42(4):530–533.
12. Cole JA, Yeaw JM, Cutone JA, et al. The incidence of abdominal and pelvic surgery among patients with irritable bowel syndrome. Dig Dis Sci 2005;50(12):2268–2275.
13. Colin-Jones D, Bloom B, Bodemar G, et al. MANAGEMENT OF DYSPEPSIA: REPORT OF A WORKING PARTY. Lancet 1988;331(8585):576–579.
14. Collins SM. Is the irritable gut an inflamed gut? Scand J Gastroenterol Suppl 1992;192:102–105.
15. Drossman DA. The functional gastrointestinal disorders and the Rome III process. Gastroenterology 2006;130(5):1377–1390.
16. Drossman DA, Li Z, Andruzzi E, et al. U.S. householder survey of functional gastrointestinal disorders. Prevalence, sociodemography, and health impact. Dig Dis Sci 1993;38(9):1569–1580.
17. Everhart JE, Renault PF. Irritable bowel syndrome in office-based practice in the United States. Gastroenterology 1991;100(4):998–1005.
18. Farre R, Vanheel H, Vanuytsel T, et al. In functional dyspepsia, hypersensitivity to postprandial distention correlates with meal-related symptom severity. Gastroenterology 2013;145(3):566–573.

19. Filippatos TD, Derdemezis CS, Gazi IF, et al. Orlistat-associated adverse effects and drug interactions: a critical review. Drug Saf 2008;31(1):53–65.
20. Fosnes GS, Lydersen S, Farup PG. Constipation and diarrhoea - common adverse drug reactions? A cross sectional study in the general population. BMC Clin Pharmacol 2011;11:2.
21. Francis CY, Duffy JN, Whorwell PJ, Morris J. High prevalence of irritable bowel syndrome in patients attending urological outpatient departments. Dig Dis Sci 1997;42(2):404–407.
22. Francis CY, Whorwell PJ. Bran and irritable bowel syndrome: time for reappraisal. Lancet 1994;344(8914):39–40.
23. Gonsalkorale WM, Perrey C, Pravica V, et al. Interleukin 10 genotypes in irritable bowel syndrome: evidence for an inflammatory component? Gut 2003;52(1):91–93.
24. Grandjean EM, Aubry JM. Lithium: updated human knowledge using an evidence-based approach: part III: clinical safety. CNS Drugs 2009;23(5):397–418.
25. Halvorson HA, Schlett CD, Riddle MS. Postinfectious irritable bowel syndrome--a meta-analysis. Am J Gastroenterol 2006;101(8):1894–1899; quiz 1942.
26. Harris AM, Orav EJ, Bates DW, Barsky AJ. Somatization increases disability independent of comorbidity. J Gen Intern Med 2009;24(2):155–161.
27. Harvey R, Salih SY, Read A. ORGANIC AND FUNCTIONAL DISORDERS IN 2000 GASTROENTEROLOGY OUTPATIENTS. Lancet 1983;321(8325):632–634.
28. Hata T, Kato M, Kudo T, et al. Comparison of gastric relaxation and sensory functions between functional dyspepsia and healthy subjects using novel drinking-ultrasonography test. Digestion 2013;87(1):34–39.
29. Herschbach P, Henrich G, von Rad M. Psychological factors in functional gastrointestinal disorders: characteristics of the disorder or of the illness behavior? Psychosom Med 1999;61(2):148–153.
30. Hu WH, Wong WM, Lam CL, et al. Anxiety but not depression determines health care-seeking behaviour in Chinese patients with dyspepsia and irritable bowel syndrome: a population-based study. Aliment Pharmacol Ther 2002;16(12):2081–2088.
31. Kassinen A, Krogius-Kurikka L, Makivuokko H, et al. The fecal microbiota of irritable bowel syndrome patients differs significantly from that of healthy subjects. Gastroenterology 2007;133(1):24–33.
32. Keszthelyi D, Jansen SV, Schouten GA, et al. Proton pump inhibitor use is associated with an increased risk for microscopic colitis: a case-control study. Aliment Pharmacol Ther 2010;32(9):1124–1128.
33. Koloski NA, Jones M, Kalantar J, et al. The brain--gut pathway in functional gastrointestinal disorders is bidirectional: a 12-year prospective population-based study. Gut 2012;61(9):1284–1290.
34. Koloski NA, Talley NJ, Boyce PM. Epidemiology and health care seeking in the functional GI disorders: a population-based study. Am J Gastroenterol 2002;97(9):2290–2299.
35. Kroenke K, Spitzer RL, Williams JB. The PHQ-15: validity of a new measure for evaluating the severity of somatic symptoms. Psychosom Med 2002;64(2):258–266.
36. Kruis W, Thieme C, Weinzierl M, et al. A diagnostic score for the irritable bowel syndrome. Its value in the exclusion of organic disease. Gastroenterology 1984;87(1):1–7.
37. Levy RL, Jones KR, Whitehead WE, et al. Irritable bowel syndrome in twins: heredity and social learning both contribute to etiology. Gastroenterology 2001;121(4):799–804.
38. Levy RL, Whitehead WE, Von Korff MR, Feld AD. Intergenerational transmission of gastrointestinal illness behavior. Am J Gastroenterol 2000;95(2):451–456.
39. Locke GR, 3rd, Weaver AL, Melton LJ, 3rd, Talley NJ. Psychosocial factors are linked to functional gastrointestinal disorders: a population based nested case-control study. Am J Gastroenterol 2004;99(2):350–357.
40. Locke GR, 3rd, Zinsmeister AR, Talley NJ, et al. Familial association in adults with functional gastrointestinal disorders. Mayo Clin Proc Mayo Clin 2000;75(9):907–912.
41. Lomer MC, Parkes GC, Sanderson JD. Review article: lactose intolerance in clinical practice--myths and realities. Aliment Pharmacol Ther 2008;27(2):93–103.
42. Longstreth GF, Thompson WG, Chey WD, et al. Functional bowel disorders. Gastroenterology 2006;130(5):1480–1491.
43. Longstreth GF, Wolde-Tsadik G. Irritable bowel-type symptoms in HMO examinees. Prevalence, demographics, and clinical correlates. Dig Dis Sci 1993;38(9):1581–1589.
44. Manabe N, Wong BS, Camilleri M, et al. Lower functional gastrointestinal disorders: evidence of abnormal colonic transit in a 287 patient cohort. Neurogastroenterol Motil 2010;22(3):293-e282.
45. Manning AP, Thompson WG, Heaton KW, Morris AF. Towards positive diagnosis of the irritable bowel. Br Med J 1978;2(6138):653–654.
46. Maxwell PR, Rink E, Kumar D, Mendall MA. Antibiotics increase functional abdominal symptoms. Am J Gastroenterol 2002;97(1):104–108.

47. Mearin F, Badia X, Balboa A, et al. Irritable bowel syndrome prevalence varies enormously depending on the employed diagnostic criteria: comparison of Rome II versus previous criteria in a general population. Scand J Gastroenterol 2001;36(11):1155–1161.
48. Moayyedi P, Soo S, Deeks J, et al. Eradication of Helicobacter pylori for non-ulcer dyspepsia. Cochrane Database Syst Rev 2003(1):CD002096.
49. Moore RA, McQuay HJ. Prevalence of opioid adverse events in chronic non-malignant pain: systematic review of randomised trials of oral opioids. Arthritis Res Ther 2005;7(5):R1046–1051.
50. Mukherjee S. Diarrhea associated with lansoprazole. J Gastroenterol Hepatol 2003;18(5):602–603.
51. Nobaek S, Johansson ML, Molin G, et al. Alteration of intestinal microflora is associated with reduction in abdominal bloating and pain in patients with irritable bowel syndrome. Am J Gastroenterol 2000;95(5):1231–1238.
52. North CS, Downs D, Clouse RE, et al. The presentation of irritable bowel syndrome in the context of somatization disorder. Clin Gastroenterol Hepatol 2004;2(9):787–795.
53. Owens DM, Nelson DK, Talley NJ. The irritable bowel syndrome: long-term prognosis and the physician-patient interaction. Ann Int Med 1995;122(2):107–112.
54. Pike BL, Porter CK, Sorrell TJ, Riddle MS. Acute gastroenteritis and the risk of functional dyspepsia: a systematic review and meta-analysis. Am J Gastroenterol 2013;108(10):1558–1563; quiz 1564.
55. Pilichiewicz AN, Horowitz M, Holtmann GJ, et al. Relationship between symptoms and dietary patterns in patients with functional dyspepsia. Clin Gastroenterol Hepatol 2009;7(3):317–322.
56. Pimentel M, Chow EJ, Lin HC. Normalization of lactulose breath testing correlates with symptom improvement in irritable bowel syndrome. a double-blind, randomized, placebo-controlled study. Am J Gastroenterol 2003;98(2):412–419.
57. Prior A, Wilson K, Whorwell PJ, Faragher EB. Irritable bowel syndrome in the gynecological clinic. Survey of 798 new referrals. Dig Dis Sci 1989;34(12):1820–1824.
58. Rammer M, Kirchgatterer A, Hobling W, Knoflach P. Lansoprazole-associated collagenous colitis: a case report. Z Gastroenterol 2005;43(7):657–660.
59. Ringel Y. Brain research in functional gastrointestinal disorders. J Clin Gastroenterol 2002;35(1 Suppl):S23–25.
60. Rodríguez LAG, Ruigómez A. Increased risk of irritable bowel syndrome after bacterial gastroenteritis: cohort study. BMJ 1999;318(7183):565–566.
61. Saito YA. The role of genetics in IBS. Gastroenterol Clin North Am 2011;40(1):45–67.
62. Scott A, Mihailidou A, Smith R, et al. Functional gastrointestinal disorders in unselected patients with non-cardiac chest pain. Scand J Gastroenterol 1993;28(7):585–590.
63. Serra J, Azpiroz F, Malagelada J-R. Impaired transit and tolerance of intestinal gas in the irritable bowel syndrome. Gut 2001;48(1):14–19.
64. Simpson K, Jarvis B. Lisinopril: a review of its use in congestive heart failure. Drugs 2000;59(5):1149–1167.
65. Spiegel BM, Farid M, Esrailian E, et al. Is irritable bowel syndrome a diagnosis of exclusion?: a survey of primary care providers, gastroenterologists, and IBS experts. Am J Gastroenterol 2010;105(4):848–858.
66. Talley NJ, Zinsmeister AR, Schleck CD, Melton LJ, 3rd. Dyspepsia and dyspepsia subgroups: a population-based study. Gastroenterology 1992;102(4 Pt 1):1259–1268.
67. Thabane M, Simunovic M, Akhtar-Danesh N, et al. Clustering and stability of functional lower gastrointestinal symptom after enteric infection. Neurogastroenterol Motil 2012;24(6):546–552, e252.
68. Thompson WG, Irvine EJ, Pare P, et al. Functional gastrointestinal disorders in Canada: first population-based survey using Rome II criteria with suggestions for improving the questionnaire. Dig Dis Sci 2002;47(1):225–235.
69. Thompson WG, Longstreth GF, Drossman DA, et al. Functional bowel disorders and functional abdominal pain. Gut 1999;45(suppl 2):II43-II47.
70. Thomson RD, Lestina LS, Bensen SP, et al. Lansoprazole-associated microscopic colitis: a case series. Am J Gastroenterol 2002;97(11):2908–2913.
71. Van Oudenhove L, Demyttenaere K, Tack J, Aziz Q. Central nervous system involvement in functional gastrointestinal disorders. Best Pract Res Clinical Gastroenterol 2004;18(4):663–680.
72. Wallander MA, Johansson S, Ruigomez A, et al. Dyspepsia in general practice: incidence, risk factors, comorbidity and mortality. Family Pract 2007;24(5):403–411.

CHAPTER 19

Anorectal Dysfunction and Chronic Pain

Marc Beer-Gabel

INTRODUCTION

The anus and the rectum are two different parts of the large intestinal tract, which have distinct physiology, function, and innervation. Their physiological role consists of controlling continence and defecation during bowel movement, a complex function that involves the activity of other pelvic organs and nearby muscles. The normal function of the anorectum is mainly unconscious, regulated by the autonomic nervous system, except for the final phase of defecation, which involves a conscious action via the central nervous system (CNS). Alteration of anorectal function can result in pain, which may be mechanical, chemical or neuropathic and can originate in the pelvic viscera or the pelvi-perineal muscles, whose innervations project to the same spinal cord segments. Chronic pain only develops when anorectal dysfunction occurs most of the time or during a prolonged period of time. In this context, neuroplastic changes in the nervous system ensue owing to stimulation of pain receptors (nociceptors) by innocuous inputs, which activate pain circuits, resulting in less inhibition and central amplification of pain-derived signals. The dysfunction may be mechanical, chemical or neuropathic. The pain may originate in the pelvic viscera or the pelvi-perineal muscles, whose innervations project to the spinal cord segments. Because pain is a subjective and complex experience with sensitive, cognitive, emotional and motivational elements, it should be considered real and be treated whether the dysfunction is based on mechanical or psychological dysfunction.

In this chapter, we will discuss chronic pain derived from anorectal dysfunction and the development of painful dysfunction from a normal anorectal state. An introduction to the normal anatomy and physiology of the anus and the rectum will help us describe its connection with the CNS and other pelvic organs to explain in detail the onset and development of chronic pain, its reciprocal effect on anorectal function and potential treatments.

BASIC ASPECTS

Anatomy of the Anorectum

The Anus

The anal canal is 4–5 cm in length and is the distal part of the colon, extending from the anorectal junction to the anal margin [5]. It contains two sphincters that overlap in the mid-anal canal and keep the lumen closed during continence. .The external anal sphincter is a voluntary, cylindrical striated muscle located distally in the anus and is about 4 mm thick as measured by endoluminal ultrasound. Whereas its posterior fibers connect to the tail bone through the anococcygeal ligament, some of the anterior fibers decussate into the superficial transverse perineal muscles and perineal body to attach the anal canal to the pubic bone. The proximal external sphincter is intimately related to the puborectalis muscle, which creates a posterior sling. The internal anal sphincter is an involuntary, smooth muscle structure located in the proximal 2/3 of the anus and the distal end of the inner circular muscle layer of the rectum [45].

The anus is normally closed to prevent leakage of fluids or gas. The internal anal sphincter, the external sphincter, and the haemorrhoidal cushion contribute to the permanent resting pressure in the anus (55%, 30%, and 15%, respectively) [21]. The puborectal muscle displays some resting tone; however, it contracts as a reflex in response to a brisk increase in intra-abdominal pressure thereby preventing incontinence. The external sphincter is a muscle under voluntary control that predominantly consists of slow-twitch fibers, capable of prolonged contraction. Its innervation comes from the inferior rectal branch of the pudendal nerve located in S2 and S3, and the perineal branch of the fourth sacral nerve. It has a dual somatic innervation by the levator ani nerve on its superior surface (S3-S4) and by the pudendal nerve.

In contrast to the colorectum, the anal canal is extremely sensitive to touch, pin prick, temperature and movements within the lumen [31]. Specific sensory receptors are therefore numerous, with the afferent nerve pathway for anal sensation coming from inferior hemorrhoidal branches of the pudendal nerve to S2–S4.

The Rectum

The rectum, which is located in the pelvis, begins at the level of the sacral promontory and extends distally to the anus, thus representing the end of the colon. The rectum has three submucosal folds called the valves of Houston, and acts as a reservoir for stool and as a pump to defecate. It has a double innervation through the pelvic plexuses on both sides of the rectum with the sympathetic innervation originating from lumbar regions L1–L3 and the parasympathetic nerves coming from sacral S2-S4 (nervi erigentes). The pelvic plexus then innervates not only the rectum but also the urinary and genital organs with both parasympathetic and sympathetic fibres.

Rectal sensation is transmitted by various receptors at different levels of the rectal wall. For example, rectal intraganglionic laminar endings (rIGLEs) are mechanoreceptors that respond to tension and rapid distension; other mucosal afferents that are both mechano and chemosensitive have been described [32].

Normal Anorectal Function

Continence and Defecation

Anal continence is achieved by a complex mechanism involving sphincters, pelvic muscles, visceral sensation and operates under the control of the autonomic and central nervous system. At rest, the anal pressure, which is higher than the rectal pressure, is responsible for continence. There is a causal relation between the post prandial increase of food residue and elevation of the abdominal pressure. Immediately before abdominal pressure is elevated and during contraction of the distal colon while propelling the stool to the rectum, the anus closure is enhanced through elevation of the pressure of the external sphincter and the puborectalis to maintain the continence. This normal anorectal sensation must be preserved to learn to postpone the urge to defecate when needed.

Once the rectal reservoir is stretched, the rectal pressure increases and the defecation process can begin. Upon relaxation of the internal sphincter (recto anal inhibitory reflex), the rectal contents progress into the upper anal canal, which allows the discrimination of solid from liquid and gaseous luminal contents. This process is finally followed by the conscious need to defecate, which is allowed by stimulation of the parasympathetic nerves, indicating that the rectal function involves a complex sensory-motor coordination.

Coordination of Pelvic Organs During Complex Functions: The Horizontal Links

Complex functions involving different organs and structures, such as defecation, micturition and sexual intercourse, are possible due to a higher level of cooperation between the different organs involved and the integration of signals by the CNS. The coordination needed for these functions emphasizes the importance of crosstalk between the pelvic organs. The pelvic organs are selectively activated according to the function they exert; for instance, the anus closes during sexual intercourse. During urination in humans, rising of the intraluminal pressure of the urinary bladder produces contractions of the anal sphincter, preventing defecation [4]; similarly, the urinary system is inhibited during defecation in humans, as functional stimulation of the anal sphincter inhibits detrusor muscle contraction which is involved in bladder emptying [13].

Because of this level of interactions and functional coordination between various systems, a pathological condition in one pelvic or visceral organ can affect the normal function of another organ. For example, some patients who suffer from irritable bowel syndrome have micturition problems, such as urinary incontinence [53]. Both the peripheral nervous system and CNS probably mediate the neural mechanisms underlying the interactions between the various pelvic and visceral organs. These complex visceral functions are controlled by viscerovisceral convergence within the CNS, both in the spinal cord itself, in which different viscera are stimulated by afferent dichotomized nerves [37] as well as in the brain.

DESCRIBING THE SUBJECT

Integration of Anorectal Sensations in The CNS: The Vertical Links

As previously described, the rectum and the anus have different innervation patterns but also differ in sensitivity. The afferent innervation of the rectum consists of C fibres and A-delta fibres which are only sensitive to distension [39]. A-delta fibres are spread in the rectal mucosa [47] and respond to changes in rectal distension [33], whereas the C fibres endings are mainly located within the muscular wall of the rectum and are activated by the intensity of rectal distension. The rectum and internal anal sphincter have an autonomic innervation through the inferior hypogastric plexus. Sensations from the rectum are poorly localized, often referred to somatic structures and result in greater autonomic response than with somatic sensation [39,47].

The external anal sphincter and levator ani muscle in the anal canal are under the control of the peripheral somatic nervous system (pudendal nerve) [38]. The presence of a high density of specialized receptors and afferent pathways allows for discrimination between different types of sensation, resulting in well-localized sensations at the level of the anal canal, in contrast to the rectum. These differences between rectal and anal sensation are partly based on the differences in their peripheral innervation and possibly to differences in their cortical representation [15].

The brain areas that control and process ano-rectal sensations, include those involved in spatial discrimination (primary and secondary somatosensory cortices SI and SII) and those that process affective and cognitive aspects of sensation (anterior cingular cortex, insula and prefrontal cortex) [16]. However, there are differences between the areas of somatosensory cortex responsible for processing the visceral and somatic components of sensation. The visceral sensation is processed in the inferior part of the SI, whereas somatic sensation is located in higher areas of the SI. The SII, which receives afferents from the SI [42], is activated by both rectal and anal stimulation; however, when the rectal stimulation is not painful the anterior cingulate cortex (ACC) is activated. The differences explained above may explain why a visceral stimulation induces autonomic reactions, whereas somatic stimulation triggers conscious reactions [39].

From Normal Function to Dysfunction and Pain

Normal Function and Some Alterations are Innocuous

The anus and the rectum are both active during continence and defecation, without any pain in the physiological situation. Most of the time the gastrointestinal sensory-motor functions are unconscious, although they can also be painful depending on certain factors such as acidity levels, intestinal contraction, and food composition. Only a few sensations, including postprandial fullness and the urge to defecate upon increased stool accumulation, become conscious, maybe because of their behavioral consequences. For instance, the feeling of incomplete defecation will trigger recurrent defecation efforts even when the rectum is actually empty.

Dysfunctions such as constipation, diarrhea and incontinence are occasionally painful, although different mechanisms can lead to functional alterations [14,35,30]. In a group of 67 patients with constipation, 24% had functional constipation, 27% showed pelvic floor dysfunction, and 49% were diagnosed with irritable bowel syndrome with constipation (IBS-C) [14]. Notably, there are often changes in diagnosis of this type of dysfunction; thus, after 12 months, a third of functional constipated patients developed IBS-C and a third of IBS-C reverted to functional constipation [54]. Anorectal dysfunctions can therefore vary over time within the same patient and may be associated with or without pain.

From Innocuous to Noxious Sensations and Development of Pain

In 1973, Ritchie J first described pain after mechanical distension of the rectum in patients with IBS, by showing that a balloon of 60 ml in the rectum caused pain in 55% of patients with IBS compared to 6% of the controls [44]. These results have been confirmed in many other studies [8,34,52].

The low threshold for pain is considered a hallmark of IBS in 20–90% of the cases [12,34]. Repetitive rectal stimulation in patients with IBS induces rectal hyperalgesia and viscerosomatic referral [36], suggesting that rectal hypersensitivity induced by repetitive distension, could be a reliable marker for IBS [40]. Pain, during repetitive rectal mechanical stimulation can differentiate patients with IBS from functional abdominal pain patients, as the latter do not have visceral hypersensitivity. Balloon distension of the colon or contraction of the muscle by a spasm distends the mechanoreceptors located in the intestinal circular muscle layer and can elicit firing of impulses by these receptors which are transmitted via sensory afferent fibres. This may explain the pain that occurs in the postprandial period when the bowel is distended by the bolus as well as the pain during a bowel spastic reaction upon stress, which may mimic an urge to defecate and induce recurrent need to strain.

Visceral hypersensitivity in IBS is not related to abnormal distensibility of the gut wall but rather to a lower threshold for pain. The pain detection thresholds to electrical stimuli at the rectosigmoid junction were lower in the IBS patients compared to control subjects [19]. The enhanced perception of innocuous peripheral stimuli or pain at a lower threshold for mechanical or electrical stimulation in patients with IBS suggests abnormal processing of sensory information at the peripheral level or in the CNS. Use of local rectal anaesthetics reduces rectal and somatic pain in IBS patients, hinting at the possibility that visceral hyperalgesia and secondary cutaneous hyperalgesia in IBS could be owing to central sensitization dynamically maintained by input from the gastrointestinal tract [51]. Hypersensitivity in IBS patients may involve the whole gastrointestinal system, from the oesophagus [50] and the stomach [56] to the small bowel [1]. For instance, distal oesophageal acid instillation in healthy patients resulted in increased rectal sensitivity upon balloon distension [22]

Hypersensitivity may also affect organs other than the gut and an extension of pain or dysfunction may be seen in other pelvic organs, supporting again the crosstalk between these organs. For example, sigmoid colon hypersensitivity has been shown in women with dysmenorrhea [10] and numerous patients with IBS complained of pain in body regions distant from the gut, including the head and neck [53]. Several recent studies have also demonstrated widespread somatic hyperalgesia in patients with IBS [9,43,51]. Conditions that have a common etiology of central sensitization, such as chronic fatigue, low back pain, chronic tension-type headache, migraine, temporomandibular joint disease, major depression, panic attacks and post-traumatic stress disorder are found in patients with IBS more often than expected [2,49,46,29].

Pathophysiology of Anorectal Pain

Sensitization: The Name of the Game

After injury, an acute pain ensues, which is transient and lasts until the wound is healed. This is considered a nociceptive pain caused by activation of nerve endings or nociceptors (pain receptors), which are normally characterized by a high threshold to stimulation. Chronic pain is different, as it is associated with either, peripheral tissue damage and inflammation or with lesions to the nervous system. During chronic pain, there is a persistent hypersensitivity, due to central sensitisation even in the absence of any obvious current peripheral stimulus, that enhances the responsiveness of nociceptors to a painful stimulus, such as the urge to defecate, post prandial fullness or acid reflux (hyperalgesia), and reduces the sensory threshold so non-noxious function becomes painful, such as defecation (allodynia). This is considered sensitization of the periphery and the CNS.

Two parallel pathways normally transmit the sensory input from the periphery to the CNS: nerves that transmit low intensity stimuli that elicit innocuous responses and high intensity stimuli that activate nociceptors at the site of damage and transmit these signals to the CNS, leading to pain. During central sensitization in sensory pathways, there is an amplification of the pain response of neurons to noxious stimuli, so that signals from low threshold sensory fibers can also activate the pain circuit. The two parallel sensory pathways converge in the posterior dorsal horn [55] so normal function and dysfunction can become painful.

Peripheral noxious stimuli can elicit pain via nociceptors, which are often polymodal and can thus be activated by mechanical (spasms) or chemical (released inflammatory mediators e.g. substance P, cytokines, histamine, potassium, prostaglandins and free radicals) stimuli. Due to the effect of the 'inflammatory soup' in the periphery, silent c-fibers will become sensitive to mechanical stimuli for instance. This process of sensitization results in viscerosomatic convergence [7] and the pain is now perceived to originate from a somatic area that projects on the same dorsal roots as the visceral afferent fibers innervating the affected organs. Afferent fibers to the dorsal horn fire antidromically (towards the injured organs) inducing a state of neuroinflammation in the periphery [41]. Another effect of the up-regulation of these silent visceral nociceptors is the pelvic viscera crosstalk between those organs that have shared innervation via a spinal cord reflex, an inflamed organ could cause neuroinflammation in a neighboring viscera [26].

During distention of a hollow organ such as the rectum or the sigmoid colon, there are also abnormal visceromuscular reflexes, which result in contraction of muscles of the abdomen, trunk and the limbs. This may explain why a patient can develop muscular pain as a result of visceral sensitization. In this context, if the pain persists in the viscera, a myofascial pain syndrome may develop with trigger points in referred muscles, which can complicate the pain sensation in the patient. Even after the visceral pain disappears, the muscular hyperalgesia can persist. Conversely, hyperactivity of the pelvic floor can give rise to visceral dysfunction, such as urinary urgency, constipation, and dyspareunia [11].

Levator Ani Syndrome Contributes to Anorectal Pain

A chronic muscular pain is similar to visceral pain in that it is poorly localized, becomes severe if the dysfunction of the muscle persists and extends to other muscles and may be referred to viscera. In 1859, Simpson JY first described the levator ani syndrome, which is a type of chronic proctalgia that includes tenderness during posterior traction of the puborectalis muscle and a painful sensation that is acutely perceived in the pelvis. It was also called levator spasm, puborectal syndrome because of its relation to muscle spasm as described later by Thiele GH [48]. The pain is dull and involves a sensation of the presence of a ball in the rectum, which is exacerbated by prolonged sitting. In the general population, the prevalence of such symptoms is about 6.6%, although it is more frequent among middle age women and symptoms decrease in individuals over 45.

Although its aetiology remains unclear, clinical examination in patients suffering from levator ani syndrome have shown that it may be owing to inflammation of the tendon arc of the levator ani muscle or to a myofascial pain syndrome. Often, palpation shows taut bands and trigger points related to pain associated to this syndrome. The syndrome is diagnosed if the pain is chronic or recurrent, pain episodes last for more than 20 minutes and if other causes of organic anorectal pain are excluded. If the posterior traction of the puborectalis muscle does not lead to pain, the functional anorectal pain is unspecified.

The type of pain caused by levator ani syndrome is classified as 'rectal pain' however, this is misleading as it is a muscular pain, not a visceral pain. Rectal pain is commonly felt in the left abdomen although it may also be projected in the sacral S3 area in healthy individuals [44,20]; in IBS, the pain may reach the thoracic area on the right side [44]. In levator ani syndrome, the pain is frequently localized in the muscle itself, although it often extends to other perineal and gluteal muscles. Anorectal pain is called proctalgia in the rome III classification. This pain is related to myofascial pain (levator ani syndrome). Chronic proctalgia is divided by the rome III criteria into two subtypes, namely levator ani syndrome (las) and unspecified functional anorectal pain. The diversion is based on the presence or absence of a sensation of tenderness when the levator muscle is palpated during digital rectal examination. So the term "rectal pain" used by the patient often represents a muscular pain. Rectal pain that is perceived as a result of distension of a balloon in the rectum is projected in different territories (visceral pain).

Direct trauma, regional surgery, and stress that induce chronic muscle contraction may trigger the syndrome. The musculoskeletal dysfunction that develops as a consequence of the prolonged contraction may be the primary factor of chronic pelvic pain [3]; however, these muscular pains may also be associated with pelvic organ dysfunctions. In fact, an association between levator ani syndrome and interstitial cystitis has been shown [6], and IBS is linked to chronic pelvic pain and myofascial pain. A visceromuscular convergence of different nerves at the same dorsal horn level may account for the type of visceral pain caused by the levator ani syndrome.

Aside from levator ani syndrome, unspecified functional anorectal pain may also be related to other muscle conditions that refer pain to the pelvic floor, such as sacroiliac joint dysfunction, piriformis syndrome, pubococcygeus overactivity, coccyx pain syndrome or prostate pain syndrome.

Impaired Defecation Worsens Anorectal Pain

Patients incapable of relaxing the perineal muscles or suffering from prolonged contraction of the puborectalis and the external anal sphincter during defecation, need to engage abdominal muscles to add pressure to the abdomino-pelvic cavity and overcome the high anal pressure [28]. This can cause muscular lesions during which muscle fibre contractions can compress local blood vessels, impairing the arterial flow, the supply of oxygen, calcium, and nutrients necessary to meet the high energy demands required by sustained muscle contraction. Inflammatory mediators and histamine are released locally, which sensitize the muscle nociceptors group III (A delta) and IV (C) afferent fibres so their mechanical activation threshold is reduced. As a result progressive muscle hyperalgesia and mechanical allodynia ensue, innocuous pressure or normal muscle contraction is perceived as painful. There is a vicious cycle leading to muscle shortening, causing further deterioration of the oxygen supply resulting in myofascial trigger points and referred pain.

Clinically, the pain occurs shortly after defecation and may persists for hours. Often the pain worsens in a sitting position. The same positional factor is noted in cases of pudendal neuralgia. Sitting may stretch the nerve on ligaments or boney structures. The painful sensation is often maximal at the end of the day. Musculoskeletal dysfunction or certain positions can aggravate the pain and if the situation persists, individuals may complain of outlet blockage, such as obstructive defecation, bloating, abdominal distension and emptying disorders.

The Relevance of Viscero-Muscular Convergence in Anorectal Pain

Visceral distension may elicit muscular pain. As previously mentioned, when a balloon was inflated in the rectum of IBS patients, pain was referred to different areas such as the, hypogastrium (40%), iliac fossae (31%), rectum (21%) (dermatome S3 or perineal area) and to other areas (8%) [44]. Most patients with IBS point to aberrant sites for sensations (abdominal projections to dermatomes T8 to L1) [18,20]. In these patients, the referred pain can be perceived in wider areas compared to healthy subjects. For example, the dermatomes involved can reach the thoracic area and pain can be perceived in some areas of the abdominal wall because of the convergence of afferent visceral nerves with somatic efferents. The expansion of the somatic area of referred pain in IBS patients is a manifestation of secondary hyperalgesia.

Bladder pain syndrome, prostate pain syndrome and IBS often are associated with trigger points in the abdominal wall and pelvic floor muscles [17]. In myofascial pain syndromes, trigger points appear in the muscle in response to visceral pain such as that caused by Bladder pain syndrome / interstitial cystitis, prostate pain syndrome and endometriosis [27]. Trigger points can therefore cause referred pain syndromes that may mimic visceral pain [24]. Visceral pain from pelvic organs and myofascial pain syndrome from muscle trigger points share similar characteristics [23]. Notably, because the referred pain syndrome can continue in the absence of the initiating event, diagnosis of the initial problem may become difficult [25].

PRACTICAL IMPLICATIONS

Chronic anorectal pain is a complex phenomenon. It is part of the chronic pelvic pain syndrome and frequently associated with other visceral pain syndromes such as BPC/IC, endometriosis, male chronic pelvic pain and irritable bowel syndrome. It can be associated to fibromyalgia, vulvar pain syndrome, pelvi-perineal myofascial pain and pudendal neuralgia. It may also originate in the rectum or in the pelvi-perineal muscles. It can be the cause or the consequence of a chronic obstructive defecation syndrome.

Chronic anorectal pain is a dysfunctional pelvi-perineal syndrome. It is generated by a state of visceral and or muscle hypersensitivity. The central sensitization explains the viscero-visceral and viscero-somatic convergence, resulting in the state of persistent low threshold pain. The pain lasts more than 6 months. Since pain shares the same mechanisms in the different syndromes, the end organ classification of chronic pelvic pain could be replaced by phenotyping the patient with abdominal and pelvic pain.

LOOKING AT THE FUTURE

An organ dysfunction suggests in fact a dysregulation of the function of this organ inside an homeostatic circuit. This dysregulation is a complex phenomenon. It can be the cause of sensory, transduction, perception, integration, autonomic dysregulation, inflammation processes. Chronic pain is the expression of a convergence between low and high threshold nerves. Since the function of organs is integrated in complex systems whose aims is to maintain homeostasis one should keep in mind the cross talk between intra-pelvic organs , between these organs and musculoskeletal structures and between intra-pelvic and abdominal organs.

The understanding, the management of these situations gives a place to specialized multidisciplinary clinics.

TAKE HOME MESSAGES

- The dysfunction of intra-pelvic organs is not automatically painful. To be painful there must be other mechanisms such as the convergence of high and low threshold nerves in the posterior dorsal horn and repetitive mechanical stimulation or persistence of inflammation or nerve injury

- Anal pain of somatic origin and rectal pain which is visceral may be associated but are different. A chronic anal or rectal pain is often express in the pelvi-perineal muscles and shall be recognized to be treated adequately

REFERENCES

1. Accarino AM, Azpiroz F, Malagelada JR. Selective dysfunction of mechanosensitive intestinal afferents in irritable bowel syndrome. Gastroenterology. 1995;108(3):636–43.
2. Aggarwal VR, McBeth J, Zakrzewska JM, et al. The epidemiology of chronic syndromes that are frequently unexplained: do they have common associated factors? Int J Epidemiol. 2006;35(2):468–76.
3. Backer P. Contemporary management of chronic pelvic pain. 1993; 20(4): 719–742.
4. Basinski C, Fuller E, Brizendine EJ, Benson JT. Bladder–anal reflex. Neurourol Urodyn. 2003;22:683–686.
5. Beets-Tan RGH, Morren GL, Beets G, et al. Measurement of anal sphincter muscles: endoanal US, endoanal MR imaging, or phased array MR imaging? A study with healthy volunteers. Radiology 2001;220:81–9.
6. Berger RE. Chronic prostatitis/chronic pelvic floor syndrome. BMC Urology; 2007; 7(17): 1–7.
7. Bielefeldt, K, Lamb K, Gebhart F. Convergence of sensory pathways in the development of somatic and visceral hypersensitivity. Am J Physiol Gastrointest Liver Physiol 2006;291: G658–G665
8. Bouin M, Plourde V, Boivin M, et al. Rectal distention testing in patients with irritable bowel syndrome: sensitivity, specificity, and predictive values of pain sensory thresholds. Gastroenterology. 2002;122(7):1771–7.
9. Bouin M. Hypersensitivity: A Complex Marker for a Complex Disease. J Pain 2006;7(8): 536–538.
10. Brinkert W, Dimcevski G, Arendt-Nielsen L, et al. Dysmenorrhoea is associated with hypersensitivity in the sigmoid colon and rectum. Pain. 2007;132(Suppl 1):S46–51.
11. Butrick CW. Discordant urination and defecation as symptoms of pelvic floor dysfunction. In: Howard F, Perry CP, Carter JE, El-Minawi AM (eds). Pelvic Pain: Diagnosis and Management. Philadelphia, PA: Lippincott Williams & Wilkins; 2000:279–99.
12. Camilleri M, McKinzie S, Busciglio I, et al. Prospective study of motor, sensory, psychologic, and autonomic functions in patients with irritable bowel syndrome. Clin Gastroenterol Hepatol. 2008;6(7):772–81.
13. Cheng HY, Pitcher GM, Laviolette SR, et al. DREAM is a critical transcriptional repressor for pain modulation. Cell. 2002;108:31–43.
14. Chitkara DK, Bredenoord AJ, Cremonini F, et al. The role of pelvic floor dysfunction and slow colonic transit in adolescents with refractory constipation. Am J Gastroenterol. 2004;99(8):1579–84.
15. Hobday DI, Neil Thacker QA, Hollander I, et al. A study of the cortical processing of ano-rectal sensation using functional MRI. Brain 2001;124(2):361–368.
16. Derbyshire SWG. Visceral Afferent Pathways and Functional Brain Imaging. Sci World J 2003;3:1065–1080
17. Doggweiler-Wiygul R. Urologic myofascial pain syndromes. Curr Pain Headache Rep. 2004;8(6):445–51.
18. Dorn SD, Palsson OS, Thiwan SI, et al. Increased colonic pain sensitivity in irritable bowel syndrome is the result of an increased tendency to report pain rather than increased neurosensory sensitivity. Gut. 2007;56(9):1202–9.
19. Drewes AM, Petersen P, Rossel P, et al. Sensitivity and distensibility of the rectum and sigmoid colon in patients with irritable bowel syndrome. Scand J Gastroenterol 2001;36:827.
20. Faure C, Wieckowska A. Somatic referral of visceral sensations and rectal sensory threshold for pain in children with functional gastrointestinal disorders. J Pediatr. 2007 Jan;150(1):66–71.
21. Ferrara A, Pemberton JH, Levin KE, et al. Relationship between anal canal tone and rectal motor activity. Dis Colon Rectum 1993;36(4):337–42.
22. Frøkjaer JB, Andersen SD, Gale J, et al. An experimental study of viscero-visceral hyperalgesia using an ultrasound-based multimodal sensory testing approach. Pain. 2005;119(1–3):191–200.
23. Gerwin, Robert D. Myofascial and Visceral Pain Syndromes: Visceral-Somatic Pain Representations. J Musculoskel Pain 2002;10(1/2): 165–175.
24. Giamberardino MA. Referred muscle pain/hyperalgesia and central sensitisation. J Rehabil Med. 2003; (41 Suppl):85–8.
25. Giamberardino MA, Affaitati G, Lerza R, et al. Relationship between pain symptoms and referred sensory and trophic changes in patients with gallbladder pathology. Pain. 2005;114(1–2):239–49.
26. Giamberadino MA, Berkley KJ, Affetati G, et al. Influence of endometriosis on pain behaviors and muscle hyperalgesia induced by a ureteral calculosis in female rats. Pain; 2002; 95:247257.
27. Jarrell J, Giamberardino MA, Robert M, Nasr-Esfahani M. Bedside testing for chronic pelvic pain: discriminating visceral from somatic pain. Pain Res Treat. 2011;69:2102.

28. Kawimbe BM, Papachrysostomou M, Binnie NR, et al. Outlet obstruction constipation (anismus) managed by biofeedback. Gut. 1991;32(10):1175–9.
29. Kindler LL, Bennett RM, Jones KD. Central sensitivity syndromes: mounting pathophysiologic evidence to link fibromyalgia with other common chronic pain disorders. Pain Manag Nurs. 2011; 12(1): 15–24.
30. Knowles CH, Martin JE. Slow transit constipation: a model of human gut dysmotility. Review of possible aetiologies. Neurogastroenterol Motil. 2000;12(2):181–96.
31. Li L, Li Z, Huo HS, et al Sensory nerve endings in the puborectalis and anal region of the fetus and newborn. Dis Colon Rectum. 1992; 35(6):552–9.
32. Lynn PA, Olsson C, Zagorodnyuk V, et al. Rectal intraganglionic laminar endings are transduction sites of extrinsic mechanoreceptors in the guinea pig rectum. Gastroenterology 2003;125:786–94.
33. Mayer EA, Gebhart GF. Basic and clinical aspects of visceral hyperalgesia. Gastroenterology. 1994;107 (1):271–93.
34. Mertz H, Naliboff B, Munakata J, et al. Altered rectal perception is a biological marker of patients with irritable bowel syndrome. Gastroenterology. 1995;109(1):40–52.
35. Mertz H, Naliboff B, Mayer EA. Symptoms and physiology in severe chronic constipation. Am J Gastroenterol. 1999;94(1):131–8.
36. Munakata J, Naliboff B, Harraf F, et al. Repetitive sigmoid stimulation induces rectal hyperalgesia in patients with irritable bowel syndrome. Gastroenterology 1997;112:55–63.
37. Nadelhaft I, Vera PL. Separate urinary bladder and external urethral sphincter neurons in the central nervous system of the rat: simultaneous labeling with two immunohistochemically distinguishable pseudorabies viruses. Brain Res. 2001;903:33–44.
38. Ness TJ, Gebhart GF. Characterization of neurons responsive to noxious colorectal distension in the T13-L2 spinal cord of the rat. J Neurophysiol 1988;60:1419–1438.
39. Ness TJ, Gebhart GF. Visceral pain: a review of experimental studies. Pain 1990;41:167–230.
40. Nozu T, Kudaira M, Kitamori S, Uehara A. Repetitive rectal painful distention induces rectal hypersensitivity in patients with irritable bowel syndrome. J Gastroenterol. 2006;41(3):217–22.
41. Pinter E , Szolcsanyi J. Plasma extravasation in the skin and pelvic organs evoked by antidromic stimulation of the lumbosacral dorsal roots of the rat. Neuroscience 1995;68(2):603–614.
42. Pons TP, Garraghty PE, Friedman DP, Mishkin M. Physiological evidence for serial processing in somatosensory cortex. Science 1987;237(4813):417–20.
43. Price DD, Zhou Q, Moshiree B, Robinson ME, Verne GN. Peripheral and central contributions to hyperalgesia in irritable bowel syndrome. J Pain. 2006;7(8):529–35.
44. Ritchie J. Pain from distension of the pelvic colon by inflating a balloon in the irritable colon syndrome. Gut. 1973;14(2):125–32.
45. Rociu E, Stoker J, Eijkemans MJC, et al. Normal anal sphincter anatomy and age- and sex-related variations at high spatial resolution endoanal MR imaging. Radiology 2000;217:395–401.
46. Schur EA, Afari N, Furberg H, et al. Feeling bad in more ways than one: comorbidity patterns of medically unexplained and psychiatric conditions. J Gen Intern Med. 2007;22(6):818–21.
47. Sengupta JN, Gebhart GF. Characterization of mechanosensitive pelvic nerve afferent fibers innervating the colon of the rat. J Neurophysiol. 1994;71(6):2046–60.
48. Thiele GH. Tonic spasm of the levator anicoccygeus and piriformis muscles: its relationship to coccygodynia and pain in the region of the hip and down the leg. Trans Am Proctol Soc 1936; 37:145.
49. Tietjen GE, Brandes JL, Peterlin BL, et al. Allodynia in Migraine: Association With Comorbid Pain Conditions. Headache 2009;49:1333–1344.
50. Trimble KC, Douglas S, Heading RC. Twenty-four hour esophageal pH monitoring: technique and application. Gastroenterologist. 1995;3(3):187–98.
51. Verne GN, Robinson ME, Vase L, Price DD. Reversal of visceral and cutaneous hyperalgesia by local rectal anesthesia in irritable bowel syndrome (IBS) patients. Pain. 2003;105(1–2):223–30.
52. Whitehead WE, Holtkotter B, Enck P, et al. Tolerance for rectosigmoid distention in irritable bowel syndrome. Gastroenterology. 1990;98(5 Pt 1):1187–92.
53. Whorwell PJ, Lupton EW, Erduran D, Wilson K. Bladder smooth muscle dysfunction in patients with irritable bowel syndrome. Gut. 1986;27:1014–1017.
54. Wong RK, Palsson OS, Turner MJ, et al. Inability of the Rome III criteria to distinguish functional constipation from constipation-subtype irritable bowel syndrome. Am J Gastroenterol. 2010;105(10):2228–34.
55. Woolf CJ. Central sensitization: implications for the diagnosis and treatment of pain. Pain. 2011;152(3 Suppl):S2–15.
56. Zighelboim J, Talley NJ, Phillips SF, et al. Visceral perception in irritable bowel syndrome. Rectal and gastric responses to distension and serotonin type 3 antagonism. Dig Dis Sci. 1995;40(4):819–27.

PART 3

Management Aspects

SPECIFIC TREATMENT AND MANAGEMENT

Chapter 20 **Primary Care Management of Abdominal and Pelvic Pain**

Chapter 21 **Physiotherapy in Assessment and Management of Pain**

Chapter 22 **Psychology in Assessment and Management of Pain**

Chapter 23 **Neuromodulation of Abdominal and Pelvic Pain**

Chapter 24 **Pharmacotherapy in Neuropathic Pain**

PAIN PATIENT PATHWAYS

Chapter 25 **European Association of Urology Algorithms**

Chapter 26 **British Pain Society Patient Pathways**

THE FUTURE OF ABDOMINAL AND PELVIC PAIN MANAGEMENT

Chapter 27 **Developing a Structure for Delivery of Care**

Chapter 28 **Generating the Evidence-Base for Pelvic Pain in the Future**

Chapter 29 **The Future of Abdominal and Pelvic Pain Management**

Chapter 30 **The Role of the Patient Organizations**

CHAPTER 20

Primary Care Management of Abdominal and Pelvic Pain

Huibertien Oosterlee

INTRODUCTION

In the Netherlands, the General Practitioner (GP) is seen as the gatekeeper to the health care system. Essentially all patients have to pass via the GP to gain access to specialist care. Access to GP's is free of charge leaving no financial barricades in seeking his or her help. All patients with abdominal pain are seen by a GP, other specialists (if necessary) for treatment, or when they remain in chronic pain for which no diagnosis is found. During all stages of treatment or follow-up, GP's will be involved either directly or indirectly.

This chapter deals with basic aspects of abdominal pain as seen in primary practice. The occurrence of abdominal pain and the most common diagnoses are explored as well as when and to whom to refer. Finally the management of chronic abdominal pain is dealt with.

The family doctor due to his role and relationship with the patient is pivotal in the whole process of diagnosis, treatment and support of patients with (chronic) abdominal-pelvic pain.

BASIC ASPECTS

The term used in general practice to describe abdominal-pelvic pain is 'abdominal pain'. This might seem rhetoric but quite often no clear diagnosis is made during the first contact. During follow-up abdominal pain can be specified (e.g. Inflammatory Bowel Disease). However, more often than not the term used to describe the patients complaint remains abdominal pain. The terms pelvic pain and abdominal pain are often used to describe the same phenomena.

Epidemiology of Abdominal Pain in Primary Practice in the Netherlands

Abdominal pain comes in many forms and is a common complaint in all ages and both sexes. It can be presented as localized pain or a more general complaint; furthermore, it can be episodic or more chronic.

On average, one fifth of all people have a period of abdominal pain each year. A mere quarter of these patients will actually visit a doctor. An average GP with a population of 2,300 patients will see slightly more than 100 people with acute abdominal pain each year. Women are seen twice as often as men [1].

In 80% of the cases, the final diagnosis of an episode of acute abdominal pain is found to have its origin in the gastro-intestinal system. The majority is a "symptom" diagnosis like Irritable Bowel Syndrome or constipation. Approximately 10% of abdominal pain is a urinary system diagnosis [1].

To illustrate the treatment of patients with (sub) acute abdominal pain by Dutch GP's a case study concerning Johanna will be presented.

Johanna, a case study

Johanna is a 22 year old woman. You have known her for 15 years as a generally healthy individual. You have seen her once for an ear infection and as a high school attendee she suffered from menstrual pains for which you prescribed anti-inflammatories. You have lost sight of her during the last few years as she started studying psychology in a nearby town.

She is suffering from lower abdominal pain for the last few days and is additionally slightly constipated. The pain is more or less continuous. Her last period started almost a week ago and was slightly less productive than she is used to. She has no further health complaints. She is a student and has no steady relationship. She is heterosexual. She stopped using oral contraceptives 6 months ago. For the occasional sexual encounter she uses condoms. She has had no untoward sexual experiences in the past.

She is concerned about the pain and wonders if it has anything to do with her period.

Upon examination, you find a slightly tender lower abdomen whereby the left side is more tender. There are no signs of acute inflammation. On vaginal examination there is some discharge and you can feel a fecal mass in the rectal pouch. She has no fever. Her urine is clean. Her CRP is < 5. You have taken vaginal swabs for PCR testing on Chlamydia as there is a likelihood of a sexually transmitted disease, even though there are no real signs of pelvic inflammatory disease upon investigation. After a few days you get the results back and no Chlamydia was detected.

After considering your findings the most likely diagnosis in Johanna's case is dysmenorrhea, possibly due to endometriosis. Constipation could possibly also play a part.

You decide to treat her constipation with advice and possibly laxatives. You restart oral contraceptives, which will also solve the problem of unreliable contraception. Obviously the risk of PID will only be reduced by using barrier contraception.

You instruct her to come back if there is no improvement in the condition and sooner than planned if alarm-symptoms like fever, rectal blood loss or general feeling of illness arise. In three months' time, you decide to review her.

DESCRIBING THE SUBJECT

SOEP Methodology

GP's in the Netherlands use the so called SOEP (Subjective, Objective, Evaluation, Plan) methodology. This helps to structure the consultation and makes a uniform registration possible and can easily be done within ten minutes.

- The "S" stands for subjective; essentially history-taking. As well as inquiring to the history of the current complaint other involved systems also are inquired into. In the case of abdominal/pelvic complaints this includes the gastro-intestinal and urogenital systems. In the case of menstrual complaints it is important not to forget to ask about previous sexual experiences. There is a significant correlation between untoward sexual experiences and menstrual complaints [9].

  It is particularly important to be aware of the patients own interpretation of the origin of their complaints. Doctors tend to overestimate the knowledge people have regarding their bodies. Despite this, it is still helpful to be aware of their conclusions pertaining to their abdominal pain.

- It all becomes more apparent during the "O" of objective, which stands for examination both physical and or laboratory, x-ray etc. How the patient enters the consultancy room gives information regarding the level of painfulness and general health. The abdomen is examined whereby attention is paid to scars from earlier operations and any herniation of the abdominal wall. The abdomen is auscultated to check the bowel sounds. Percussion masses and possibly air in the bowels can be detected. Finally, palpation is important to check where the exact pain is. Hereby signs of acute inflammation are checked which will make referral to specialist care more imminent. The patient is asked to sit upright from a supine position to rule out any pain coming from the abdominal wall.

  If indicated a vaginal and rectal examination is performed. In the above mentioned case, a vaginal examination is important to rule out the possibility of Pelvic Inflammatory Disease. Check for signs of inflammation like discharge or pain. While doing a vaginal examination it is advisory to check the function of the pelvic floor muscles. A rectal examination can be necessary to determine if there are haemorrhoids, fissures, or fecal masses.

  After physical examination, there are a number of investigations which can be done in primary practice. Most practices can do urine analysis to detect infection and hematuria. Furthermore, urine specimens can be checked to rule out pregnancy. Commonly it is also possible to do some simple blood tests like, hemoglobin (Hb), C-reactive protein (CRP), and Blood Sedimentation Rate (BSR). More extensive blood tests can be done in nearby laboratories of which the results are available within a couple of days. Fluor analysis can be done by the GP for the more benevolent problems like Candida. Further tests, like PCR for Chlamydia and Gonorrhea, can be done in laboratories.

- The "E" is for evaluation viz. diagnosis and working hypothesis.

  As mentioned earlier, in the majority of cases of abdominal pain the GP practice ends up being a symptom diagnosis. In adolescents, 90% of the cases have no clearly identifiable cause of abdominal pain [4].

- Finally, the "P" of plan. This can be a prescription, referral to specialist care, further investigations, or most importantly in Dutch primary care, reassurance!

  The GP instructs the patient to contact them in the case of alarm symptoms including: rectal blood loss, bowel complaints as a new complaint in people over 50 years of age, unintentional weight loss, postmenopausal pain, heavy and totally irregular menses, post-coital blood loss and thoughts of suicide.

Dutch GP's refers 4% of all their contacts on average [5]. There are no clear figures on the number of patients that are referred upon the first consultation with acute abdominal pain.

Scandinavian research shows that three- quarters of patients with acute abdominal pain are handled by the general practitioner [2].

It is vital to differentiate between serious diseases, which will need immediate referral, and mild complaints. In the aforementioned case it shows how easily this differentiation can be done. Additionally, the first contact is an opportunity to prevent chronic complaints by reassurance and thorough explanation of possible pathways within the treatment of abdominal pain. When patients are confident that their doctor listens to them and that their doctor is competent in distilling their complaints into treatable diseases, they will easily be reassured concerning the benign nature of their pain.

Chronic Abdominal Pain

Chronic pelvic pain is defined as continuous or intermittent non-cyclic pain over six or more months duration localized in the anatomic pelvis, anterior abdominal wall at or below the umbilicus, the lumbosacral back or the buttocks, and is of sufficient severity as to cause functional disability or lead to medical care [7].

This part of the chapter focuses on those patients who remain with chronic pain and for whom there is no further referral or investigation needed. These are often the patients who turn to their GP for help [8].

All chronic complaints start with a first episode. It is not well known how frequently acute abdominal pain ends up being chronic pelvic or abdominal pain. Pain in the lower abdomen exists in around 25% of women in the general population. If these complaints are experienced for more then three months then 25% of these women will visit the family doctor [10]. This means that the majority of women have found a way to cope with chronic pain. However, there is a group of patients who continuously and repeatedly return to the GP for the same symptoms.

This raises the question, "What does a patient with chronic pain actually want from their doctor?". Patients want to be taken seriously, be listened to and have recognition of their complaints. A misperception is that they want to be referred or be medicated. Basically they want support.

This can be achieved by listening to what they have to say. Statements like "it is all in your head" are known to be counterproductive. Exploration of what the complaint means to the patient is especially important. This can be structured by using the SCEBS methodology (Somatic, Cognitive, Emotional, Behavioral and Social).

Once again, allowing the patient to deliberate on their symptoms is vital in them feeling that they are being listened to. Exploring their own views of the origins of their pain is also vital. Ask what they expect from their doctor. How do they feel emotionally? Are they concerned, do they feel guilty? Are there any behavioral changes like not working or seeking medical help in various places or alternative medicine? Finally, how does the patients' social network react? Do they feel supported and is their family also concerned?

The doctor should have an eye for the cues, which are there in almost every consultation. Listening is an important tool. It seems that doctors in the majority of cases miss the cues that can help them in finding a solution [3].

The problem needs to shift from being the patients' problem to one of joint-possession. There is strong evidence to suggest that looking for "common ground" together with empathy and care helps patients address their symptoms in a different way. It may be the case that health professionals presume that patients want to be referred or want to receive medication. It appears that listening and empathy is what they want and need [6].

GP's cannot prevent chronic abdominal or pelvic pain. However there may well be a way to prevent fixation on that pain. Due to the long-term GP-patient relationship and the personal nature of this relationship, GP's obviously know their patients better than most specialists. It is this relationship that can be a tool in preventing fixation on that pain. Abdominal pain is a challenge for each doctor and can be rewarding when solved. Fortunately this is quite often the case. As a GP, you are in the unique position to be aware of your patient's backgrounds, knowledge of the family, where they come from, their social status, and other current social issues (e.g. health of their children, care for elderly parents, working problems). All of these factors can play a major role in their sense of well-being.

The continuity of GP care allows a comprehensive approach to our patients' well-being. It is important to see a patient not as a patient who has pain but as a patient who is experiencing pain. Support the patient without necessarily looking for a solution.

PRACTICAL IMPLICATIONS

A Structured Approach Gives the Most Rewarding Results

In the acute phase of abdominal pain, this needs to be treated and serious diseases are to be ruled out. In the chronic phase, it remains important to be vigilant for new disease. Give support and prevent over-medicalization due to unnecessary repeated referral. Continue to listen to the patient as a "joint-possessor" of the problem. Having a shared view that the pain is there without an explanation for it being there may possibly help the patient in living with the pain.

The GP is the health professional to whom the patient is most likely to return.

LOOKING AT THE FUTURE

Within the Dutch health care system, a multi-disciplinary approach to abdominal-pelvic pain is resulting in the arrival of so-called 'Pelvic Care Centers'. These centers are a co-operation between the fields of urology, gynecology, gastroenterology, surgery, psychology, and physiotherapy and promise to see an improvement in diagnosing and in treating problems related to different aspects of the abdomen and pelvic area. This will; however, not prevent the incidence of chronic abdominal pain, as there is not always a solution for all types of pain. This is why the role of the GP as a listener, supporter, empathizer and joint-possessor remains the cornerstone in the treatment of chronic abdominal and pelvic pain.

TAKE HOME MESSAGES

- The strength of the General Practitioner lies in the continuity of the relationship with the patient.
- Listening, support, and empathy remain useful tools in the care for people with chronic abdominal pain.
- Most cases of acute abdominal pain can be diagnosed and treated in primary practice.

ACKNOWLEDGEMENT

With courtesy to Anja De Vries, GP in Maassluis, the Netherlands, for the use of her lecture on treatment of chronic abdominal pain in Primary Practice; and to Darren Cornish, GP in Dedemsvaart, the Netherlands, for his advise on the English language.

REFERENCES

1. van Boven C. Abdominal pain. Bijblijven 2012;28(7):9–13.
2. Brekke M, Krogh Eilertsen R. Acute abdominal pain in general practice: tentative diagnoses and handling. Scand J Prim Health Care, 2009;27:137–140.
3. olde Hartman TC, van Ravesteijn HJ. "Well, doctor, it is all about how life is lived": cues as a tool in the medical consultation. Ment Health Fam Med. 2008;5(3):183–187.
4. Holland-Hall CM, Brown RT. Evaluation of the adolescent with Chronic Abdominal or Pelvic Pain. J Pediatr Adolesc Gynecol 2004;17:23–27.
5. Nationaal Kompas Volksgezondheid, versie 4.10, 13 december 2012 M, Bilthoven / Disclaimer. © RIV.
6. Salmon P, Ring A, Dowrick CF, Humphris GM. What do general practice patients want when they present medically unexplained symptoms, and why do their doctors feel pressurized? J Psychosom Res 2005;59 (4): 255–260.
7. Samray GPN, Kuritzki L, Whit Curry Jr R. Chronic Pelvic Pain in Women, Evaluation and Management in Primary Care. Comprehens Ther 2005;31(1):28–39.
8. Verhaak PFM, Meijer SA, Visser AP, Wolters G. Persistent presentation of medically unexplained symptoms in general practice. Fam Pract 2006;23:414–20.
9. Vink CW, Labots-Vogelesangh SM, Lagro-Janssen ALM. Menstruation Disorders more frequent in women with a history of sexual abuse. Ned Tijdschr geneeskd. 2006;150:1886–90.
10. Weijenborg PTM, ter Kuile MM, Gopie JP, Spinhoven P. Reduction in chronic pelvic pain in women with less catastrophising pain. Ned. Tijdsch. Geneeskd. 2010;154:A2109.

CHAPTER 21

Physiotherapy in Assessment and Management of Pain

Rebecca McLoughlin, Katrine Petersen, and Suzanne Brook

INTRODUCTION

This chapter describes the approach to assessment and management of chronic abdominal pelvic pain (CAPP) used by physiotherapists working within an interdisciplinary pain management centre. We discuss why pain management physiotherapists work in the way they do, look at the evidence-base for our practice, and describe how we utilise knowledge from relevant evidence in clinical practice. We hope this will provide insights into both current research and clinical strategies and skills.

BASIC ASPECTS

Evidence-Based Pain Management Physiotherapy

Evidence-based medicine is espoused by many governments and healthcare organisations [28] and has been recognised as a concept of growing importance for physiotherapy [21]. As the underlying neurophysiological mechanisms of CAPP reflect those of other chronic pain syndromes, it has been stated that CAPP syndromes should be managed with the same general approach as is used for other pain syndromes [3]. Therefore, pain management physiotherapy approaches, for which there is strong evidence in other forms of chronic pain, can be utilised in the management of CAPP and outcomes measured in order to improve the evidence-base.

Pain management physiotherapy is delivered within a cognitive behavioural therapy (CBT) framework. Evidence suggests that rehabilitation and exercise programmes delivered using a CBT approach produce better long term outcomes than other approaches [17, 26, 34]. Therefore, CBT provides an ideal framework for the delivery of physical rehabilitation [32].

A recent systematic review of psychological therapies for the management of chronic pain [43] confirmed that the evidence-base is dominated by studies of treatment stemming from behavioural or cognitive behavioural theories. Of these two approaches, CBT is more effective in reducing pain-associated disability [43]. It should be noted that there is a distinction between physiotherapists utilising the principles of CBT, and formal delivery of a cognitive behavioural intervention by a trained cognitive behavioural therapist. Few physiotherapists are trained cognitive behavioural therapists. The approach that we describe is not a cognitive behavioural therapy intervention; it is physiotherapy delivered within a CBT framework and utilising cognitive behavioural principles alongside and within other physiotherapy interventions.

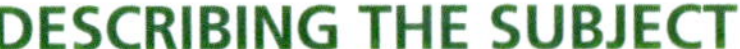

DESCRIBING THE SUBJECT

Pain Management Physiotherapy Assessment

Physiotherapy within a CBT pain management model has a core aim of increasing patients' ability to manage their own pain and become more active despite it [2]. In order to support patients in achieving this, it has been suggested that the clinician's role 'is that of a teacher or guide, who's main responsibility is to encourage or assist the patient in learning and making better use of pain self-management skills' [20]. Therefore, pain management physiotherapy assessments focus on listening to the patient's experience of pain, their beliefs about the nature and mechanism of their pain and the journey that has brought them to the clinic. The clinician might say, "I know that you might have told this story many times before, but it's really helpful for me to hear from you about what has happened since your pain began". The patient might later be asked to describe the impact that their pain has on their life in terms of daily activity, work, family and social interactions, intimate relationships and valued activities. An impression of the patient's thoughts and beliefs about movement and activity can be elicited from this explanation. Additional information might be gleaned from a question like: "Are there any movements that you think you should not do because of your pain? What do you think will happen if you move in that way or do that movement?" The specific content of a pain management physiotherapy assessment will vary according to the needs and goals of the individual patient, but the assessment is led by the patient's answers. The physiotherapist can demonstrate understanding and empathy by posing questions in an order that follows the patient's fears, concerns and questions [3]. Some typical physiotherapy specific questions included in an assessment are shown in Table 1, however, this should not be considered as a complete assessment outline. In Table 1, an explanation is given as to why each topic is discussed and suggestions for the type of open question that might elicit the most complete and useful answer are provided.

A CBT guided assessment concludes with the clinician highlighting or summarising what she thinks she has heard and what she hopes she and the patient can work on together, using phrases and key words from the conversation with the patient. The final decision about whether to engage in further sessions and begin working towards identified goals must come from the patient, rather than being assumed by the clinician. As mentioned above, ensuring goals are meaningful to the patient, based around functional activities rather than being pain reduction-based can help patients engage in a pain management physiotherapy approach. It is also helpful to support the discussion from the assessment with relevant resources that the patient can read prior to the next appointment, or copies of diagrams or images that were used in explanation during the session.

Pain Management Programmes (PMP) and Individual Pain Management Physiotherapy

CBT guided physiotherapy can be delivered in one-to-one sessions, but it is more commonly delivered within interdisciplinary pain management programmes (PMPs). Interdisciplinary PMPs have been identified by the British Pain Society as the treatment of choice

TABLE 1 Physiotherapy Specific Questions in Assessment

Topic	Reason	Suggestions
Expectations of pain management physiotherapy	Opportunity to identify unrealistic/ inaccurate expectations and discuss if patient wants to engage in a CBT focused self-management approach.	"What are your hopes or expectations of pain management physiotherapy and your appointment today?"
Pain History	To gain an understanding of what the patient has experienced, how their pain has changed, and where they are in terms of needing, wanting, undergoing investigations or treatments. This is not an acute assessment of nature, irritability, and severity as this will be misleading in chronic pain.	"Please tell me about your pain, when you think it started, and how it has been over the past... years?" "Who have you seen for treatment or advice about your pain?" "Do you think you need more investigations"
Previous experience of physiotherapy	Open discussion about previous difficult or helpful experiences.	"I've obviously read through your notes, but I couldn't tell whether you've had any physiotherapy in the past..."
Previous investigations/ explanations/ treatments	To get an impression of the patient's understanding of investigations and treatments that they've had in the past and why they did or didn't help.	"What do you think your investigations show?" "Was it explained to you?" "Is there anything else that you think should be looked at?"
Perception of pain: what is the cause of the patient's pain	To gain insight into what the patient believes is causing their pain, the reasons it persists, and possibly, what this means for the future. Elicit beliefs about pain, for example pain being a sign of injury or damage. At a later appointment this information can help the physiotherapist to provide alternative models and explanations if the patient's beliefs are based on inaccurate information.	"What do you think is causing your pelvic pain?
Impact of pain: 24 hours/ weekly routine	To get an impression of the relationship between pain and activity. Is the person avoiding activity, or pushing to their limit and having to recover with hours/ days of rest? Pain can often be unhelpfully used by a patient as a guide to dictate whether they should do more or less activity.	"What's a normal day like for you?" "Do you have days which are better than others or days of more pain than others? If so, what you do on a good pain day and on a bad pain day?"
Avoided movements/ activities	Links with beliefs about pain and injury or damage and can lead to insight into where beliefs come from. For example, a patient might say, "After surgery 4 years ago, the doctor told me not to bend, so I try not to bend because it's bad for me."	"Are there any movements or activities that you think you should avoid because of your pain?"

Table continued on following page

TABLE 1 **Physiotherapy Specific Questions in Assessment (Continued)**

Topic	Reason	Suggestions
Exercise	Increase understanding of relationship with exercise before and alongside pain and possible thoughts about increasing exercise.	"Do you think exercise is helpful in managing pain?" "Is exercise something that you enjoy? Is it part of your routine at the moment? Would you like it to be?"
Helpful strategies	Identify positive/helpful coping strategies that the patient is using to reinforce what they are doing well and to engage the patient in building on their current strategies. Rest and avoidance are not considered helpful but for the patient they may avoid increases in pain in the short term.	"Are there things that you can do that help with your pain or help you to cope with living with pain?"
Medication use	Gain insight into beliefs about the role of pain medication and information about benefits of medication and side effects. Also understand how pain medication is taken.	"Do you take any medication for your pain?" "Is it helpful?" "How do you take it?"
Past medical history/ other health conditions	Gain insight into additional health challenges that might interact with experience of CAPP, impact on activity or impact on management of CAPP.	"Do you have any other health conditions?" "Does it impact on your abdominal and pelvic pain?" "How do you manage it?"
Social situation	Understanding of home and social challenges, work, financial situation, litigation, etc.	"Are you working at the moment?" "Are there people in your life who depend on you?"
Support	Gain insight into the network that the person lives within and the degree of support they feel they have within that network.	"Do you have family/friends around you?" "Do you think they're supportive? How?"
Mood	Identify if the individual is at risk or requires urgent assessment of mood. Identify the impact of pain on mood and subsequent relationship between mood, thoughts, and behaviour.	"Do you think that your pain has affected your mood? It would be understandable if you felt that it does or had."
Values	Begin to identify actions/ behaviours/ activities that are particularly important to the individual, their identity and quality of life. This is a big topic and there are numerous resources and exercises that can help someone explore and connect with their values – this is an initial starting point.	"We all have some things - activities, behaviours or characteristics - that we really value. What would you say are the things that come to mind that you particularly value?"
Goals	Begin to identify specific targets that they would like to work towards in pain management physiotherapy.	"Are there particular things that you'd like to be able to do differently or do more of?"

for people with persistent pain which adversely affects their quality of life [8]. The multidisciplinary approach is supported in the literature of female chronic pelvic pain [24]. The overall aim of physiotherapy in a PMP is 'to reduce the disability and distress caused by chronic pain, by teaching sufferers physical, psychological and practical techniques to improve their quality of life, [19]. Whether working with a patient within a group or individually, pain management physiotherapy does not focus on pain reduction as a principle aim of treatment, the focus of pain management physiotherapy is to facilitate return to normal daily activities even if the pain is not completely resolved [15]. Physiotherapists have a key role in supporting patients in improving function through behavioural change, including reduction of; avoidance, pain and illness behaviours, and increasing well behaviours [19]. This can support a shift away from behaviour that is contingent on pain or providing pain relief, and promote development of behaviour that is contingent on goal achievement related to the values of the individual with pain [43].

Despite guidelines advocating group pain management over one-to-one work, it is important that one-to-one physiotherapy is available for patients who do not speak the same language as the clinician (interpreters can then be utilised) or would not benefit from group work for other reasons such as visual or hearing impairment, significant social anxiety, or other limiting health conditions such that attendance at a group will be difficult.

The content of pain management physiotherapy sessions within both pain management programmes and individual work varies dependent on the patient's individual needs, but some consistent themes are seen. Well established, and evidenced, components of pain management physiotherapy sessions include pain education, desensitisation, stretches and exercise. These approaches are discussed in more detail in relation to management of CAPP. Additional approaches not discussed within this chapter include: exploring the relationship between activity and pain; graded re-introduction of avoided or feared movement and activity; understanding and management of flare-ups; and the use of relaxation or meditation strategies (see [2] for further reading).

Pain Management Physiotherapy Treatments for CAPP

Pain Education

Traditional physiotherapy education focused on informing patients about anatomy, posture and ergonomics, with less focus on pain experience and science, and the broader impact of pain on physical activity, function, emotional wellbeing, social interaction and relationships. In recent years increasing evidence to support the role of neuroscience education in pain management has emerged. Pain education should routinely be included in physiotherapy management of chronic pain conditions including CAPP, as discussed above. Exclusion of such information from treatment is contrary to evidence-based medicine principles, which require that the best available evidence from basic and clinical sciences is incorporated into management [30].

The content and delivery of pain education has changed significantly in recent decades after the value of traditional educational approaches was challenged [7]. Evidence supporting the role of neuroscience education in management of chronic pain conditions (although not specifically CAPP) has been available for over a decade [31] and early positive findings have been corroborated by more recent systematic review and meta-analysis [11, 27]. Neuroscience education aims to describe how the nervous system, through peripheral nerve sensitisation, central sensitisation, synaptic activity and brain processing, interprets information from the tissues and that neural activation, as either up regulation or down regulation, has the ability to modulate the pain experience [27]. Neuroscience education attempts to effect change through reconceptualisation of pain [30]. This aim reflects the aim of education within pain management programmes, which is viewed as a cognitive event: the giving of information which, it is hoped, will lead to cognitive reappraisal and finally behavioural change, with the application of new knowledge to relevant situations [19].

Desensitisation

The term desensitisation is often used in other chronic pain conditions such as Complex Regional Pain Syndrome (CRPS) where the desensitising strategy is recommended to gradually normalise the response to a movement or stimuli causing abnormal unpleasant sensations [40]. Some urology studies indicate physiological similarities between CAPP and CRPS [22]. Nickel [35] highlighted that patients with CAPP exhibit the same heightened response to noxious stimuli as patients diagnosed with CRPS. Other similarities include abnormalities in the autonomic nervous system i.e. noticeable links to stress and neurogenic inflammation [5]. This strategy of desensitising is especially helpful if the patients have goals such as: returning to or increasing sexual function; reducing urinary urgency; improving sitting tolerance and tolerating contact from clothing (e.g. trousers, underwear and belts). Pain management physiotherapy aims to increase confidence and tolerance to return to these activities in a graded and systematic way. This approach is based on knowledge of pain mechanisms.

For bladder urgency, it is well known that patients with CAPP often experience abnormal sensations in response to normal stimuli such as pain on bladder filling and a perceived increased urge to void as part of central sensitisation [3,12]. Zanette [44] also found that avoidance behaviour and fear has a measurable effect on excitability of the motor cortex, indicating that unhelpful behavioural responses can further sensitise the central nervous system. This supports the importance of addressing patients' fears and aim to restore normal function through education and a graded approach to decreasing the sensitivity.

In order to help someone reduce their urgency when linked to pain increases, we would encourage patients to slowly and consistently increase the time (seconds then minutes) before they try to empty their bladder. Often, patients tell us that despite the feeling that their bladder is full and needs emptying when they do try to empty their bladder there is no urine. But if they try to delay going to the toilet and hold, the pain increases. By using a steady and paced approach, patients report to that the feeling of bladder fullness linked to pain reduces. If this happens at night, patients also say that their sleep improves as they are less disturbed.

To help patients feel more confident to start a programme of desensitising they need to be clear about what they want to do and by when, setting realistic goals is key to a successful outcome. Clinical experience informs us that many patients have returned to valued activities experiencing reduced sensitivity and fear [4].

Stretches

Stretches are a key part of a pain management physiotherapy approach. The main aim is to help patients feel more confident to move, to be less avoidant and, as a knock-on effect, help move towards achieving their more physically-based goals, be that cycling, shopping, walking up hills or cooking a meal. FitzGerald [16] demonstrated that myofascial treatments, combined with exercises and relaxation, have a beneficial impact on CAPP when compared to massage alone, and stretches can be an active way of self-managing long term. One study found that nurses with low back pain reported a greater degree of self-efficacy using stretches than other forms of treatment [10].

The approach to stretch is not based on stretching just the muscle where pain is felt, as it is known that CAPP can cause lower pain thresholds and greater tenderness in non-pelvic locations [14]. The introduction of general static stretches can be a useful way of building up patients' confidence in movement and exercise. The stretch can focus on specific goals, such as bending the spine to enable the patient to pick things up from the floor, or the patient may choose to work on stretching muscles around the pelvis to achieve a relaxation effect using breathing techniques. Law [23] found that daily stretches performed by a group of patients with chronic low back pain, does not necessarily improve muscle extensibility but does improve the patients' tolerance to a greater range of movement.

Bretischwerdt [6] demonstrated that stretching can have a hypoanalgesic effect in distant areas through descending inhibitory pathways. This supports the benefit of stretching to address a complex sensitised central nervous system rather than focusing specifically on muscles around the uro-genital-abdominal area. This is also useful for patients who have high levels of fear as it can have a positive effect to start stretching exercises by performing stretches in a non- or less-painful area, gradually gaining confidence to move all areas of the body.

Exercise

It has been assumed that chronic pain leads to reduced activity levels. Patients are deconditioned, have poor posture and lack of muscle strength therefore contribute to the patients' pain [42]. However, several studies found that deconditioning and poor physical status in chronic pain have proved to be unsubstantiated [26, 41]. A recent systematic review of physiotherapy management of CAPP did not find any research on exercise as a stand-alone treatment [25]. Stones [39] reported similar findings and they were not able to include any studies on exercise in their Cochrane review of treatment of CAPP. Both reviews recommended a Multidisciplinary Team (MDT) approach including physiotherapy, and exercise is recommended as a key component of managing chronic pain conditions [8, 33, 34].

Exercise fits well into a CBT model and the emphasis of exercise as part of a pain management approach is on gaining the health benefits and providing a self-management strategy that empowers patients to feel in control of their physical health and function [28,29]. Exercise is also a key component of participating in a social life [13]. Gondoh [18] also showed that aerobic exercises may inhibit loss of grey matter and increase brain-derived neurotrophic growth factors which stimulate neural plasticity.

The key to exercise progression or prescription is that the patient is in control of setting a starting point. Many patients report that they are given sets of ten exercises to repeat three times a day. For many patients, returning to this level of exercise will result in a significant increase in pain. As a consequence they may stop doing any exercise. A pain management approach will focus on supporting the patient to find a realistic and manageable baseline to exercises and thereby gaining more control of their pain management. It is also important to address any fears and previous experiences of exercises, utilising a cognitive behavioural approach, which has been shown to increase and facilitate long-term adherence in chronic pain [36,37]. These neuroanatomical and physiological changes combined with appropriate pain management education may help to explain why graded exercise has been found to be effective in treating conditions such as fibromyalgia [9], but further studies are needed to establish the link in CAPP.

There should be no need to reiterate the multiple general health benefits of exercise. More recently, exercise has also been linked with better outcomes in those with mild to moderate depression, which is a common co-morbid factor in chronic pain [38, 1]. Epidemiologic studies strongly suggest that functional disability is inversely related to physical activity levels or physical fitness in various domains [3] so it will play a key part in helping patients manage their pain.

LOOKING AT THE FUTURE

Pain management physiotherapy is delivered within an evidence-based framework, however, the evidence-base for pain management physiotherapy specifically within management of CAPP remains limited. For continued debate and extending the treatment and management of patients with CAPP this needs to be addressed. Equally the way in which pain education is thought about by professionals needs to be addressed.

A study investigating the ability of health professionals and patients to understand neurophysiology of pain [30] demonstrated that both professionals and patients can understand pain neuroscience. Both groups showed improved performance in knowledge tests after education about neurophysiology of pain. However, the study also revealed that health professionals underestimated patients' ability to understand information about pain, thus creating a barrier to reconceptualisation of the problem of chronic pain away from a structural-pathology model. Moseley highlighted that therapists must believe that their patients can understand pain science, through acknowledgement of the evidence to support this, in order for the therapist to then guide the patient in creating an accurate and helpful model of their pain.

Effective pain management physiotherapy relies on the physiotherapist being able to reflect on his/her own practice, be up to date with new evidence [21] for the model of provision of physiotherapy for chronic pain patients. Physiotherapists must also be aware of their limitations if working independently from other pain professionals (doctors, psychologists, nurse specialists). Physiotherapists need to continually challenge themselves and not continually work with this patient group in an acute tissue-based model but to integrate the evidence-based chronic pain work. The challenge for the future is for these two models to be integrated in practice rather than only on paper.

TAKE HOME MESSAGES

- Pain Management programmes and MDT approaches to managing CAPP are strongly recommended in the literature (supported by our CAPP pain management programme (LINK) data).
- There is little evidence for individual physiotherapy techniques in isolation for managing CAPP.
- Exercise and movement are an important component of long-term pain management, but there is no evidence supporting specific exercises over general exercises.

FURTHER READING

BPS: The British Pain Society (2007) Recommended guidelines for pain management in adults. Available at: http://www.britishpainsociety.org/book_pmp_main.pdf (accessed 24/12/2012)

Williams A, Eccleston C, Morley S Psychological therapies for the management of chronic pain (excluding headache) in adults. Cochr Database Syst Rev 2012;11:CD007407

Hayden J, van Tulder M, Malvivaara A, Koes B. Exercise therapy for treatment of non-specific low back pain. Cochr Database Syst Rev 2005;3:CD000335

REFERENCES

1. Arnow B, Nunkler E, Blasey C, et al. Comorbid depression, chronic pain, and disability in primary care. Psychosom Med 2006;68:262–8.
2. Brook, S. Improving fitness and function in complex regional syndrome. In: Gifford, L.S. (ed) Topical issues in Pain 3. Falmouth: CNS Press; 2002:161–175.
3. Chin M, Fillingim R, Ness T (ed). Pain in Women. London: Oxford University Press, 2013:220–222.
4. Baranowski PA, Mandeville AL, Edwards S, et al. Male chronic pelvic pain syndrome and the role of interdisciplinary pain management. World J Urol 2013;31:779–784.
5. Baranowski AP. Chronic Pelvic Pain. Best Pract Res Clin Gastroenterol 2009;23(4):593–610.
6. Bretischwerdt C, Rivas-Cano L, Palomeque-del-Cerro L. Immediate Effect of Hamstring Muscle Strengthing on Pressure Pain Sensitivity and Active Mouth Opening in healthy subjects. J Manip Physiol Ther 2010;33:42–47.
7. Brox J, Storheim K, Grotle M, et al. Systematic Review of back schools, brief education and fear-avoidance training for chronic low back pain. Spine J 2008;8:948–958.
8. BPS: The British Pain Society (2007) Recommended guidelines for pain management in adults. Available at: http://www.britishpainsociety.org/book_pmp_main.pdf (accessed 24/12/2012)
9. Busch AJ, Barber K, Overend TJ, et al. Exercise for Fibromyalgia. Curr Pain Headache Rep 2011;15:358–367.
10. Chen H-M, Wang H-H, Cheng H, Hu H. Effectiveness of a Stretching Exercise Programme on Low Back Pain and Exercise Self-Efficacy Among nurses in Taiwan: A Randomised Clinical Study. Pain Manag Nurs 2012;6:1–9.
11. Clarke C, Ryan C, Martin D. Pain neurophysiology education for the management of individuals with chronic low back pain: A systematic review and meta-analysis. Manual Ther 2011;16:544–549.
12. Collett B. Chronic pelvic and vulvar pain in women, Rev Pain 2008; 2:8–15.
13. Damsgaard E, Dewar A, Roe C, Hamran T. Staying active despite pain: Pain beliefs and experiences with activity-related pain in patients with chronic musculoskeletal pain. Scand J Caring Sci 2011;25:108–116.
14. Davies S, Maykut CA, Binik Y, et al. Tenderness as Measured by Pressure Pain Threshold Extends Beyond the Pelvis in Chronic Pelvic Pain Syndrome in Men. J Sex Med 2010;8:232–239.
15. Farquhar, C, Latthe P. Chronic Pelvic Pain: Aetilogy and Therapy. Rev Gynaecol Perin Pract 2006;6:177–184.
16. FitzGerald MP, Payne CK, Lukatz CS, Yang CC. Randomised muliticentred feasibility trial of myofascial physical therapy for the treatment of urological chronic pelvic pain syndromes. J Urology 2012;187:2113–8.
17. Fordyce WE, Brockway JA, Bergman JA, Spengler D. Acute back pain: a control-group comparison of behavioral vs traditional management methods. J Behav Med 1986;9:127–140.
18. Gondoh Y. Effect of aerobic exercise training on brain structure and psychological well-being in young adults. J Sport Med Phys Fit 2009;49:129–135.
19. Harding VH, Williams ACdeC. Extending physiotherapy skills using a psychological approach, cognitive-behavioural management of chronic pain. Physiotherapy 1995;81:681–688.
20. Hanson, RW, Gerber, KE. Coping with Chronic Pain; A guide to patient self-management. New York: The Guildford Press;1990:44–46.
21. Iles. R, Davidson M. Evidence based practice: a survey of physiotherapist's current practice. Phys Res Int 2006;11:93–103.
22. Janicki TI. Chronic Pelvic Pain as a form of Complex Regional Pain Syndrome. Clin Obstet Gynecol 2003;46:797–803.
23. Law R, Harvey L, Nicholas MK, et al. Stretch Exercises Increase Tolerance to Stretch in Patients With Chronic Musculoskeletal Pain: A Randomized Controlled Trial. Phys Ther 2009;89:1016–1026.
24. Loving S, Nordling J, Jaszczak T, Thomsen T. Does Evidence Support Physiotherapy Management of Adult Female Chronic Pelvic Pain? A Systematic Review. Scand J Pain 2012;3:70–82.

25. Lin, CW, McAuley JH, Macedo L, et al. Relationship between physical activity and disability in low back pain: A systemic review and meta-analysis. Pain 2011;152:607–613.
26. Lindstrom I, Ohlund C, Eek C, Wallin L, et al. The effect of graded activity on patients with subacute back pain: a randomised prospective clinical study with an operant behavioural approach. Phys Ther 1992;72:279–293.
27. Louw A, Diener I, Butler D, Puentedura E. The effect of Neuroscience education on pain, disability, anxiety and stress in chronic musculoskeletal pain. Arch Phys Med Rehabil 2011;92:2041–2056.
28. Mattsson M, Wikman M, Dahlgren L, Mattsson B. Physiotherapy as Empowerment - treating women with chronic pelvic pain. Adv Phys 2000;2: 125–143.
29. Morley S, Williams A, Hussain S. Estimating the effectiveness of cognitive behavioural therapy in the clinic: Evaluation of a CBT informed pain management programme. Pain 2004;137:670- 680.
30. Moseley L. Evidence for a direct relationship between cognitive and physical change during an education intervention in people with chronic low back pain. J Pain 2003;4:184–189.
31. Moseley L. Combined physiotherapy and education is efficacious for Chronic low back pain. Aust J Phys 2002;48:297–302.
32. Muncey H. Topical Issues in Pain 4. Falmouth: CNS Press. 2000. p.148.
33. NICE. Early Management of Persistent Non-Specific Low Back Pain 2009. Available at: www.nice.org.uk/CG88 accessed 19/12/2012
34. Nicholas M. Chronic Pain Principles and Practice of Relapse Prevention. New York: Guildford Press, 1995: 255–289.
35. Nickel JC, Baranowski AP, Pontari M, et al. Management of men diagnosed with chronic prostatitis/chronic pelvic pain syndrome who have failed traditional management, Med Rev 2007;9: 63–72.
36. Redondo JR, Justo CM, Moraleda FV, et al. Long Term Efficacy of Therapy in Patients with Fibromyalgia: A Physical Exercise-Based Programme and a Cognitive Behavioural Approach. Arthritis Care Res 2004;51: 184–192.
37. Rimer J, Dwan K, Lawlor D, et al. Exercise for depression. Cochr Database Syst Rev 2013;9:CD004366
38. Singh MA. Exercise to prevent and treat functional disability. Clin Geriatr Med 2002;18:431–462.
39. Stones W, Cheong YC, Howard FM. Interventions for treatment of chronic pelvic pain in women, Cochrane Database Syst Reviews 2005;2:CD000387
40. Turner-Stokes L, Goebel A. on behalf of the guideline development group. Complex regional pain syndrome in adults: concise guidance. Clin Med 2011;11:596–600.
41. Verbunt JA, Smeeets RJ, Wittink HM. Cause or effect? Deconditioning or chronic low back pain. Pain 2010;149:428–430.
42. Watson P. Physical activity programme content. In: Main CJ, Spanwick CC (eds) Pain management: an interdisciplinary approach. Edinburgh: Churchill Livingstone, 2000: 285–301.
43. Williams ACDeC, Eccelston C, Morley S. Psychological therapies for the management of chronic pain (excluding headache) in adults. Cochrane Database Syst Rev 2012;11:CD007407.
44. Zanette G, Manganotti P, Fiaschi A, Tamburin S. Modulation of motor cortex excitability after upper limb immobilization. Clin Neurophysiol 2004;115:p.1264–1275.

CHAPTER 22

Psychology in Assessment and Management of Pain

Sarah Edwards, Katherine Herron, and Amanda C de C Williams

INTRODUCTION

Psychological considerations are important in both assessment and management of chronic abdominal and pelvic pain (CAPP), ideally by a multi-disciplinary team (MDT) including a psychologist. As in all chronic pain, CAPP has an emotional and cognitive impact in addition to functional limitations [4], and its effects extend to relationships with family, friends, social life, work, and study [57].

BASIC ASPECTS

The biopsychosocial model of pain describes a complex interaction between pain, behaviour, cognition, emotion, and social context [25]. This model underpins problem formulation and integrated care delivered by the MDT. It is, importantly, shared with patients and related to an individual's particular pain experiences. Psychological components of pain management are included in the evidence-based treatment guidelines of the British Pain Society (BPS) [8] and the European Association of Urology (EAU) [22]. This chapter focuses on how clinicians can incorporate psychological elements into their assessment and treatment.

The term CAPP is used throughout the chapter, applying psychology irrespective of CAPP subtype while recognizing the need to shape it around the patient's problems and situation.

DESCRIBING THE SUBJECT

Integrating Psychology

Pain experience is modulated through interaction between the brain and afferent and efferent pathways, thus cognitive, emotional, and social networks influence the processing and experience of pain. In the short term, negative emotions and thoughts act to facilitate pain signalling and to reduce its inhibition; these dynamics are subserved by anatomical differences in pathways which may be established over the long term [9], such that the longer the individual has had pain, the more emotional its processing [2]. Social and environmental variables, particularly stressors, are represented in these cognitive and emotional networks [28]. Brain imaging studies show that persistent pain is associated with structural, chemical, and functional changes in the brain [5,56].

There is therefore no simple relationship between physical findings, pain experienced, and resulting distress and change in activity [46, 56]. Secondary to pain and the problems it causes, depression and anxiety are common [23,61], further exacerbating pain, feelings of helplessness and difficulty coping [31,53,57]. In all chronic pain, sexual and relationship difficulties occur [1], but particularly in CAPP.

Despite the widely used notion of 'somatisation', the evidence for this in chronic pain is very weak [13]. While longstanding emotional difficulties are likely to predispose to problems managing pain [28], this is far from a straightforward cause and effect relationship, given the complexity of pain as described above. Instruments intended to measure 'somatisation' in fact quantify symptoms, attention to them and concern about them, all unsurprising in the context of unresolved and distressing pain [12]. One study found that a third of women with pelvic pain rated anxiety about the cause of pain as the most troubling aspect [61], anxiety represented in some women by distressing mental images of (imagined) causes such as 'tearing', 'ripping' or 'falling out' of internal organs [7].

Aversive sexual experiences, particularly in childhood, are often suggested as major risk factors for CAPP [16, 28], with implications for patients' and health professionals' attributions about cause. However, methodological shortcomings mean that effects of sexual abuse cannot be segregated from other possible risks [16, 28], and the incidence of sexual abuse is similar in other chronic pains [44]. Most studies use retrospective accounts by women in clinical settings, and use varied definitions of sexual abuse, sometimes combined with physical and emotional abuse. The only prospective study of young women with previously established sexual abuse showed no relationship with CAPP [44].

The main evidence-based psychological models, which we believe can be integrated with biomedical formulations of pain, are behavioural and cognitive. The behavioural model focuses on avoidance of activities which are feared to exacerbate pain or cause injury, such as sexual activity. In the long-term this avoidance restricts activity and worsens fear, often exacerbated by hypervigilance to pain and pain-related cues [12]. The cognitive model posits that many of the behavioural and emotional phenomena described by pain patients are mediated by changes in processing or content of thoughts, such as catastrophising (interpreting internal or external information as threatening and unmanageable) [27] or holding beliefs about the pain or its meaning which add to distress and disability, such as the images described above, or having little confidence in being able to cope with pain [3]. Although described before the imaging studies cited above, the model has been strengthened by these findings [56].

These phenomena and the psychological models which underpin them are described in some detail because they make sense of how people with CAPP present to health services, and the problems they describe in their lives outside healthcare. Historically, theories of 'psychogenic' pain impute moral weakness or motivational deficits as the explanation. For instance, women with pelvic pain commonly report high levels of distress compared to women with no pain, and this was cited as evidence that they were neurotic or exaggerating, often to avoid sexual activity. Once they were compared with women with chronic non-pelvic pain, those differences disappeared: distress is common in any chronic pain [46].

For the individual with CAPP, the experience of unremitting pain whose cause cannot be identified is often frightening and confusing, with fears based on models of acute, not chronic, pain. The hope of finding a treatable cause of pain and eliminating the pain persists in patients and in those who treat them [11, 51], with serial investigations for possible causes. A study of women with chronic pelvic pain receiving negative laparoscopy results found that "women and the professionals with whom they have contact appear to be operating within a medical system designed for acute illnesses" [47]. How test results are delivered to the patient is important: being told that "nothing is wrong" can be seen as a denial of pain, and usually destroys the therapeutic relationship [34]. Test results need to be contextualised within the question, the risk profile, and the entire pathway.

When the symptoms are not eliminated by interventions (often more appropriate for acute pain), patients are understandably distressed and frustrated. Both patient and clinicians may experience a sense of failure, and clinicians may use quasi-psychological explanations [35], such as 'medically unexplained symptoms', interpreted by patients as scepticism or disbelief about the pain [47]. These experiences tend to strengthen the patient's search for validation by diagnosis, still within an acute and predominantly medical framework.

A more helpful framework for conceptualising the emotional, behavioural and cognitive changes associated with chronic pain is a "normal psychology of pain" [19]. Worry about health problems is normal, but particularly distressing when about pain [18]. The recourse to medical help is also normal, given its frequent success for acute pain. Serial consultation is not 'doctor-shopping' or 'dependence' so much as persistence in seeking a solution to something which has seriously disrupted normal life [14]. Reluctance to accept that the problem is chronic and unresolvable is also understandable.

A key task for the clinician is to help the patient to understand chronic pain within a fuller biopsychosocial model, recognising that thoughts, emotions, and behaviour influence the pain and its impact, and that the wider socio-cultural context may also be unsupportive. This reassures patients that they are believed rather than 'making it up', that they are not 'going mad', and inclines them towards accepting advice and treatment from that clinician.

Assessment

A detailed assessment is essential to working successfully with patients with persistent pain, and to understanding their preferences and decisions about treatment. Psychologists tend to conceptualise assessment and intervention as overlapping rather than distinct processes, with ongoing assessment taking place during intervention sessions as a therapeutic alliance develops and the patient becomes more able to divulge their deeper fears or more intimate difficulties. This leads to a formulation of the patient's pain experience and its impact on life, shared between patient and clinician, set in the broader context of the patient's ways of thinking about the world, emotional changes, social circumstances, life events and relationships. On this foundation, treatment goals are identified, and risk and abuse history can be assessed. We describe below how other clinicians can use these assessment principles when opportunities arise.

Beyond symptom assessment, asking how the patient's life has changed because of pain, such as in activities, mood, sleep, work, and close relationships, enables the clinician to appreciate the impact of pain. Specific worries about ability to cope with exacerbations of pain are common, and are often combined with negative cognitive bias. For instance, "I won't be able to work if my pain is this bad, and if I keep missing work I'll lose my job", describes a genuine concern but with catastrophic thinking that pain precludes work, and that job loss (and the consequences of that) is inevitable. Such thinking is typically associated with emotional distress such as sadness, shame, or frustration. Helping to explore the other possibilities and resources which will avoid the catastrophe alleviates distress; recognizing the pattern of thinking enables the individual better to identify it and counter it.

Asking about worries and ideas about what is causing pain, including images, provides the opportunity to give accurate, realistic and personalized information. A question such as "After talking to so many different specialists over the years, what is *your* understanding of why you have pain?" can start this process. Clinicians may be concerned that eliciting these worries will add weight to them, but on the contrary this conversation generally unburdens the patient and legitimises his or her feelings [47]. Patients who are particularly anxious and find it hard to dismiss their worries, despite negative investigations, will benefit from a biopsychosocial explanation of pain and provision of self-management strategies from the outset (see next section), as these help to contain anxiety. This explanation also lays the ground for a more active role for the patient in self-management, even if only reading more about what chronic pain is and is not. It is useful to provide or direct the patient to good quality information, as there is much of poor quality [49].

Questionnaires can be used to elicit more detail, or to gather information from patients who struggle to talk about particular subjects. The Pain Catastrophising Scale [54] effectively identifies catastrophic thinking; the Pain Self-Efficacy Questionnaire [59] measures confidence in engaging in being active despite pain. Assessing mood is complex and often poorly captured by questionnaires, as symptoms such as disrupted sleep and reduced activity are associated with mood and with chronic pain, and some with medication. Publications by the Initiative on Methods, Measurement, and Pain Assessment in Clinical Trials (IMMPACT) group give further guidance on measuring mood as an outcome in chronic pain [57]. Where there is concern about suicide risk [55], or patients report thoughts of self-harm, clinicians need to ascertain if the patient has made plans or attempted to harm themselves. Such patients may not necessarily appear depressed, so assessment requires specific questioning. Clinical experience suggests that specific questions on avoidance of sexual behaviours, and the sexual anxiety subscale of the Multidimensional Sexuality Questionnaire [50], provide a helpful starting point for interventions around sexual activity.

It is also important for clinicians to consider the role of sexual abuse as part of the wider picture in CAPP. Assessing sexual abuse history is a sensitive subject, and requires a trusting therapeutic alliance. Disclosure may not occur at the first visit to the clinic or the first time the question is asked, because of shame, anticipation of negative judgments, or fear of the perpetrator. Open questions about the possible cause of pain, or "Is there anything in your history that you feel may have contributed to your pain?" are consistent with exploring the patient's understanding of pain. It can also be approached by normalising the experience in people with CAPP, for example, "Some of our patients have had traumatic sexual experiences – is that something you have experienced?" For some patients, disclosure may depend on knowing there is sufficient time, privacy, and a supportive context in the consultation, whoever the clinician is. It is crucial to ascertain whether the abuse is ongoing, as this is likely to impact on ability to apply pain management strategies and should be immediately passed onto the appropriate social or healthcare services.

Using those close to the patient, such as family members or friends, can supplement information and involve them in supporting the patient's self-management. It is important that this follows the patient's own account and is not given precedence, and that if an accompanied patient shows signs of reticence about answering questions, the clinician asks for time alone with the patient.

PRACTICAL IMPLICATIONS

Treatment

As difficult as it is to relieve chronic pain, the nervous system is plastic and treatment can focus on reversing some, at least, of these changes. Cognitive and behavioural techniques mainly aim to reverse the impact of pain, but the experience of pain usually also improves. A biopsychosocial assessment is the start [15,22]; then cognitive behavioural therapy (CBT), as a group or individual programme, is usually combined with reactivation involving physical therapist education and guidance, and alongside or following medical management.

A CBT approach aims to help patients reduce distress and disability associated with persistent pain. This is achieved by learning skills such as managing emotional responses which exacerbate or are triggered by pain, changing unhelpful beliefs about pain, learning the most productive way of approaching activities, and re-engaging in feared activities using a graded exposure approach. There is strong evidence for efficacy of CBT in helping people to manage chronic pain [60]. In-depth mood management and cognitive work requires psychological training, but other members of the MDT using CBT methods can facilitate a wide range of changes for patients at behavioural, cognitive and emotional levels, which then impact positively on the pain experience. Particularly in explaining pain, normalising worries about it, and discussing risks and benefits of extending activity towards goals, all clinicians can contribute significantly. Normalisation of the emotional, behavioural, and cognitive changes linked with CAPP, by reassuring the patient that they are "not the only one" going through these, and explaining them in terms of a "normal" reaction to pain [19], can go a long way to reducing anxiety and the sense of isolation which patients with CAPP feel.

The value of education about pain mechanisms, individualised to the patient's particular symptoms and history, cannot be overestimated, and is often what CAPP patients most want from their first appointment [43]. It may also help the clinician to elicit the "what if?" worries about and images of cancer or other serious diseases, and fears about pain prognosis, the correction of which is an essential part of CBT work. When working with patients with a history of sexual abuse, the clinician should consider the possibility that the patient believes that the abuse caused irreparable damage which generates pain, providing an obvious target for education.

Patients with any type of persistent pain may struggle to maintain sexual intimacy [36, 48], and this is particularly true for CAPP patients [26]. In addition to the pain, the clinician should consider medication side-effects [24] and relationship problems. Most self-help texts for sexual problems are written for those in good health, but have useful material challenging myths about sexual desire, performance, and satisfaction which only add to anxiety. In addition, systematic desensitisation, communication, and a paced approach to building up sexual contact, such as sensate focus techniques, are key in rebuilding sexual activity.

There are few good quality trials of CBT for CAPP [22]. The only randomised controlled trial compared an integrated approach (although with little psychological contribution) with standard treatment for women with pelvic pain, and found that the integrated approach improved more [42]. A small pilot study of group CBT adapted for men with CAPP showed significant decreases in disability, catastrophic thinking and pain level [58]. Data from our pelvic pain management programme at the National Hospital for Neurology and Neurosurgery in London shows reductions in pain intensity, disability, unhelpful thinking about pain, and anxiety about sexual activity, and improvements in mood and pain-related confidence for both men and women [6, 20]. These gains meet or exceed the treatment benchmark for PMPs for general pain [37].

A more recent psychological treatment is Acceptance and Commitment Therapy (ACT) [59]. ACT focuses on increasing acceptance of pain and value based actions which lead to positive behavioural experiences, reducing avoidance of valued activities [32]. Unlike CBT, ACT makes fewer attempts to directly manage pain. A combined systematic review and meta-analysis for mixed chronic pain, but including uncontrolled studies, showed that ACT was not superior to CBT but provided a useful alternative, for example, for patients with widespread patterns of avoidance and little conviction in meaning of life [59].

Finally, it is important for the team to communicate frequently and effectively about patients, particularly those with complex problems, at risk of suicide or self-harm, or with many components to treatment. Apart from skills in assessing risk, and the overall psychological contribution to treatment, the psychologist can helpfully enable the team to think psychologically about all aspects of treatment, and to realise their potential in bringing about positive changes for the patient.

LOOKING AT THE FUTURE

Increasing use of neuroscience to enable us to integrate psychological understandings, often expressed in abstract but accessible terminology, with the complexity of chronic pain neurophysiology, will provide us with better models with which genuine patient-clinician partnerships can be built. Integrating those explanations into our everyday work with patients, normalising their experience for them, ourselves and fellow clinicians, reduces the gap between clinician and patient into which many genuine efforts to help disappear without trace. It also enables us to minimise the extent to which the patient is rendered a helpless body on which medical procedures are performed, after which, when those procedures fail to relieve the pain, the patient is told to 'self-manage'. Psychologists with expertise in pain are in short supply everywhere, and some of the psychologically therapeutic work we have described requires their training. But models of joint work and consultation can enhance clinicians' psychological skills and understanding, to the benefit of all their patients, and usually to the clinicians' greater satisfaction [38].

We have written mainly for clinicians in specialist care, but only a minority of patients reach specialist pain services, and primary healthcare is often poorly informed about chronic pain in general, despite its prevalence. Additionally, other healthcare providers whom the CAPP patient may encounter in their healthcare journey, such as gynaecologists and urologists, have an important role in understanding and communicating understanding of pain to their patients.

In specialist settings, we look forward to seeing more trials of CBT and ACT specifically for CAPP, but there is no reason why the literature on mixed chronic pain populations would not apply, so the issue is more of maximizing usefulness rather than evaluating efficacy. In addition to direct clinical work, there is a lack of books, websites and other resources which do not largely or exclusively refer to musculoskeletal pain; there are few designed for people with CAPP. As well as bolstering limited clinical resources, these can help patients to feel more confident in managing their own pain, initiating changes themselves which will improve quality of life (see Further Reading). Such resources need to be accessible across many languages, and for those with limited reading skills. Web-based interventions have the potential for being a cost- and time-effective way of delivering pain management, and can be helpful for some patients as part of an overall treatment package [30].

TAKE HOME MESSAGES

- Psychological considerations including behavioural, emotional, and cognitive factors are well-evidenced aspects of the biopsychosocial model of chronic pain and are recommended in best-practice management of CAPP.
- A detailed assessment eliciting information directly from the patient about these factors will maximise clinician understanding of the patients pain experience.
- Individualizing the biopsychosocial model to the patient's own difficulties, thereby integrating the biomedical, cognitive, behavioural, social, and emotional changes experienced, helps to reduce patient anxiety and encourage self-management.
- Psychological elements of pain management can be incorporated into interventional work by any clinician, by delivering education about pain mechanisms, normalising the cognitive and emotional changes seen in pain, and discussing activity re-activation.
- As well as carrying out mood management and cognitive work, psychologists have a key role in indirect patient work via team discussions and supervision facilitating colleagues in thinking psychologically about CAPP patients.

FURTHER READING

For psychologist practitioners or other clinicians interested in broadening their knowledge of cognitive-behavioural principles, "CBT for Chronic Illness and Palliative Care" [45] is a useful guide to using CBT to manage chronic health conditions which can be applied in CAPP.

Clinicians are encouraged to suggest self-help materials to build on patients' knowledge, as appropriate to their individual needs. Some suggestions include a general CBT-based text for managing pain, which can also be applied to CAPP [10, 40]; a text focussed in increasing function [52]; websites which provide information and support networks for CAPP sufferers (in the UK, the Pelvic Pain Support Network [41] or Endometriosis UK [21]); or, for a non-CBT-based approach, a text on using ACT to manage pain [29].

REFERENCES

1. Ambler N, Williams AC, Hill P, et al. Sexual difficulties of chronic pain patients. Clin J Pain 2001;17:138–45.
2. Apkarian AV, Hashmi JA, Baliki MN. Pain and the brain: specificity and plasticity of the brain in clinical chronic pain. Pain 2011;152:S49–S64.
3. Asghari A, Nicholas MK. Pain self-efficacy beliefs and pain behaviour: a prospective study. Pain 2001; 94:85–100.
4. Ashburn MA, Staats PS. Pain: management of chronic pain. Lancet 1999;353:1865–69.
5. As-Sanie S, Harris RE, Napadow V, et al T. Changes in regional gray matter volume in women with chronic pelvic pain: a voxel-based morphometry study. Pain 2012;153:1006–14.
6. Baranowski PA, Mandeville AL, Edwards S, et al. Male chronic -pelvic pain syndrome and the role of interdisciplinary pain management. World J Urol 2013;31:779–84.
7. Berna C, Vincent K, Moore J, et al. Presence of mental imagery associated with chronic pelvic pain: a pilot study. Pain Med 2011;12:1086–93.
8. British Pain Society (BPS). Recommended guidelines for pain management programmes for adults. BPS © 2007. URL: http://bps.mapofmedicine.com/evidence/bps/chronic_pelvic_pain_for_men_and_women_1.html Accessed October 2013.
9. Bushnell MC, Ceko M, Low LA. Cognitive and emotional control of pain and its disruption in chronic pain. Nat Rev Neurosci 2013; 14:502–11.
10. Cole F, Howden-Leach H, Macdonald H, Carus C. Overcoming Chronic Pain: A Self-Help Guide Using Cognitive Behavioral Techniques. London: Constable & Robinson, 2005.
11. Coudeyre E, Rannou F, Tubach F, et al. General practitioners' fear-avoidance beliefs influence their management of patients with low back pain. Pain 2006;124:330–7.
12. Crombez G, Van Damme S, Eccleston C. Hypervigilance to pain: an experimental and clinical analysis. Pain 2005;116:4–7.

13. Crombez G, Beirens K, Van Damme S, et al. The unbearable lightness of somatisation: a systematic review of the concept of somatisation in empirical studies of pain. Pain 2009;145:31–35.
14. Crombez G, Eccleston C, Van Damme S, et al. Fear-avoidance model of chronic pain: the next generation. Clin J Pain 2012;28:475–83.
15. Curran N. Chronic urogenital pain in men. BJP 2008;2:25–28.
16. Daniels JP, Khan KS. Clinical review: Chronic pelvic pain in women. BMJ 2010;341:772–5.
17. Dworkin RH, Turk DC, Farrar JT, et al; IMMPACT. Topical review and recommendations: Core outcome measures for chronic pain clinical trials: IMMPACT recommendations. Pain 2005;113:9–19.
18. Eccleston C, Crombez G, Aldrich S. Worrying about chronic pain: a description and an exploratory analysis of individual differences. Eur J Pain 2001;5:309–18.
19. Eccleston C, Crombez G. Worry and chronic pain: A misdirected problem-solving model. Pain 2007; 132:233–36.
20. Edwards S, Williams A, Brook S, et al. The effectiveness of specialised pain management programmes: Benchmarking against published outcomes for general pain management programmes. 2012 British Pain Society Annual Scientific Meeting, Liverpool UK, 24–27th April.
21. Endometriosis UK. URL: http://www.endometriosis-uk.org/. Accessed October 2013.
22. Engeler DS, Baranowski AP, Elneil S, et al. Guidelines on Chronic Pelvic Pain. Uroweb. 2012. Available at: http://www.uroweb.org/gls/pdf/24_Chronic_Pelvic_Pain_LR%20II.pdf Accessed October 2013.
23. Fitzgerald MP, Link CL, Litman HJ, et al. Beyond the lower urinary tract: the association of urinary and sexual symptoms with common illnesses. Eur Urol 2007;52:407–15.
24. Fleming MP, Paice JA. Sexuality and chronic pain. J Sex Educ Ther 2001;26:204–14.
25. Gatchel RJ, Peng YB, Peters, ML, et al. The biopsychosocial approach to chronic pain: scientific advances and future directions. Psychol Bull 2007;133:581–624.
26. Heinberg LJ, Fisher BJ, Wesselmann U, et al. Psychological factors in pelvic/urogenital pain: The influence of site of pain versus sex. Pain 2004;108:88–94.
27. Keefe FJ, Lefebvre JC, Egert JR, et al. The relationship of gender to pain, pain behaviour, and disability in osteoarthritis patients: the role of catastrophizing. Pain 2000;87:325–34.
28. Latthe P, Mignini L, Gray R, et al. Factors predisposing women to chronic pelvic pain: systematic review. BMJ 2006;332:749–55.
29. Lundgren T, Dahl J. Living Beyond Your Pain: Using Acceptance and Commitment Therapy to Ease Chronic Pain. Oakland: New Harbinger, 2006.
30. Macea DD, Gajos K, Daglia Calil YA, Fregni F. The efficacy of web-based cognitive behavioral interventions for chronic pain: a systematic review and meta-analysis. J Pain 2010;11:917–929.
31. McCracken LM, Vowles KE, Eccleston C. Acceptance of chronic pain: component analysis and a revised assessment method. Pain 2004;107:159–66.
32. McCracken LM. Contextual cognitive-behavioral therapy for chronic pain. Seattle: IASP press, 2005.
33. McCracken LM, Vowles KE, Eccelston C. Acceptance-based treatment for persons with complex, long standing chronic pain: a preliminary analysis of treatment outcome in comparison to a waiting phase. Behav Res Ther 2005;43:1335–46.
34. McGowan LPA, Clark-Carter D, Pitts MK. Chronic Pelvic Pain: A meta-analytic review. Psychol Health 1998;13:937–951.
35. Merskey H. Somatization: or another God that failed. Pain. 2009;145:4–5.
36. Monga TN, Tan G, Ostermann HJ, et al. Sexuality and Sexual adjustment of patients with chronic pain. Disabil Rehabil 1998;20:317–29.
37. Morley S, Williams A, Hussain S. Estimating the clinical effectiveness of cognitive behavioural therapy in the clinic: evaluation of a CBT informed pain management programme. Pain 2008;137:670–80.
38. Moseley GL, Nicholas MK, Hodges PW. A randomized controlled trial of intensive neurophysiology education in chronic low back pain. Clin J Pain 2004;20:324–330.
39. Nicholas MK. The pain self-efficacy questionnaire: taking pain into account. Eur J Pain 2007;11:153–63.
40. Nicolas, M, Molloy A, Beeston L, Tonkin L. Manage Your Pain: Practical and Positive Ways of Adapting to Chronic Pain. London: Souvenir Press 2011.
41. Pelvic Pain Support Network. URL: http://www.pelvicpain.org.uk/. Accessed October 2013.
42. Peters AAW, van Dorst E, Jellis B, et al. A randomized clinical trial to compare two different approaches in women with chronic pelvic pain. Obstet Gynecol 1991;77:740–744.
43. Price J, Farmer G, Harris J, et al. Attitudes of women with chronic pelvic pain to the gynaecological consultation: a qualitative study. BJOG 2006;113:446–52.

44. Raphael KG, Widom CS, Lange G. Childhood victimization and pain in adulthood: a prospective investigation. Pain 2001;92:283–93.
45. Sage N, Sowden M, Chorlton E, Edeleanu A. CBT for Chronic Illness and Palliative Care. Chichester: Wiley-Blackwell, 2008.
46. Savidge CJ, Slade P. Psychological Aspects of Chronic Pelvic Pain. J Psychosom Res 1997;42:433–444.
47. Savidge CJ, Slade P, Steward P, Li TC. Women's perspectives on their experiences of chronic pelvic pain and medical care. J Health Psychol 1998;3:103–16.
48. Schwartz L, Slater MA. The impact of chronic pain on the spouse; research and clinical implications. Holist Nurs Pract 1991;6:9–16.
49. Showghi NN, Williams ACdeC. Information about male chronic pelvic and urogenital pain on the internet: an evaluation of internet resources. Pain Med 2012;13:1275–83.
50. Snell WE, Fisher TD, Walters AS. The multidimensional sexuality questionnaire: An objective self-report measure of psychological tendencies associated with human sexuality. Anns Sex Res 1993;6:27–55.
51. Souza PP, Romão AS, Rosa-e-Silva JC, et al. Qualitative research as the basis for a biopsychosocial approach to women with chronic pelvic pain. J Psychosom Obs Gynecol 2011;32:165.
52. Stein A. Heal Pelvic Pain: The Proven Stretching, Strengthening, and Nutrition Program for Relieving Pain, Incontinence, & I.B.S, and Other Symptoms Without Surgery. USA: McGraw-Contemporary, 2008.
53. Stones RW, Selfe SA, Fransman S, Horn SA. Psychosocial and economic impact of chronic pelvic pain. Baillière's Best Pract Res Clin Obstet Gynaecol 2000;14:415–31.
54. Sullivan MJL, Bishop S, Pivik J. The Pain Catastrophizing Scale: development and validation. Psychol Assess 1995;7:524–32.
55. Tang NK, Crane C. Suicidality in chronic pain: a review of the prevalence, risk factors and psychological links. Psychol Med 2006;36:575–86.
56. Tracey I, Bushnell MC. How neuroimaging studies have challenged us to rethink: is chronic pain a disease? J Pain 2009;10:1113–20.
57. Tripp DA, Nickel JC, Wang Y, et al; National Institutes of Health Chronic Prostatitis Collaborative Research Networks (NIH-CPCRN) Study Group. Catastrophizing and pain-contingent rest predict patient adjustment in men with chronic prostatitis/chronic pelvic pain syndrome. J Pain 2006;7:697–708.
58. Tripp DA, Nickel JC, Katz LA. A feasibility trial of a cognitive-behavioural symptom management program for chronic pelvic pain for men with refractory chronic prostatitis/chronic pelvic pain syndrome. Can Urol Assoc J 2011;5:328–332.
59. Veehof MM, Oskam MJ, Schreurs KM, Bohlmeijer ET. Acceptance-based interventions for the treatment of chronic pain: A systematic review and meta-analysis. Pain 2011;152:533–42.
60. Williams A, Eccleston C, Morley S. Psychological therapies for the management of chronic pain (excluding headache) in adults. Cochrane Database Syst Rev 2012;14:CD007407.
61. Zondervan KT, Yudkin PL, Vessey MP, et al. The community prevalence of chronic pelvic pain in women and associated illness behaviour. Br J Gen Pract. 2001;51:541–7.

CHAPTER 23

Neuromodulation of Abdominal and Pelvic Pain

Melissa Farmer

INTRODUCTION

Over the last 50 years of pain research, we have been obsessed with peripheral nervous system mechanisms of nociception. From the chemical mediators that stimulate afferent nerve endings, to the glycinergic control of central sensitization in the spinal dorsal horn, our view of nociception has largely ignored the role of supraspinal processing. This preoccupation is surprising, given that the field has matured with Melzack and Wall's revolutionary idea that pain perception requires cortical processing [31]. We have, in essence, decapitated pain.

Chronic abdominal and pelvic pain consists of a family of visceral pain conditions initiated by organ pathology and chronically maintained by aberrant peripheral and central processes. The characteristics that define visceral pain emphasize the role of the brain in nociceptive processing. Visceral pain consists of diffusely localized pain that is inherently linked with negative emotion and autonomic reactivity. The implications of this coexistence are that the nociceptive processes underlying the chronification of visceral pain must be accompanied by sustained negative emotion, such as anxiety and/or depression, as well as ongoing autonomic arousal, which may parallel the elevated arousal that characterizes chronic stress, both of which recruit extensive cortical processing [37]. Furthermore, the co-occurrence of visceral pain and negative emotion may enhance the formation of pain-related memories. It has been hypothesized that memory formation relies on arousal mechanisms to modulate memory strength [10,30] such that memories encoded during emotion-laden situations will be well remembered for future adaptive purposes. In turn, abdominal and pelvic pain may further dysregulate emotional circuitry, as it disrupts some of the most inherently rewarding physiological processes, including eating, sex, urination, and defecation, which are required for the survival of the organism.

This chapter explores how the brain shapes the modulation of abdominal and pelvic pain across different time scales, through changes in brain function and structure. It is argued that limbic, rather than classic nociceptive circuitry is the primary site of central reorganization in visceral pain.

BASIC ASPECTS

Chronic visceral pain, like any learned experience, is subject to the rules of memory formation and maintenance. As a result, the impact of visceral pain is etched into the synaptic patterns that have relayed nociceptive and emotional information with the repeated exposure to painful visceral stimuli. The activity of these individual synapses is not accessible via neuroimaging due to poor spatial resolution, given that a single voxel represents roughly 100,000 neurons [28]. However, in understanding the rules by which these neurons function and interact, we can extrapolate these principles to large populations of neurons that are accessible via imaging.

The Hebbian axiom, "Neurons that fire together wire together," is useful in understanding how brain function relates to anatomy. The relay of neural information is physically constrained by the properties of individual neurons (such as variations in axonal and dendritic morphology), their interactions with resident glia, the number of synaptic connections they make with neighboring neurons, and their connections with distant neuronal populations. These anatomical constraints are not fixed; rather, these properties can dynamically adapt to reflect new learning, rendering brain function and anatomy interdependent.

Brain function and structure convey a rich amount of information about the progression from acute to chronic pain. A range of imaging modalities can address unique and complementary clinical questions as to how the brain adapts to pain in the short- and long-term. Short-term changes are reflected in brain functional properties, whereas longer-term changes (as well as predispositions) associated with chronic pain are evident in gray and white matter properties, as well as through cross-sectional and longitudinal assessments of brain function related to clinical pain.

Functional activity associated with acute and chronic pain is measured using functional magnetic resonance imaging (fMRI), which infers neural activation from local variations in oxygenated blood flow [27]. Regional changes in the blood oxygen level dependent (BOLD) signal that correlate with painful stimulation or its perception have yielded consistent patterns of activity in the anterior cingulate cortex (ACC), somatosensory cortices (S1 and S2), insula (INS), thalamus (Th), and prefrontal cortex (PFC), which are collectively referred to as the acute pain "matrix" [46]. Functional activation of these regions has repeatedly correlated with clinically important aspects of pain perception (e.g., pain intensity, unpleasantness, duration, etc), potentially providing an "objective" measure of pain [49]. However, critics have questioned the sensitivity and specificity of this acute pain signature because it is also elicited by non-painful stimulation, as well as by other sensory modalities [21]. Growing evidence also suggests that the neural representation of chronic pain deviates from this acute pain matrix in condition-specific patterns [2]. The literature remains divided as to how abnormal cortical processing of nociceptive information may manifest in the chronic pain state.

A complementary view of brain functional activity is to view the brain as a conglomerate of efficiently communicating neural networks. When activity in two or more network elements (e.g., voxels, regions) consistently correlate across time they are said to be functionally connected. Network connectivity appears to reflect transient states of mind, including intrinsic and task-related states [19], as well as developmental processes and the presence of chronic disease [1,39]. This suggests that networks can manifest short- and long-term neuroplasticity by (a) adapting to brain state changes in order to optimize the representation of information, as well as (b) evolve over time based on reinforced functional connections, which may in turn promote structural changes [17]. As a result, the rich information conferred by neural networks captures activity and communication patterns that are inaccessible via traditional general linear modeling analysis of fMRI data.

Neuroimaging can differentiate broad anatomical features of the brain, such as gray (neuronal) matter and white (axonal) matter properties. Gray matter is visualized with T1-weighted anatomical images, which differentiate types of brain tissue based on their magnetic properties. Although gray matter density is often assumed to reflect regional concentrations of neurons, it may also reflect changes in vasculature, non-neuronal (glial) growth, neuron morphology (e.g., dendritic arborization and spine growth), neurodegeneration, and less often neurogenesis. The regional distribution of gray matter can capture anatomical changes that take weeks to months to occur. Regional changes in gray matter are associated with the central processes that underlie the maintenance and remission of chronic pain [4,41]. Indeed, brain morphology continues to adapt to the presence of chronic pain over the course of years [5].

White matter microstructure is deduced using diffusion tensor imaging (DTI), which measures directional water flow within the brain. Whereas the water flow within the physical confines of a neuron is uniform in all directions, the water flow along the length of myelinated axons is directionally dependent, or anisotropic. Chronic pain is typically accompanied by subtle changes in white matter integrity, and these axonal properties may change over the course of days to weeks, indicating that it is a longer-term index of brain reorganization. Alternatively, certain white matter properties may also reflect a predisposition for chronic pain development, as suggested by the first longitudinal neuroimaging study of the transition to chronic back pain [29].

DESCRIBING THE SUBJECT

Genital Pain

Vulvar pain syndrome/Vulvodynia, is the most common type of female genital pain, affecting approximately 8% of premenopausal women [36]. In healthy women, vulvar touch and pain perception evoke equivalent patterns of brain activity that are classically observed with acute pain [16]. Similarly, women with provoked vulvodynia exhibit a similar pattern of activity during experimentally-induced vulvar mechanical stimulation. Higher levels of INS and PFC activation were cited as evidence of elevated pain processing in patients, yet equivalent levels of subjective pain in healthy women were not assessed, nor was an innocuous vulvar stimulation control included in the design [35]. This activation pattern was confirmed in a recent study, however, women presenting with different subtypes of vulvodynia did not show elevated regional activity when compared to clinical (fibromyalgia) and healthy controls [20]. Despite this equivocal evidence of altered central nociceptive processing, women with provoked vulvodynia exhibit increased subcortical gray matter density in the basal ganglia and parahippocampal gyrus/hippocampus [38]. These structural changes may reflect longer-term shifts in information processing related to chronic vulvar pain. Indeed, these gray matter properties correlated with multiple clinical indices of vulvar hypersensitivity, as well as with self-reports of pain catastrophizing.

These studies indicate that provoked vulvar pain in women with vulvar pain/vulvodynia recruits the same pattern of nociceptive processing observed during acute pain perception in healthy individuals. On first glance, this finding challenges the hypothesis that abnormal vulvar pain processing plays a role in vulvar pain/vulvodynia. However, multiple methodological and sample biases, noted above, may confound these results. It is also possible that these studies may have failed to elicit clinically-relevant vulvar pain (due to vaginal penetration, for instance) and therefore have limited relevance to the actual mechanisms underlying the condition. The presence of subcortical anatomical abnormalities that correlate with clinical pain parameters, in particular, suggests the presence of either preexisting vulnerabilities that make these women more likely to develop vulvar pain/vulvodynia, or they are indicative of subcortical reorganization related to the maintenance of chronic vulvar pain.

Menstrual Pain

One of the most common forms of female pelvic pain is menstrual pain, or dysmenorrhea, which causes severe pain in 2–29% of premenopausal women [23,48]. During menstruation, pain-related brain activity does not differ between women with and without dysmenorrhea. Specifically, painful thermal lower abdominal and arm stimulation evoked similar activation patterns in the secondary somatosensory cortex (SII), premotor cortex (PMC), INS, ACC, posterior cingulate cortex (PCC), orbitofrontal cortex (OFC), and subcortical regions (e.g., putamen, thalamus (Th), caudate, and brainstem) [48].

Women with dysmenorrhea exhibit a range of cortical and subcortical anatomical changes that correlate with clinical parameters. A well-designed study of this population discovered nuanced gray matter changes during menstrual and peri-ovulatory phases [47]. Compared to menstrual phase-matched controls, women with dysmenorrhea exhibited increased gray matter in the left medial OFC, left PMC, right postcentral gyrus within S1, right precuneus (PC), and right hypothalamus, as well as decreased gray matter in S2, ACC, and dorsal PCC. Menstrual pain intensity positively correlated with increased right caudate nucleus and hypothalamus gray matter and negatively correlated with left Th gray matter density [47]. Furthermore, during menstruation, women with pain had increased gray matter density in the left orbital gyrus, left precentral gyrus within the PMC, left inferior temporal gyrus, right hypothalamus, as well as decreased gray matter in left S2 and left anterior/dorsal PCC. These findings may not generalize to other types of female pelvic pain, however, given that women with endometriosis-related pain exhibit reduced gray matter restricted to the left Th, left cingulate gyrus, right putamen, and right INS, compared to controls [3].

The Tu study [47] is significant in the visceral pain imaging field, as it demonstrates the impact of chronic, intermittent visceral pain on the brain. Specifically, rapid fluctuations in gray matter properties closely correlate with variations in clinical pain severity. These data suggest that visceral pain conditions that are characterized by cyclic exacerbations of pain may show greater cortical reorganization with increased pain frequency and severity. These short-term pain fluctuations are of particular clinical interest given our poor understanding of pain "flares," a term used to describe exacerbations of pain that may last minutes, days, or weeks [45]. Importantly, a subset of the observed anatomical changes may reflect the ongoing central maintenance of visceral pain, whereas other morphological features may signify the short-term structural changes resulting from repeated peripheral insults related to menstruation. These findings stand in stark contrast to data from musculoskeletal pain populations, who show sustained reductions in regional gray matter density across the course of months [4].

Urological Pelvic Pain

Prostate Pain Syndrome/Chronic Pelvic Pain Syndrome (PPS/CPPS) occurs in 5–8% of men [12]. PPS/CPPS is characterized by a combination of spontaneous or provoked pelvic or genital pain, as well as pain with ejaculation in approximately a third of the clinical population [14]. Symptoms may be accompanied by bladder dysfunction similar to that observed in Bladder Pain Syndrome/interstitial cystitis (BPS/IC), including pain with urination, as well as urinary urgency and frequency. No imaging studies have evaluated neural correlates of experimental or naturalistic pain in men or women with BPS/IC, yet imaging work has begun to explore neural correlates of PPS/CPPS. In an early study, men with PPS/CPPS continuously rated the intensity of their spontaneous pain during a 10 minute scan, and this activity was contrasted with activity from a sensorimotor and cognitive-evaluative control task [18]. The contrast yielded a unique map of pelvic pain-related brain activity, including the INS, dorsolateral PFC, PPC, SI, primary motor cortex (M1), and precuneus regions. Anterior INS activity and gray matter density were associated with the magnitude of pelvic pain, whereas anterior ACC gray matter density increased with longer pain duration. In addition to regional alterations, the relationship between whole-brain gray and white matter was disrupted, which is suggestive of large-scale cortical reorganization [18]. In a separate PPS/CPPS cohort, significant reductions in anterior ACC volume, which correlated with pain severity, were identified [33]. However, these findings are difficult to interpret given that the presence of distinct PPS/CPPS subtypes within these samples may increase sample variability and reduce statistical power. Despite the preliminary nature of these findings, these studies provide intriguing initial evidence of local and global brain changes in PPS/CPPS that reflect the severity and duration of pelvic pain.

The use of spontaneous pain ratings to extract pain-relevant brain activity in men with pelvic pain highlights the methodological and clinical biases that are characteristic of the pain imaging field. First, these findings confirm that ongoing, naturalistic pelvic pain shows limited functional overlap with acute pain-related activity, and this conclusion would not have been reached with the experimental pain induction tasks used elsewhere in the literature. Rather, chronic pelvic pain recruits a unique pattern of brain activity that likely reflects neural mechanisms specific to the condition. Second, this study emphasizes the intrinsic temporal variability of the pelvic pain experience. This variability is not adequately captured with a single visual analog scale number, which is widely used by clinicians.

Abdominal Pain

The most common functional gastrointestinal disorder is irritable bowel syndrome (IBS), which may be characterized by a combination of abdominal pain, cramping, bloating, constipation and diarrhea. The majority of IBS pain imaging studies, have evaluated brain activity during acute visceral pain induction using experimentally-induced rectal distension, which admittedly has limited relevance to the clinical state. These studies have yielded mixed support for the hypothesis that chronic abdominal pain is propagated by abnormal nociceptive and descending inhibitory processes. On one hand, nonpainful and painful rectal distension activates a common set of brain regions in IBS and healthy populations, including the ACC, INS, PFC, Th, and brainstem [6,7,15,26,32,34,44,50]. Despite the claims that greater activations in these regions are evidence of abnormal nociceptive processing in IBS, a meta-analysis of 16 studies with comparable methodology concluded that only anterior INS (antINS) activity and its connectivity with other key regions (e.g. posterior INS, Th, PCC, ACC, PFC) is consistently greater in IBS [42]. Given that the antINS regulates interoception (including emotional awareness, based on its rich connectivity to limbic regions) as well as visceral and autonomic responses, these functions may be critically disrupted in IBS.

Specific regions are implicated in the top-down modulation of IBS pain. One study found that greater IBS related functional activity in the ACC and PFC was no longer statistically significant when anxiety and depression were controlled for and these regions may therefore preferentially mediate the affective responses to IBS pain [15]. Reduced activation of the PFC, in particular, is associated with heightened negative emotion [8], potentially suggesting an impaired capacity for top-down control of pain perception. Sex differences in distension-related brain activity, driven by emotion circuitry, appear to mediate this dissociation between sensory and affective aspects of chronic abdominal pain [24,25].

Structural changes related to IBS remain controversial. Cortical thinning of gray matter in the midcingulate cortex, ACC, and INS has been replicated across multiple laboratories [9,13,22,25]. The INS structural abnormalities are corroborated by a report of increased white matter integrity adjacent to the postINS and antINS, which correlated with pain severity, unpleasantness, and duration [11]. Reports of regional changes in gray matter volume have been less consistent and have included evidence of increased hypothalamic volume and reduced anterior/medial Th volume [9,13]. In contrast, the largest IBS study conducted to date determined that, after controlling for anxiety and depression, only increased gray matter in the PFC and PPC remained statistically significant [40], again highlighting the importance of segregating sensory and affect related structural abnormalities.

PRACTICAL IMPLICATIONS

One of the most intriguing findings from visceral pain neuroimaging is that the extent of brain functional and structural reorganization can reflect clinically meaningful pain properties, such as subjective pain intensity, duration, and even emotional dimensions of pain. After years of living with pain, these neural adaptations have far-reaching influences on how an individual perceives herself and her world. The sufferer has learned that certain activities such as sex, eating, and excretion will reliably elicit visceral pain. She has learned to avoid behaviors that exacerbate this pain, so perhaps she no longer dines in public for fear of abdominal discomfort and its consequences. Perhaps she no longer desires sexual contact or seeks physical closeness with her partner because it will inevitably lead to painful intercourse. She has also learned to carefully adopt physical postures that minimize discomfort, leading to restricted movement and heightened pelvic floor muscle tension. Our traditional focus on end-organ pathology is woefully inadequate to explain these physiological, behavioral, and psychological consequences of chronic visceral pain.

The field has evolved with the assumption that suspected etiology, based on an initial identifiable peripheral injury, should play a primary role in phenotyping and treatment efforts. This fallacy is conceptually and practically counterproductive because it ignores the role of ongoing peripheral and central interactions that determine how the body adapts to the persistence of pain, that is, it neglects critical aspects of the disease process. Central mechanisms of pain maintenance are necessarily part of this process.

Clinicians and researchers are acutely aware of the need for a paradigm shift in how abdominal and pelvic pain is assessed, diagnosed, and treated. A prominent conceptual issue that must be resolved is the problem of accurate clinical phenotyping. Because many of these idiopathic pain conditions are defined by a collection of symptoms rather than clearly defined disease processes, the current diagnostic classifications are based on heterogeneous patient samples that may include a variety of mechanistically-distinct subtypes. Accumulating clinical and basic science research confirms that these subtypes will vary in the respective roles of peripheral and central processes in both the initiation and maintenance of chronic visceral pain. Therefore, the identification of brain functional and anatomical biomarkers that covary with clinically relevant symptoms should be a priority for these classification efforts.

For instance, even the increasingly popular UPOINT classification system for pelvic pain (*U*rinary symptoms, *P*sychosocial dysfunction, *O*rgan-specific findings, *I*nfection, *N*eurologic/systemic, *T*enderness of skeletal muscles) does not currently acknowledge the contribution of brain reorganization in chronic pelvic pain [43]. The UPOINT psychosocial domain, which is restricted to cognitive-emotional responses that can be dissociated from chronic pain, does not reference the cortical processing of nociceptive information. The neurologic/systemic domain refers to pelvic versus extra-pelvic pain, with the implication that extra-pelvic pain may reflect central sensitization, a spinal phenomenon. Inclusion of brain functional and structural abnormalities within the neurologic/systemic domain would be an appropriate amendment to these criteria.

LOOKING AT THE FUTURE

The priority for visceral pain neuroimaging is the thorough assessment of brain functional and structural abnormalities, or biomarkers, that characterize the natural course of pain development and maintenance. Although visceral pain conditions may share similar patterns of brain reorganization, such as large-scale shifts in subcortical function and structure, the identification of the neural biomarkers that distinguish these diagnoses is necessary. As demonstrated with cyclic menstrual pain, a longitudinal characterization of brain structure is required to dissociate mechanisms underlying chronic pain initiation versus maintenance. The key in translating these findings to the clinic is to identify behavioral proxies of these biomarkers that can be rapidly and accurately assessed by clinicians. Ideally, such proxies can guide early interventions in those who are vulnerable to develop persistent pain and can direct the therapeutic use of centrally acting agents and/or psychotherapy in patients who are most likely to respond.

TAKE HOME MESSAGES

- Central mechanisms underlying abdominal and pelvic pain are accessible via brain imaging techniques.
- Brain functional and structural reorganization reflects pain-related neuroplasticity.
- The chronification of abdominal and pelvic pain is characterized by central nociceptive and emotional abnormalities.
- Condition-specific brain reorganization takes place at the regional and global levels.

FURTHER READING

Bodnar RJ, Commons K, Pfaff DW (eds), Central neural states relating sex and pain. Baltimore, MD: John Hopkins University Press, 2002.

Bailey A, Bernstein C (eds). Pain in women: A clinical guide. New York, NY: Springer, 2013.

REFERENCES

1. Alexander-Bloch AF, Vertes PE, Stidd R, et al. The anatomical distance of functional connections predicts brain network topology in health and schizophrenia. Cerebral cortex 2013;23(1):127–138.
2. Apkarian AV, Hashmi JA, Baliki MN. Pain and the brain: specificity and plasticity of the brain in clinical chronic pain. Pain 2011;152(3 Suppl):S49–64.

3. As-Sanie S, Harris RE, Napadow V, et al. Changes in regional gray matter volume in women with chronic pelvic pain: a voxel-based morphometry study. Pain 2012;153(5):1006–1014.
4. Baliki MN, Petre B, Torbey S, et al. Corticostriatal functional connectivity predicts transition to chronic back pain. Nature Neurosci 2012;15(8):1117–1119.
5. Baliki MN, Schnitzer TJ, Bauer WR, Apkarian AV. Brain morphological signatures for chronic pain. PloS one 2011;6(10):e26010.
6. Berman SM, Naliboff BD, Suyenobu B, et al. Reduced brainstem inhibition during anticipated pelvic visceral pain correlates with enhanced brain response to the visceral stimulus in women with irritable bowel syndrome. J Neurosci 2008;28(2):349–359.
7. Bernstein CN, Frankenstein UN, Rawsthorne P, et al. Cortical mapping of visceral pain in patients with GI disorders using functional magnetic resonance imaging. Am J Gastroenterol 2002;97(2):319–327.
8. Bishop SJ. Trait anxiety and impoverished prefrontal control of attention. Nature Neurosci 2009;12(1):92–98.
9. Blankstein U, Chen J, Diamant NE, Davis KD. Altered brain structure in irritable bowel syndrome: potential contributions of pre-existing and disease-driven factors. Gastroenterology 2010;138(5):1783–1789.
10. Cahill L, McGaugh JL. The neurobiology of memory for emotional events: adrenergic activation and the amygdala. Proc West Pharmacol Soc 1996;39:81–84.
11. Chen JY, Blankstein U, Diamant NE, Davis KD. White matter abnormalities in irritable bowel syndrome and relation to individual factors. Brain Res 2011;1392:121–131.
12. Clemens JQ, Meenan RT, O'Keeffe-Rosetti MC, et al. Prevalence of prostatitis-like symptoms in a managed care population. J Urol 2006;176(2):593–596; discussion 596.
13. Davis KD, Pope G, Chen J, et al. Cortical thinning in IBS: implications for homeostatic, attention, and pain processing. Neurology 2008;70(2):153–154.
14. Davis SN, Binik YM, Amsel R, Carrier S. A subtype based analysis of urological chronic pelvic pain syndrome in men. J Urol 2013;190(1):118–123.
15. Elsenbruch S, Rosenberger C, Enck P, et al. Affective disturbances modulate the neural processing of visceral pain stimuli in irritable bowel syndrome: an fMRI study. Gut 2010;59(4):489–495.
16. Farmer FA, Baria A, Maykut C, et al. Network-based differentiation of vulvar touch and pain. Pain Submitted.
17. Farmer MA, Baliki MN, Apkarian AV. A dynamic network perspective of chronic pain. Neurosci Lett 2012;520(2):197–203.
18. Farmer MA, Chanda ML, Parks EL, et al. Brain functional and anatomical changes in chronic prostatitis/chronic pelvic pain syndrome. J Urol 2011;186(1):117–124.
19. Gusnard DA, Raichle ME, Raichle ME. Searching for a baseline: functional imaging and the resting human brain. Nature Rev Neurosci 2001;2(10):685–694.
20. Hampson JP, Reed BD, Clauw DJ, et al. Augmented central pain processing in vulvodynia. J Pain 2013;14(6):579–589.
21. Iannetti GD, Mouraux A. From the neuromatrix to the pain matrix (and back). Exp Brain Res 2010;205(1):1–12.
22. Jiang Z, Dinov ID, Labus J, et al. Sex-related differences of cortical thickness in patients with chronic abdominal pain. PloS one 2013;8(9):e73932.
23. Ju H, Jones M, Mishra G. The prevalence and risk factors of dysmenorrhea. Epidemiol Rev 2014;36(1):104–113.
24. Labus JS, Gupta A, Coveleskie K, et al. Sex differences in emotion-related cognitive processes in irritable bowel syndrome and healthy control subjects. Pain 2013;154(10):2088–2099.
25. Labus JS, Naliboff BN, Fallon J, et al. Sex differences in brain activity during aversive visceral stimulation and its expectation in patients with chronic abdominal pain: a network analysis. NeuroImage 2008;41(3):1032–1043.
26. Larsson MB, Tillisch K, Craig AD, et al. Brain responses to visceral stimuli reflect visceral sensitivity thresholds in patients with irritable bowel syndrome. Gastroenterology 2012;142(3):463–472 e463.
27. Logothetis NK. The neural basis of the blood-oxygen-level-dependent functional magnetic resonance imaging signal. Philos Trans R Soc London B Biol Sci 2002;357(1424):1003–1037.
28. Logothetis NK. What we can do and what we cannot do with fMRI. Nature 2008;453(7197):869–878.
29. Mansour AR, Baliki MN, Huang L, et al. Brain white matter structural properties predict transition to chronic pain. Pain 2013;154(10):2160–2168.
30. McGaugh JL. Memory--a century of consolidation. Science 2000;287(5451):248–251.
31. Melzack R, Wall PD. Pain mechanisms: a new theory. Science 1965;150(3699):971–979.
32. Mertz H, Morgan V, Tanner G, et al. Regional cerebral activation in irritable bowel syndrome and control subjects with painful and nonpainful rectal distention. Gastroenterology 2000;118(5):842–848.
33. Mordasini L, Weisstanner C, Rummel C, et al. Chronic pelvic pain syndrome in men is associated with reduction of relative gray matter volume in the anterior cingulate cortex compared to healthy controls. J Urol 2012;188(6):2233–2237.

34. Naliboff BD, Berman S, Suyenobu B, et al. Longitudinal change in perceptual and brain activation response to visceral stimuli in irritable bowel syndrome patients. Gastroenterology 2006;131(2):352–365.
35. Pukall CF, Strigo IA, Binik YM, et al. Neural correlates of painful genital touch in women with vulvar vestibulitis syndrome. Pain 2005;115(1–2):118–127.
36. Reed BD, Harlow SD, Sen A, et al. Prevalence and demographic characteristics of vulvodynia in a population-based sample. Am J Obstet Gynecol 2012;206(2):170 e171–179.
37. Rodrigues SM, LeDoux JE, Sapolsky RM. The influence of stress hormones on fear circuitry. Ann Rev Neurosci 2009;32:289–313.
38. Schweinhardt P, Kuchinad A, Pukall CF, Bushnell MC. Increased gray matter density in young women with chronic vulvar pain. Pain 2008;140(3):411–419.
39. Seeley WW, Crawford RK, Zhou J, et al. Neurodegenerative diseases target large-scale human brain networks. Neuron 2009;62(1):42–52.
40. Seminowicz DA, Labus JS, Bueller JA, et al. Regional gray matter density changes in brains of patients with irritable bowel syndrome. Gastroenterology 2010;139(1):48–57 e42.
41. Seminowicz DA, Wideman TH, Naso L, et al. Effective treatment of chronic low back pain in humans reverses abnormal brain anatomy and function. J Neurosci 2011;31(20):7540–7550.
42. Sheehan J, Gaman A, Vangel M, Kuo B. Pooled analysis of brain activity in irritable bowel syndrome and controls during rectal balloon distension. Neurogastroenterol Motil 2011;23(4):336–346, e158.
43. Shoskes DA, Nickel JC, Dolinga R, Prots D. Clinical phenotyping of patients with chronic prostatitis/chronic pelvic pain syndrome and correlation with symptom severity. Urology 2009;73(3):538–542; discussion 542–533.
44. Silverman DH, Munakata JA, Ennes H, et al. Regional cerebral activity in normal and pathological perception of visceral pain. Gastroenterology 1997;112(1):64–72.
45. Sutcliffe S, Colditz GA, Pakpahan R, et al. Changes in symptoms during urologic chronic pelvic pain syndrome symptom flares: Findings from one site of the MAPP Research Network. Neurourol Urodyn 2013 Nov 23 [Epub ahead of print].
46. Tracey I, Bushnell MC. How neuroimaging studies have challenged us to rethink: is chronic pain a disease? J Pain 2009;10(11):1113–1120.
47. Tu CH, Niddam DM, Yeh TC, et al. Menstrual pain is associated with rapid structural alterations in the brain. Pain 2013;154(9):1718–1724.
48. Vincent K, Warnaby C, Stagg CJ, et al. Dysmenorrhoea is associated with central changes in otherwise healthy women. Pain 2011;152(9):1966–1975.
49. Wager TD, Atlas LY, Lindquist MA, et al. An fMRI-based neurologic signature of physical pain. N Engl J Med 2013;368(15):1388–1397.
50. Yuan YZ, Tao RJ, Xu B, et al. Functional brain imaging in irritable bowel syndrome with rectal balloon-distention by using fMRI. World J Gastroenterol 2003;9(6):1356–1360.

CHAPTER 24

Pharmacotherapy in Neuropathic Pain

Gregory Gordon, Pei Ge, Jeffrey Segal, and Immaculada Silos-Santiago

INTRODUCTION

Neuropathic pain is a common, complex disorder caused by multiple underlying disease processes. Pharmaceutical treatment is often inadequate and is characterized by unpredictable efficacy, complicated dosing, delayed onset, and significant side effect profiles [7]. Although the clinical recognition of neuropathic pain is straightforward, relating the patient's symptoms to a defined underlying diagnosis or pathophysiologic mechanism is difficult, and no standardized diagnostic procedures exist [9]. Neuropathic pain often co-exists with other pain syndromes, further complicating effective pharmacologic management [7].

DESCRIBING THE SUBJECT

The International Association for the Study of Pain (IASP) defines neuropathic pain as pain caused by a lesion or disease of the somatosensory nervous system [10]. This includes both peripheral and central neuropathic pain. The nature of the pain can be ongoing, spontaneous or evoked pain. Evoked pain is further characterized as allodynia (pain due to a stimulus that does not normally provoke pain) or hyperalgesia (increased pain from a stimulus that normally provokes pain). Regardless of the site or initial cause of the pain, these ongoing symptoms that characterize neuropathic pain are probably a consequence of both irritation to the peripheral nervous system as well as alterations to the central nervous system [2]. Peripheral sensitization of nociceptors can involve release of cytokines, growth factors and other mediators, as well as changes in peripheral receptors, channels and cross innervation; this results in the clinical expression of chronic allodynia and hyperalgesia. Central sensitization involves increases in synaptic transmission and amplification of pain responses. There are also changes which occur centrally, whereby inhibition of pain processing is reduced or disinhibited, resulting in descending facilitation.

Current Treatments for Neuropathic Pain

To date, eight medications (six oral and two topical treatments) have been approved by the Food and Drug Administration (FDA) for conditions related to neuropathic pain. Multiple pain organizations have released consensus guidelines for the treatment of neuropathic pain [17]. Consensus treatment recommendations are complicated by the complexity and variety of the underlying diseases. Although the majority of both randomized controlled trials and regulatory approvals have occurred for post-herpetic neuralgia (PHN) and diabetic neuropathy (DN), many other indications have been explored. The extent to which results of clinical trials in one indication can be extrapolated to other indications is unclear. Additionally, treatment duration in clinical trials has generally been short, leading to a lack of understanding of the long-term risks and benefits of treatments [7]. There are few head-to-head, randomized, controlled trials [26].

The calcium channel alpha2-delta ligands, gabapentin and pregabalin, are generally considered a first-line treatment. Gabapentin has received regulatory approval for the treatment of PHN, although there is evidence of efficacy in other neuropathic pain syndromes [7]. Pregabalin has been approved for PHN, DN, fibromyalgia and spinal cord injury. Both are generally safe and have few drug-drug interactions. Dose-limiting side effects include somnolence and dizziness, which can be reduced by gradual dose titration [7]. The tricyclic (TCA) and serotonin and norepinephrine reuptake inhibitor (SNRI) antidepressants are also generally considered either first- or second-line treatments, although only duloxetine has received regulatory approval for a neuropathic pain indication (diabetic neuropathy and fibromyalgia). A number of TCAs have shown efficacy in randomized, controlled trials in different neuropathic pain indications, venlafaxine (an SNRI) has shown efficacy in DPN and painful polyneuropathy [17]. Finally, topical lidocaine is often considered a first-line agent where appropriate, specifically for localized, peripheral neuropathic pain. The other approved medications, along with opioid analgesics, are considered second- or third-line agents, due to cost, side-effect profile, or risk of addiction or abuse [17]. Over the past two years, many new analgesic drugs have been approved by the FDA, although the majority were new formulations of old drugs or new indications for approved drugs. With the exception of topical lidocaine (which targets primary afferents in the periphery), the above treatments are most likely targeting central components of neuropathic pain pathology. Moreover, the selectivity of the mechanisms being targeted is likely not very high. Thus, these treatments are typically of moderate efficacy with side effect profiles that can often limit their use. There is a need for new treatments with novel, more selective mechanisms.

Compounds in Clinical Development for Neuropathic Pain

There are a number of compounds currently in clinical development which are based on an approach of novel or more selective mechanisms of action for the treatment of neuropathic pain (Table 1).

Nerve Growth Factor

One such target is nerve growth factor (NGF). NGF expression is increased in response to tissue and nerve injury and its receptor tropomyosin-related kinase A (TrkA), is expressed in nociceptors [19]. The binding of NGF to TrkA results in activation of transient receptor potential vanilloid 1(TRPV1) channels as well as release of calcitonin gene-related peptide (CGRP) and substance P (SP) from nociceptors, collectively contributing to peripheral sensitization in the evolution of neuropathic pain. NGF levels have been shown to be increased in several distinct pain conditions with neuropathic components such as diabetic neuropathy, Bladder Pain Syndrome/interstitial cystitis (BPS/IC), and chronic pelvic pain (CPP) [19]. Thus, inhibition of NGF signaling may be a pathway to the treatment of

TABLE 1 **Drugs in clinical development for neuropathic pain**

Mechanism Of Action	Company	Drug Name	Global Status	Delivery Route
NGF antibody	Pfizer	Tanezumab	Phase II/III	Injectable
Nav1.7 Selective	Convergence	CNV1014802	Phase II	Oral
Nav1.7 Selective	Xenon/Teva	XEN402	Phase II	Oral, ointment
Nav1.7 Selective	Pfizer	PF-05089771	Phase II	Oral
NGF antibody	Johnson & Johnson	Fulranumab, JNJ-42160443	Phase II	Injectable
NGF antibody	Regeneron	REGN475	Phase II	Injectable
N-type Calcium channel blocker	Zalicus	Z160	Phase II	Oral
Angiotensin II antagonist	Spinifex Pharma.	EMA-401	Phase II	Oral
Sigma 1 receptor antagonist	Esteve	E-52862	Phase II	Oral
Erythropoietin receptor agonist	Araim Pharma.	ARA-290	Phase II	Injectable
Cannabinoid CB2 receptor agonist	Kyowa Hakko Kirin	KHK-6188	Phase II	Oral
Potassium channel agonist	Relevare Pharma.	flupirtine, CNSBio	Phase II	Oral
NMDA antagonist, Opioid receptor agonist		CNSB-015		
Orexin receptor antagonist	Merck & Co	filorexant	Phase II	Oral
		MK-4305 back up, MK-6096		
Alpha2delta calcium channel antagonist	Daiichi Sankyo	DS-5565	Phase II	Oral
Serotonin and norepinephrine reuptake inhibitor	Theravance	TD-9855	Phase I	Oral
TRPA1 antagonist	Glenmark	GRC-17536	Phase II	Inhaled
				Oral
Nitric oxide synthase inhibitor	NeurAxon	NXN-462	Phase II	Oral
TRPV1 antagonist	Daewoong	DWP-05195	Phase II	Oral
TRPV1 antagonist	PharmEste	PHE-377	Phase I	Oral
Bone formation stimulant	Newron	HF-0299	Phase I	Oral
Corticosteroid agonist				

Table continued on following page

TABLE 1 **Drugs in clinical development for neuropathic pain** (Continued)

Mechanism Of Action	Company	Drug Name	Global Status	Delivery Route
Voltage-gated sodium channel antagonist (Nav1.7 and Nav1.8 inhibitor)	Dainippon Sumitomo Pharma.	DSP-2230	Phase I	Oral
Opioid mu receptor agonist	Cytogel	Cyt-1010	Phase I	Injectable
Glycine NMDA associated antagonist	VistaGen, Neurex	AV-101, GLYX-13	Phase I	Oral Injectable
Unidentified pharmacological activity	CLL Pharma.	SYN-1002	Phase I	Unspecified
Unidentified pharmacological activity	BioLineRx	BL-1021	Phase I	Oral
Unidentified pharmacological activity	Astellas	ASP-9226	Phase I	Oral
Unidentified pharmacological activity	Astellas	ASP-8477	Phase I	Oral
Unidentified pharmacological activity	Astellas	ASP-3652	Phase II	Oral

neuropathic pain, and a number of molecules are currently undergoing clinical development, such as tanezumab, fulranumab and fasinumab (RGN475).

Tanezumab, a NGF antibody preparation, has been tested in randomized controlled trials in many pain indications, including BPS/IC [7] and neuropathic pain syndromes such as diabetic neuropathy [3]. BPS/IC is characterized by chronic discomfort attributed to the bladder, and is usually associated with worsening on bladder filling and relief with urination. The severity of the symptoms varies both within and between subjects, and the sensations that patients experience often change over time, variably described as "pain", "discomfort", "cramping" or "fullness" [6]. The etiology of the disease is unclear, and multiple underlying pathophysiologic mechanisms have been proposed, including bladder wall dysfunction, tissue and nerve injury, and mast cell degranulation [8]. Although not well understood, it is thought that the process critically involves both peripheral and central sensitization. NGF released from bladder epithelium, activated mast cells, and/or detrusor smooth cells upon stretch binds to TrkA receptors on bladder afferent neurons, likely contributing to this neuronal sensitization [18].

In a randomized, double-blind, placebo-controlled, parallel-group trial, 64 patients suffering from moderate to severe BPS/IC symptoms received a single dose of 200 mcg/kg intravenous tanezumab or placebo [8]. The patients were followed for 16 weeks, although the primary endpoint occurred at the six week study visit. At various points in the trial, patients recorded daily pain and urinary symptom scores. At the six week visit, on the primary endpoint, patients treated with tanezumab showed a trend towards decreased average daily pain scores vs. placebo. Additionally, they were more likely to report a 30% or 50% reduction in pain scores from baseline and were more likely to report moderate or marked improvement on a global response assessment questionnaire, although none of these results reached statistical significance. Patients treated with tanezumab did report a statistically significant decrease in the numbers of episodes of urinary urgency per 24-hours. Conversely, scores on other secondary outcomes, including the Interstitial Cystitis Symptom Index, number of micturitions per 24-hours, and mean volume voided per micturition did not separate from placebo. Tanezumab was generally well tolerated in this study, and the rate of treatment emergent adverse events (TEAEs) was similar between those receiving active drug and those receiving placebo. Headache was the most commonly reported adverse event in the tanezumab group. A number of patients in the tanezumab group experienced new, peripheral neurologic symptoms, such as paresthesia and hyperesthesia, although these were reported to be generally mild or moderate, and resolved by the end of the study.

Tanezumab has also been tested for the treatment of diabetic neuropathy [3]. In a trial that was initially designed as a 24-week randomized, double-blind, placebo-controlled, parallel group study, patients were scheduled to receive 20 mg of subcutaneous tanezumab every eight weeks. Due to safety concerns with the molecule, this trial was terminated early. Seventy-three patients with diabetic neuropathy had entered the trial and received at least one dose of medication at the time of discontinuation, their efficacy data was analyzed at the eight week time point. There was a significant difference between the tanezumab and placebo groups in mean change from baseline in average pain score and percentage of patients reporting improvement from baseline of 30%, 50%, and 70%. There was a non-statistically significant trend towards patients reporting a 90% improvement in pain and the patients' global improvement scores. There was no apparent effect on quantitative sensory testing thresholds or intra-epidermal nerve fiber density on distal thigh and leg biopsies. The most common treatment-emergent adverse events were other pain syndromes (e.g. arthralgia, pain in extremity, myalgia) and abnormal peripheral sensations.

Fulranumab is another NGF antibody currently undergoing clinical development. The first randomized, controlled trial results were recently published for this compound, for the treatment of patients with osteoarthritis pain [21]. The compound is also being evaluated for the treatment of various neuropathic pain indications, including BPS/IC, PHN, DN, post-trauma pain and cancer pain (www.clinicaltrials.gov). A third NGF antibody, fasinumab (RGN475), is also in development, although no clinical data have yet been published (Regeneron Pharmaceuticals website, accessed Aug 8, 2013).

The FDA suspended NGF clinical trials in 2010 due to suspected cases of osteonecrosis in patients using NGF antibody alone or with NSAIDs. A review of findings suggested a dose response relationship between NGF antibody and rapidly progressing osteoarthritis (OA), which was greater in combination with NSAIDs [22]. In 2012, the FDA recommended reinitiating clinical trials with a greater attention to abnormal joint side effects, including baseline imaging and continuous clinical evaluations [22].

Nav1.7

Regulation of voltage-gated sodium channels (Nav) is believed to play a role in neuropathic pain, and selective blockage of specific channels is currently being explored as a possible route to effective pain treatment. Sodium channels are involved in membrane excitability and the generation and propagation of action potentials that contribute to the transmission of peripheral nociceptor signaling to the central nervous system [25]. Moreover, sodium channel expression is regulated in pathological pain conditions and some of them are selectively expressed in nociceptors [6,23]. These aspects make targeting sodium channels a viable and appealing approach to treat pain, and in fact, several sodium channel blockers are analgesic including lamotrigine, carbamazepine, and lidocaine. However, these agents are non-selective sodium channel blockers and thus clinically express adverse events which limit their dosing and efficacy. The current approach being taken by many groups is to identify and develop subtype-selective sodium channel blockers, specifically those selective for nociceptive neurons and thus involved in pathological pain. One of the most highly pursued subtypes is the Nav1.7 sodium channel. Genetic changes in the SCN9A gene, which encodes for the Nav1.7 voltage-gated sodium channel, has been linked to multiple rare pain syndromes, such as congenital indifference to pain (loss of function mutations) and inherited erythromelalgia (IEM) (gain of function mutations) [11].

Patients suffering from IEM were tested in a small, four-patient, exploratory trial of Xenon Pharmaceuticals Nav1.7 voltage-gated sodium channel antagonist, XEN402 [11]. This rare autosomal dominant condition is characterized by attacks of severe, debilitating, symmetrical burning pain of the distal extremities, often associated with elevated skin temperatures and erythema [11]. The attacks can be spontaneous or evoked, with exercise, prolonged standing, exposure to heat, and changes in humidity believed to be common inciting factors. Adequate pain treatment is challenging, and often inadequate. It is theorized that hyperactivity of the Nav1.7 voltage-gated sodium channel may be the underlying pathophysiologic mechanism of the spontaneous attacks of pain, thus antagonism of this channel could lead to a decreased incidence or severity of these episodes.

The clinical trial of XEN402 had a four-patient, randomized, double-blind, placebo-controlled cross-over design. Each patient received XEN402 twice daily for two 2-day treatment periods, which were separated by a 2-day washout period. Three patients presented with episodic, spontaneous pain episodes, and six pain induction procedures were used during each two day study period in order to facilitate efficacy measurements. Pain was induced with either exposure of the distal extremities to heat or through exercise. The fourth subject presented with severe, chronic pain of her hands and feet, with episodes of acute worsening of symptoms. Due to her chronic pain, no episodes of pain induction were necessary. All four subjects reported a decrease in their pain symptoms with XEN402. The three subjects who underwent pain induction reported significant reduction in pain scores, with a reported statistically significant decrease in induced pain of 42% while treated with XEN402 compared to treatment with placebo. The fourth patient, who was in chronic pain also reported decreased chronic pain scores with XEN402 compared to placebo, although not statistically significant. Two patients experienced dizziness and somnolence with XEN402 treatment, which led to reduction of their final administered dose. No subjects discontinued from the study and no serious adverse events were reported.

Xenon Pharmaceuticals has continued the clinical development of XEN402 for the treatment of IEM as a topical medicine. Xenon Pharmaceuticals has stated that applied topically to the feet, it reduced the amount of pain and the need for rescue medication and improved sleep. (Xenon Pharmaceuticals website, accessed August 7, 2013). Topical XEN402 has also been tested in a clinical trial of PHN, and the company stated that significantly more patients had a clinically meaningful pain reduction (both a 30% and 50% reduction in pain) when treated with topically applied XEN402 compared to placebo. (Xenon Pharmaceuticals website, accessed August 7, 2013).

A number of other Nav1.7 voltage-gated sodium channel antagonists are currently in early clinical development. Convergence Pharmaceuticals has reported proof-of-concept studies in lumbosacral radiculopathy and trigeminal neuralgia for the Na1.7 voltage-gated sodium channel antagonist CNV1014802 to the Clinicaltrials.gov Clinical Trial Registry.

Pfizer has completed enrollment of a randomized, placebo-controlled trial of PF-05089771 in patients with primary (inherited) erythromelalgia (per Clinicaltrials.gov).

Angiotensin II Type receptor

The angiotensin II type 2 (AT2) receptor is also a target for the treatment of neuropathic pain. Studies have indicated that the AT2 receptor is expressed in dorsal root ganglion neurons as well as in neurons innervating the viscera [1]. Functionally, data suggests a role for the AT2 receptor in inducing neuronal excitability as well as promoting neurite outgrowth [24]. Thus it has been hypothesized that selective antagonism of the angiotensin II type 2 receptor, may be a target for decreasing neuropathic pain.

EMA-401 is a selective angiotensin type 2 receptor antagonist. Spinifex Pharmaceuticals has stated that they have completed a double-blind, placebo-controlled, randomized trial in 183 patients with PHN [20]. The clinical trial met its primary endpoint, reduction in mean daily pain score versus placebo over the last week of 28 days of treatment. Additionally a statistically significant and clinically meaningful reduction in mean pain intensity from baseline to week 4 for subjects on active treatment when compared to placebo, and a significantly greater proportion of patients on active treatment reported a more than 30% reduction in mean pain intensity score compared to baseline. The molecule is considered safe and well tolerated in this trial [20]. According to the Austrialian New Zealand Clinical Trial Registry, the company is continuing development of this molecule for the treatment of neuropathic pain following peripheral nerve injury and chemotherapy-induced neuropathic pain.

N-type Calcium Channels

Analogous to sodium channels, the regulation of voltage-gated calcium channels (VGCCs) is also believed to have a role in modulating pain. Activation of neuronally expressed N-type and T-type calcium channels propagate pain signals along afferent neurons, resulting in the release of neurotransmitters at synapses in the dorsal horn of the spinal cord, and contribute to the transmission of peripheral nociceptor signaling to the central nervous system [28]. As with sodium channels, recent efforts have focused on the identification and development of highly selective N-type calcium channel blockers. A potent and selective blocker of N-type calcium channels, ziconotide, was approved for the treatment of severe chronic pain in 2004. However, its route of administration (intrathecal) and its low therapeutic index affords the opportunity to identify new N-type calcium channel blockers with high analgesic efficacy and improved safety and tolerability relative to ziconotide.

Zalicus Pharmaceuticals has reported ongoing proof-of-concept trials to the Clinicaltrials.gov Clinical Trial Registry for the selective N-type calcium channel blocker Z160 for the treatment of lumbosacral radiculopathy and PHN. According to Zalicus Pharmaceuticals, Z160 has been considered safe and well tolerated in previous trials. In November last year, Zalicus reported that Z160 did not meet the primary endpoint in either of the Phase 2 clinical studies in patients with lumbosacral radiculopathy (LSR) and post-herpetic neuralgia (PHN) [28].

Neuropathic Pain Treatments in Clinical Development for Visceral Pain

An additional area of growth in the arena of neuropathic pain treatment involves expansion into other pain disciplines, including visceral pain. The pathophysiology of visceral pain shares many features with neuropathic pain, including contribution of peripheral and central sensitization, altered descending inhibition, and many similar molecular targets [15]. As such, treatments for neuropathic pain may have utility for visceral pain indications as well. One indication that has received recent attention as a possible clinical target for approved medications is irritable bowel syndrome (IBS). IBS is a gastrointestinal disorder that is characterized by abnormal bowel habits and chronic, visceral hypersensitivity [4,14]. Visceral hypersensitivity, represented by reduced thresholds to rectal sensation and increased sensitivity to intestinal distention, is common in patients with IBS [13,15]. Although the exact pathophysiologic mechanisms are unclear, the underlying mechanisms likely overlap with neuropathic pain, and thus, it has been proposed that medications that treat neuropathic pain may be effective in patients suffering from IBS.

Gabapentin was tested in a randomized, double-blind, placebo-controlled, parallel-group study of 43 patients with diarrhea-predominant IBS [15]. Patients were treated with five days of gabapentin (300 mg per day for the first three days, and then 600 mg per day for the next two days, in divided doses) or placebo. Patients underwent a barostat procedure to measure rectal compliance and visceral perception at baseline and at the end of the five-day treatment period. For those IBS patients treated with gabapentin, the threshold pressures for reporting bloating, discomfort, and pain significantly increased compared to baseline, a finding not seen in the placebo group. Additionally, a significant increase in the barostat pressure and wall tension needed to induce discomfort or pain of at least moderate intensity was observed in the gabapentin group, but not in the placebo group.

Likewise, pregabalin was tested in a randomized, double-blind, placebo-controlled parallel-group study of forty-one patients who had both IBS and demonstrated rectal hypersensitivity [12]. Rectal hypersensitivity was determined by meeting predefined criteria for experiencing pain below a set threshold during the initial barostat exam prior to randomization into the study. The IBS patients were treated with three weeks of pregabalin (titrated up to a maximum dose of 600 mg per day) or placebo. Patients underwent a rectal barostat at the beginning and end of the study. Additionally, patients completed a nightly Daily IBS Pain Self-Assessment diary, in which they scored the severity of their abdominal pain using an eleven-point Likert scale. In patients who were treated with pregabalin, the change in barostat pressure from baseline was significantly greater for pressure to first sensation, desire to defecate, and pain compared to those treated with placebo. Additionally, there was a non-significant trend towards improvement in self-assessed nightly reported pain scores in patients treated with pregabalin, compared to placebo. It was impossible to determine whether a relationship existed between increased sensory thresholds demonstrated by barostat and self-reported nightly pain scores, due to the small sample size and the reports of one outlier patient, which skewed the results.

These data on gabapentin and pregabalin suggest that the first line therapy for peripheral neuropathic pain may have an effect on resetting the thresholds for sensing abdominal discomfort in patients with IBS, and on decreasing the sensation of visceral pain. As this class of drugs is proven to successfully treat neuropathic pain, these findings suggest that neuropathic and visceral pain may share common pathophysiologic mechanisms. Further trials, on larger and more diverse populations of patients, suffering from both IBS and other diseases of visceral pain, are needed.

PRACTICAL IMPLICATIONS

The pathophysiology of abdominal and pelvic pain shares many features with neuropathic pain, including contribution of peripheral and central sensitization, altered descending inhibition, and many similar molecular targets. As such, treatments for neuropathic pain may have utility for visceral pain indications as well. Recent clinical trials on gabapentin and pregabalin suggest that these drugs, previously approved for the treatment of peripheral neuropathic pain, may improve abdominal discomfort in patients with IBS, and decrease abdominal pain.

LOOKING AT THE FUTURE

Further trials on larger patient populations suffering from both IBS and other abdominal and pelvic pain, are needed. Novel mechanisms are being tested in clinical trials in parallel in patients with neuropathic pain and in patients with diverse abdominal and pelvic pain. This can speed the availability of new therapeutic agents for an underserved patient population.

TAKE HOME MESSAGES

- The current treatments utilized for neuropathic pain have modest efficacy with dose limiting side effects.
- The pathophysiology of abdominal and pelvic pain shares many features with neuropathic pain.
- Drugs approved for neuropathic pain are now being tested in randomized clinical trials for abdominal and pelvic pain with promising results.
- New treatments with novel and more selective mechanisms, that might deliver better efficacy and safety profile, are now in clinical development for patients with abdominal and pelvic pain.

FURTHER READING

Engeler D, Baranowski AP, Elneil S, et al. Guidelines on Chronic Pelvic Pain. European Association of Urology 2012. http://www.uroweb.org/gls/pdf/24_Chronic_Pelvic_Pain_LR%20II.pdf

Attal N, Cruccu G, Baron R, et al. EFNS guidelines on the pharmacological treatment of neuropathic pain: 2010 revision. Eur J Neurol 2010;17: 1113–1123.

Haanpää M, Attal N, Backonja M, et al. NeuPSIG guidelines on neuropathic pain assessment. Pain. 2011;152(1):14–27.

REFERENCES

1. Anand U, Facer P, Yiangou Y, et al. Angiotensin II type 2 receptor (AT2 R) localization and antagonist-mediated inhibition of capsaicin responses and neurite outgrowth in human and rat sensory neurons. Eur J Pain 2013;17:1012–1026.
2. Baron R. Mechanisms of disease: neuropathic pain--a clinical perspective. Nat Clin Pract Neurol 2006;2:95–106.
3. Bramson C, Herrmann D, Biton V, et al. Efficacy and safety of subcutaneous tanezumab in patients with pain related to diabetic peripheral neuropathy (NCT01087203). 32nd Annual Scientific Meeting of the American Pain Society (May 8–11, 2013) 2013.
4. Camilleri M, Bharucha AE, Di LC, et al. American Neurogastroenterology and Motility Society consensus statement on intraluminal measurement of gastrointestinal and colonic motility in clinical practice. Neurogastroenterol Motil 2008;20:1269–1282.
5. Clemens JQ. Pathogenesis, clinical features, and diagnosis of interstitial cystitis/bladder pain syndrome. In: UpToDate, O'Leary, MP (Ed), UpToDate, Waltham, MA, 2013). http://www.uptodate.com/contents/pathogenesis-clinical-features-and-diagnosis-of-interstitial-cystitis-bladder-pain-syndrome
6. Cummins TR, Sheets PL, Waxman SG. The roles of sodium channels in nociception: Implications for mechanisms of pain. Pain 2007;131:243–257.

7. Dworkin RH, O'Connor AB, Backonja M, et al. Pharmacologic management of neuropathic pain: evidence-based recommendations. Pain 2007;132:237–251.
8. Evans RJ, Moldwin RM, Cossons N, et al. Proof of concept trial of tanezumab for the treatment of symptoms associated with interstitial cystitis. J Urol 2011;185:1716–1721.
9. Freynhagen R, Bennett MI. Diagnosis and management of neuropathic pain. BMJ 2009;339:b3002.
10. Geber C, Baumgärtner U, Schwab R, et al. Revised definition of neuropathic pain and its grading system: an open case series illustrating its use in clinical practice. Am J Med. 2009;122(10 Suppl):S3–12.
11. Goldberg YP, Price N, Namdari R, et al. Treatment of Na(v)1.7-mediated pain in inherited erythromelalgia using a novel sodium channel blocker. Pain 2012;153:80–85.
13. Houghton LA, Fell C, Whorwell PJ, et al. Effect of a second-generation alpha2delta ligand (pregabalin) on visceral sensation in hypersensitive patients with irritable bowel syndrome. Gut 2007;56:1218–1225.
13. Kanazawa M, Hongo M, Fukudo S. Visceral hypersensitivity in irritable bowel syndrome. J Gastroenterol Hepatol 2011;26(Suppl 3):119–121.
14. Khan S, Chang L. Diagnosis and management of IBS. Nat Rev Gastroenterol Hepatol 2010;7:565–581.
15. Lee KJ, Kim JH, Cho SW. Gabapentin reduces rectal mechanosensitivity and increases rectal compliance in patients with diarrhoea-predominant irritable bowel syndrome. Aliment Pharmacol Ther 2005;22:981–988.
16. Malykhina AP. Neural mechanisms of pelvic organ cross-sensitization. Neuroscience 2007;149:660–672.
16. O'Connor AB, Dworkin RH. Treatment of neuropathic pain: an overview of recent guidelines. Am J Med 2009;122:S22–S32.
18. Ochodnicky P, Cruz CD, Yoshimura N, Michel MC. Nerve growth factor in bladder dysfunction: contributing factor, biomarker, and therapeutic target. Neurourol Urodyn 2011;30:1227–1241.
19. Pezet S, McMahon SB. Neurotrophins: mediators and modulators of pain. Annu Rev Neurosci 2006;29:507–538.
20. Rice AS, Dworkin RH, McCarthy TD, et al; for the EMA401-003 study group. EMA401, an orally administered highly selective angiotensin II type 2 receptor antagonist, as a novel treatment for postherpetic neuralgia: a randomised, double-blind, placebo-controlled phase 2 clinical trial. Lancet. 2014;383(9929):1637–47.
21. Sanga P, Katz N, Polverejan E, et al. Efficacy, safety, and tolerability of fulranumab, an anti-nerve growth factor antibody, in the treatment of patients with moderate to severe osteoarthritis pain. Pain 2013;154:1910–1919.
22. Seidel MF, Wise BL, Lane NE. Nerve growth factor: an update on the science and therapy. Osteoarthr Cart 2013;21:1223–1228.
23. Silos-Santiago I. The role of tetrodotoxin-resistant sodium channels in pain states: are they the next target for analgesic drugs? Curr Opin Invest Drugs 2008;9:83–89.
24. Smith MT, Wyse BD, Edwards SR. Small molecule angiotensin II type 2 receptor (AT(2)R) antagonists as novel analgesics for neuropathic pain: comparative pharmacokinetics, radioligand binding, and efficacy in rats. Pain Med 2013;14:692–705.
25. Theile JW, Cummins TR. Recent developments regarding voltage-gated sodium channel blockers for the treatment of inherited and acquired neuropathic pain syndromes. Front Pharmacol 2011;2:54.
26. Watson CP, Gilron I, Sawynok J. A qualitative systematic review of head-to-head randomized controlled trials of oral analgesics in neuropathic pain. Pain Res Manag 2010;15:147–157.
27. Zalicus. Press Release: Zalicus reports results from Phase 2 clinical trials of Z160 in chronic neuropathic pain. http://phx.corporate-ir.net/phoenix.zhtml?c=148036&p=irol-newsArticle&ID=1874737&highlight= (accessed July 2014)
28. Zamponi GW, Lewis RJ, Todorovic SM, et al. Role of voltage-gated calcium channels in ascending pain pathways. Brain Res Rev 2009;60:84–89.

CHAPTER 25

European Association of Urology Algorithms

Bert Messelink

INTRODUCTION

The European Association of Urology (EAU) started working on a guideline about Chronic Pelvic Pain in 2003. Although the EAU is an association of urologists, the guideline panel was multidisciplinary from the beginning. In the later years, the panel expanded with more disciplines joining the meetings and participating in the research and writing. The most recent version of the guideline was published in 2014. The biggest rewriting and restructuring was done for the 2012 version. At this time, the EAU guideline panel was working on the future developments in the world of guidelines and of chronic pain. Many members of this panel were also involved in the work of the International Association for the Study of Pain, especially in the taxonomy reports.

The following disciplines are represented in the EAU guideline CPP panel: gastroenterology, gynaecology, pain medicine, psychology, sexology, and urology.

In 2013 the panel published an article to describe how they had been doing over the past 10 years. It is titled: "The 2013 EAU Guidelines on Chronic Pelvic Pain: Is Management of Chronic Pelvic Pain a Habit, a Philosophy, or a Science? 10 Years of Development" [1]. This chapter is fully based on this article and on the EAU guideline on CPP version 2014 [2].

BASIC ASPECTS

From the start it has been clear to the panel that multidisciplinary and multidimensional are the basic words in looking at chronic pelvic pain. The panel has been working on the development of that concept from the beginning. The process of phenotyping has consequently become more manifest in this guideline and was supported by the outcome of research done by other groups [5]. As an example: the U-point classification has been used in studies on prostate pain syndrome and on bladder pain syndrome. This system was used to better target the therapy in every specific patient [4]. Phenotyping helps to start therapy in the best possible way, often by using combinations of treatment. This is more successful then empirical sequential monotherapy. Dealing with CPP patients starts with a basal question: is the pain a symptom of a well known disease or is it pain in own rights. The first algorithm in the guideline (Fig. 1) starts with this question and directs the clinician to two different pathways, depending on the answer that is given. It is helpful for both patient and clinician to have a clear statement about the subject you are dealing with.

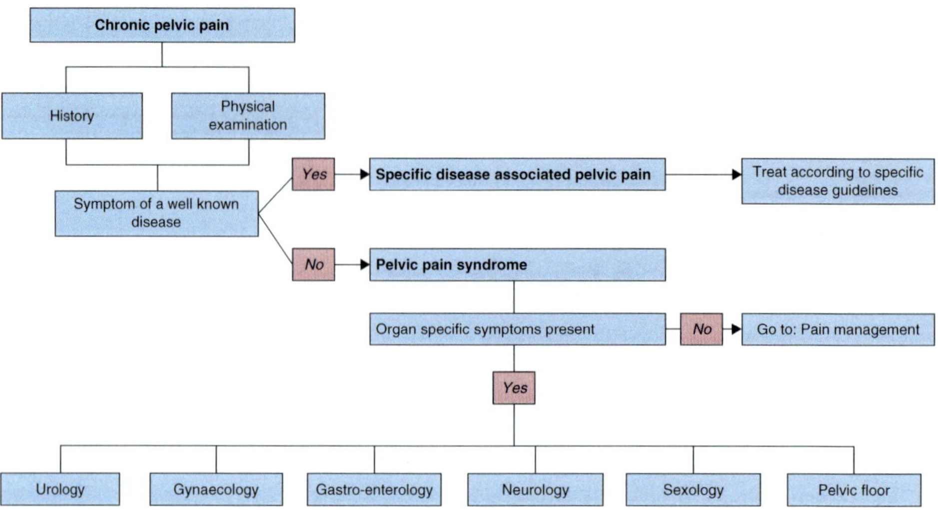

FIGURE 1 The basic algorithm in caring for patients with chronic pelvic pain.

DESCRIBING THE SUBJECT

The above-mentioned basic choice is important, but of course there is more to say. It is also a dilemma. Doing comprehensive somatic investigation and then drawing the conclusion that nothing serious is wrong and that no disease causing the pain is found, might satisfy both patient and clinician. On the other hand, it has the intrinsic risk of giving the patient the idea that the pain is somatic and needs to be seen in a biomedical perspective. This may interfere with the next step: developing a pain management programme in which there is no biomedical solution offered. Looking the other way round, there is the possible risk of harm when not doing investigations. Two kinds of harm can be mentioned. The first one is missing a well known or serious disease causing the pain and yielding a treatable cause. The other one is the ongoing discussion between patient and clinician about this subject. This may be based on important anxieties unaddressed in the patient and even in the clinician. This uncertainty can be a large obstacle in pain management and can have huge consequences for the patient-clinician relationship. As a clinician, one might lose contact with the patient who will then go to the next doctor to get his questions answered. This risk versus harm dilemma makes us clear that it is of utmost importance to work closely together with your patient as a team. The assessment done, the therapy proposed and the evaluation of the results, all should be performed with consent of both clinician and patient. In these team meetings the relatives (partner, children, parents) should be invited to take part in the discussion. Looking at chronic pain using a bio-psycho-social model will lead to the involvement of all three compartments. One might say that the 'clinician-patient-relatives' model is the practical application of the model. The earlier in the whole process the integrated model of pain is introduced, the more options will be available for negotiations with the patient and the stronger the team will become. Combining is the word that should be remembered by all dealing with chronic pelvic pain patients. Do not go for a purely somatic approach. Do not go for a purely psychological approach. Apply both from the very beginning. Consequence of this saying is that medical doctors need to have a form of psychological training allowing them to understand the needs of the patient. On the other hand the psychologist should be aware of the somatic items involved with CPP. For now in practice this means that patients with CPP are seen in a multidisciplinary practice by a team of experts in pain management.

Medical doctors often seem to hesitate introducing the role of psychology and consequently the psychologist, when talking about chronic pelvic pain. For those clinicians it might help to start talking about these aspects from the very beginning and in the same manner as talking about the physical aspects. Starting to ask the patient what his beliefs about the pain are and then build the plan on this beliefs will provide the basis for an explanation of functional changes in the pain system that constitute chronic pain.

Assessment

Diagnosing a patient with chronic pelvic pain, without appropriate investigations is unacceptable. In every patient a thorough history should be taken and physical examination must be done. When taking a history it is important to pay attention to the function of all the tracts that are represented in the pelvis: lower urinary, anorectal, gynaecological, neurological, and sexual. The psychological aspects are also addressed in the history taking. Including childhood and development, the family in which the patient has grown up along with the current social situation. Are there any losses in life (relatives, jobs); is there any trauma (physical, sexual, emotional) that need to be discussed further?

The physical examination should be focused on, but not limited to, the pelvis. Inspection and palpation are the most applicable testing methods. Inspection of the skin and mucosal tissue is the starting point. In women, a quantification of pelvic organ prolaps is mandatory. After inspection palpation of the internal and external pelvic organs is performed. In women a vaginal and sometimes rectal examination is done to palpate the pelvic organs including bladder, uterus and anal canal. In men, the external genitalia should be palpated and the prostate and bladder should be screened by performing a rectal exam. In both men and women the pelvic floor muscles should be palpated and testing of the function should be done. Classification of the pelvic floor muscle function is preferably done according to the International Continence Society (ICS) system [3].

The methods of further investigations should be chosen taking into account the risks and benefits of each test. Within the applicable tests, it is advisable to start with the least invasive one. Repeating investigations should only be considered when the presentation of the pain has changed significantly.

Management plan

Based on a shared model of pain, a management plan will address different items.

First of all, managing pain requires talking about and working on the recovery of activity. In chronic pain, there has often developed a relation between pain and certain organ systems, leading to dysfunction. In pelvic pain, this is mostly related to micturition, defecation, and sexual activities. Relief of pain does not mean recovery of function. Patients know that certain activities cause pain and they will avoid them even if the pain has gone and the remaining dysfunction may then in itself, be the source of recurrence of the pain.

The second item is what the main target is in the management plan. It is advised to focus on quality of life more than focusing on relief of pain. For every patient, the targets will be personally chosen. If sleep deprivation is a problem, restoring a good night rest may be the first target. If the patient is young and has a developing relationship, the loss of sexual function may be mentioned as most important. The clinician should ask the patient what his targets would be and give all the space to mention everything that comes up in their mind.

The third aspect is the environment. As mentioned before, the pain patient lives in an environment and the other persons are involved in the pain process. People with chronic pain may even have lost members of their environment, like partners, colleagues and friends. Restructuring life and rebuilding normal activities can be part of the pain management program. The environment can be of great help in achieving those targets.

The last item in discussing the plan is the use of algorithms. The clinician can follow the algorithms that are provided by the EAU guideline (see practical implications). This helps in finding the most evidence based practices which can then be shared with the patient. Showing the algorithms to the patient may help to deepen the feeling of a cooperative enterprise, making the management plan. Providing good and reliable information (on the web or on paper) about treatment and management could be the final stage of the first consultation.

PRACTICAL IMPLICATIONS

The EAU guideline has an increasing number of algorithms that were constructed to make a graphical representation of the road that can be followed when making a plan with the patient. The first algorithm (Fig. 1) is the basic one which is founded on the differentiation between disease associated pain and pain in own rights. In the current version of the guideline pain in its own right is denoted as pelvic pain syndrome. In the case of pelvic pain syndrome the next step is to look for symptoms that can be related to pelvic organ dysfunctions. If present, than the guideline refers to the different chapters in which the organ related symptoms are discussed. Another aspect of this algorithm is that it recommends early referral to a multidisciplinary pain team for general pain management.

The guideline also uses figures in which recommendations for assessment and treatment are presented in text boxes. The level of evidence and the grade of recommendations are presented here. As an example, you can see the one on prostate pain syndrome (Fig. 2).

In the chapter on bladder pain syndrome, phenotyping is an important item. Especially regarding whether there is a problem with the bladder. The European Society for the Study of BPS has set up a classification about this bladder pathology. In the EAU algorithm, treatment arms are based on the presence or absence of these bladder problems (Fig. 3).

The bladder pain syndrome algorithm is similar to the algorithm on chronic anorectal pain. The endoscopy is also the most important instrument used here. With the endoscopy, it is differentiated between specific disease associated pain and anorectal pain syndrome (Fig. 4).

The last algorithm in the guideline is dealing with general pain management and especially with the use of analgesic drugs in chronic pelvic pain (Fig. 5).

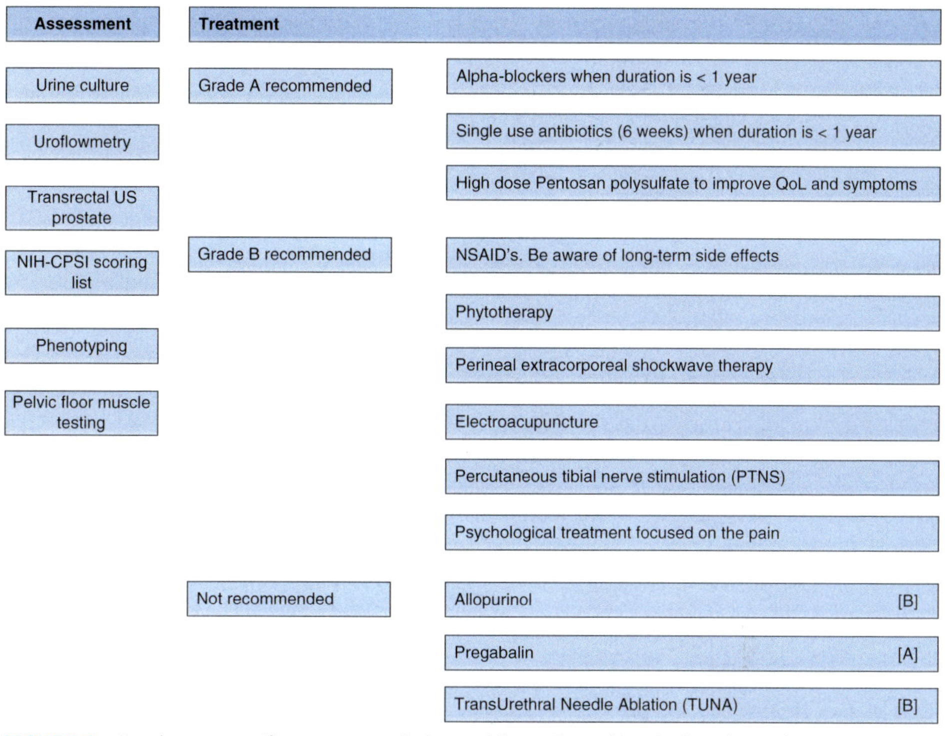

FIGURE 2 Syndrome specific recommendations with grade and level of evidence for Prostate Pain Syndrome.

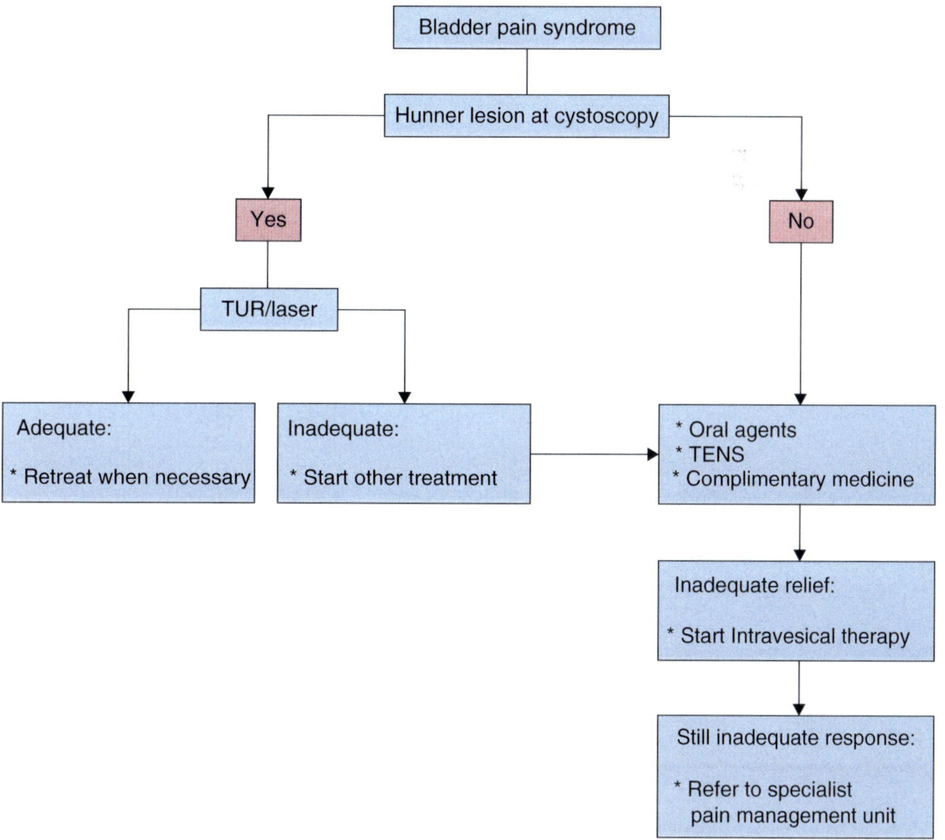

FIGURE 3 Treatments based on phenotype aspects for Bladder Pain Syndrome.

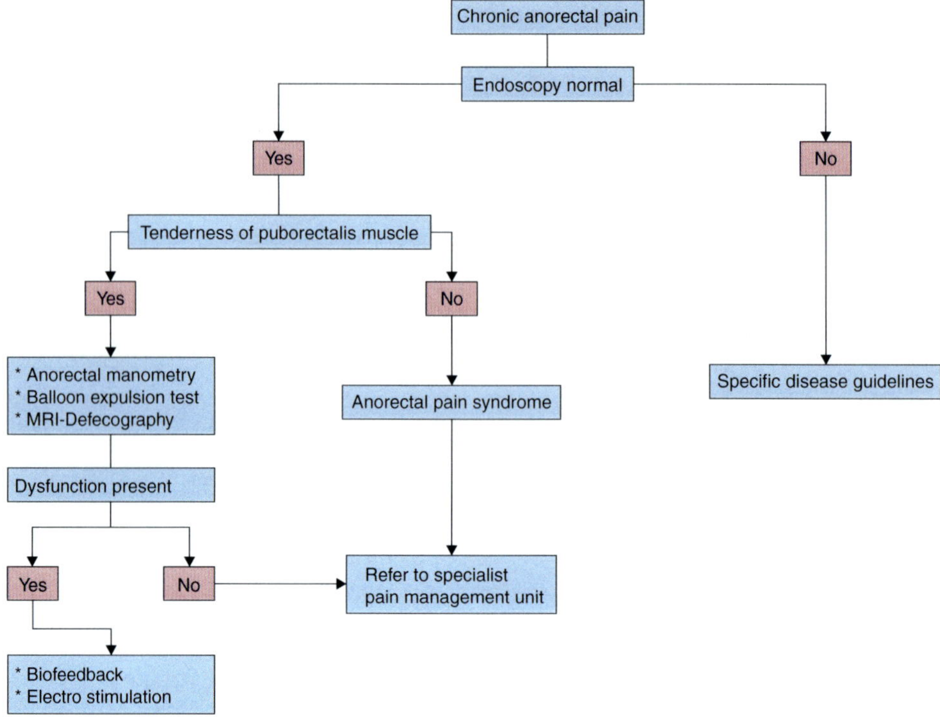

FIGURE 4 Treatments based on phenotype aspects for Chronic Anorectal Pain.

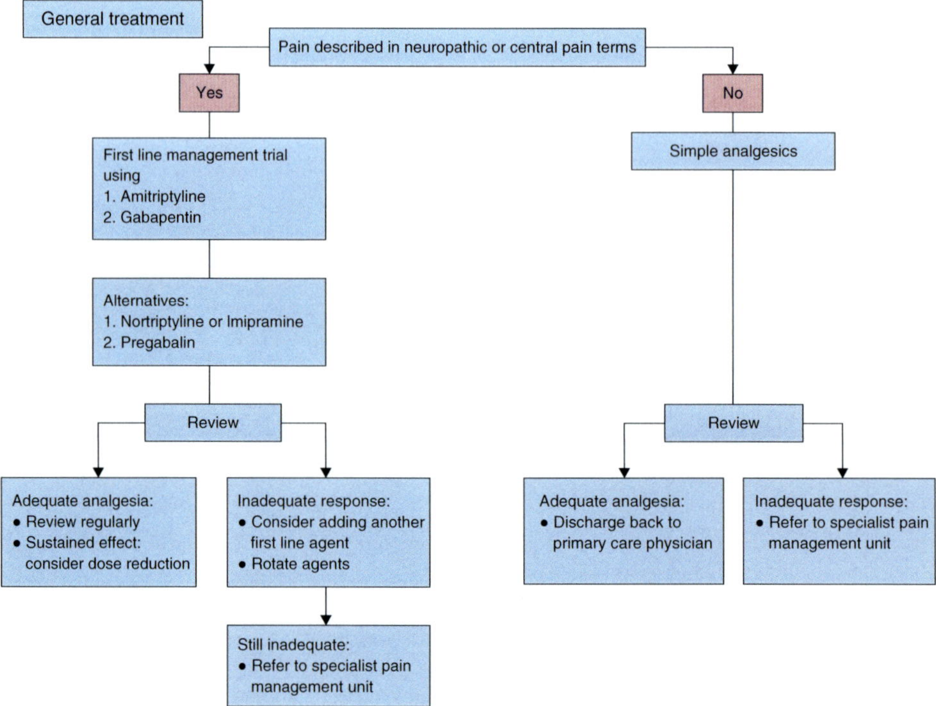

FIGURE 5 Algorithm for general pain management, especially for analgesic drugs, in chronic pelvic pain.

LOOKING AT THE FUTURE

Over recent years, there has been a clear shift in looking at chronic pelvic pain. In more and more situations, the modern terminology and philosophy has found its way. The people who are working on this new approach have done a good job. Now we need to move forward and spread the news more widely. It is not easy for clinicians to change their way of thinking and of dealing with patients. Most care givers are trained to cure patients. Physicians, especially, are used to looking for curable diseases and subsequent treatment options. In that view, it is not remarkable that in the field of chronic pelvic pain many treatments have been used without even real evidence. Clinicians need to do investigations and to offer a solution. The number of options in the world of investigations has increased quite substantially. The patient with chronic pelvic pain wants to have a diagnosis and is desperately seeking care. This makes clinicians feel obliged to keep on doing investigations and continue the search for causes. Clinicians need to realise that not only treatments, but also investigations, do have their negative effects (often called side-effects). New tests will raise expectations of finding a cause of the pain. The aspiration of the clinician is contrary to the reality because we hardly ever find such a cause. Physicians need to accept pain in its own right and must accept that no investigation will find the cause; they must accept that pain is just what it is. By doing this, they can start to help the patient and set up a good pain management plan.

TAKE HOME MESSAGES

- Guidelines on chronic pelvic pain should be multidisciplinary in its content and in the composition of the panel.
- Phenotyping is an important tool to make a more personal pain management plan for each patient.
- Ruling out treatable conditions that cause pain is as important as accepting pain in its own rights if no such conditions are found.
- Making a pain management plan is a co-operative action between clinician, patients, and relatives.
- Start talking about pain in all its aspects from the very first consultation, thereby providing the patient with a complete picture for the rest of the process.
- The use of algorithms can help the clinician in finding the best possible way to move forward in assessment and treatment of chronic pelvic pain patients.

FURTHER READING

European Urology Guideline on Chronic Pelvic Pain. http://www.uroweb.org/gls/pdf/26%20Chronic%20Pelvic%20Pain_LR.pdf

Butler DS, Lorimer G. Moseley. Explain Pain 2nd edition. Adelaide Australia: Noigroup Publications, 2013.

Flor H, Turk DC. Chronic pain, an integrated biobehavioral approach. Seattle USA: IASP Press, 2011.

REFERENCES

1. Engeler DS, Baranowski AP, Dinis-Oliveira P, et al. The 2013 EAU guidelines on chronic pelvic pain: is management of chronic pelvic pain a habit, a philosophy, or a science? 10 years of development. Eur Urol. 2013;64(3):431–9.
2. Engeler DS, Baranowski AP, Dinis-Oliveira P, et al. The EAU guideline on chronic pelvic pain 2014 edition. http://www.uroweb.org/gls/pdf/26%20Chronic%20Pelvic%20Pain_LR.pdf
3. Messelink EJ, Benson T, Berghmans B, et al. Standardization of terminology of pelvic floor muscle function and dysfunction: report from the pelvic floor clinical assessment group of the International Continence Society. Neurourol Urodyn. 2005;24(4):374–80.
4. Nickel JC, Shoskes D. Phenotypic approach to the management of chronic prostatitis/chronic pelvic pain syndrome. Curr Urol Rep 2009;10:307–12.
5. Shoskes DA, Nickel JC, Dolinga R, et al. Clinical phenotyping of patients with chronic prostatitis/chronic pelvic pain syndrome and correlation with symptom severity. Urology 2009;73:538–42.

CHAPTER 26

British Pain Society Patient Pathways

Gareth Greenslade

INTRODUCTION

After describing the background in the English National Health Service that led to the British Pain Society setting up working groups to produce pain patient care pathways, the author describes the methodologies used to produce the care pathways with particular reference to the map for chronic pelvic pain (for men and women). The role of care pathways in helping us to reach more patients with chronic pelvic pain is discussed, along with how care pathways can increase the benefit obtained from limited resources. The Map of Medicine Pathways, produced by the British Pain Society's working groups, provide guidance on best practice for clinicians managing patients with pelvic pain from primary care through to secondary care outpatient services and pain clinics. They also help us to identify the patients who should be referred to a specialist urogenital pain management unit.

In a health service with unlimited resources, all patients with chronic pelvic pain would be seen in a centre specialising in that problem. In the real world, the number of specialists is tiny when compared with the mass of people suffering from chronic pelvic pain—urogenital pain is reported by 7.6% of men [4] and 15% of women report chronic pelvic pain [6]. To put these figures into perspective, around 8% of the UK adult population suffers with asthma [1].

It is unlikely that resources will be found to expand the network of specialist pelvic pain centres to provide care for all these patients. The alternative is to equip the non-specialist, including primary care physicians, with the tools that they need to provide effective treatment in local settings. Good patient care pathways make it more likely that patients will receive timely, evidence-based care. Good pathways also reduce the use of unnecessary tests and investigations and they reduce the risk of iatrogenic harm. Overall, they reduce waste and improve patient outcomes [7].

In any healthcare system where non-specialist purchasers (government bodies, medical insurance companies, etc.) decide what will be offered to patients, clear, authoritative, evidence-based information on patient management can maintain and improve the standards of patient care. Without this information, there is a risk that ineffective or harmful treatments will be purchased and that patients will be denied effective care.

TABLE 1 British Pain Society working group

Executive Working group
Andrew P. Baranowski, Consultant in Pain Medicine specialising in pelvic pain (Chair)
Richard Langford, President of the British Pain Society
Martin Johnson, Pain Champion, Royal College of General Practitioners
Cathy Price
Members of The British Pain Society's (BPS) Map of Medicine® Chronic Pelvic Pain Patient Pathway Map (male and female) Working Group
John Hughes (Pain Medicine)
Andrew P. Baranowski (Pain Medicine)
Ms. Judy Birch (Patient)
Suzzanne Brook (Physiotherapy)
Beverly Collett (Pain Medicine)
Suzy Elneil (Urogynaecology)
Anton Emmanuel (Gastroenterology)
Alex Freeman (GP)
Judith Lee (Physiotherapy)
Katy Vincent (Gynaecologist)
Amanda C de C Williams (Psychology)

BASIC ASPECTS

This is a patient treatment pathway designed by an expert panel assembled by the British Pain Society (Table 1).

The care map is accredited at two levels. The clinical content of the care map is accredited by the British Pain Society and the editorial methodology used is accredited by the Chief Knowledge Officer of the NHS.

DESCRIBING THE SUBJECT

In July 2010, the Secretary of State for Health in the UK published the NHS White Paper "Equity and Excellence: Liberating the NHS" [8]. One of the main features was the setting out of the Government's plans for GP-lead commissioning (Clinical Commissioning Groups or CCGs). The aim of this development was to allow local primary care physicians to specify the services that would be provided by their local hospitals, including how these services would be configured. The budgets for hospital services in the local commissioning areas would be handed to the CCGs who would then pass the money to the services that they had commissioned. The Government felt that the local primary care physicians understood their patient's needs and were the best people to decide what should be bought in their local area.

There are several risks to this approach (the political implications will not be discussed here) but the main clinical risk is that the CCG purchasers may lack the knowledge needed to make the best decisions for some of their patient groups. They are *general* practitioners, so it is not reasonable to assume that they have in-depth knowledge of all the specialties they have to commission. Faced with these challenges, the British Pain Society (BPS) decided to allocate significant resources to produce up-to-date, evidence-based patient management pathways. The BPS saw this as a way to safeguard the quality of patient care by informing the CCG teams. It was also an opportunity to help all patients to receive consistent, evidence-based care, wherever they lived in the country.

The BPS set up working groups to produce pain patient care pathways in the form of maps. The aim was to establish evidence-based and expert consensus-based best practice guidance for the management of 5 major areas where chronic pain is common so that these maps could then be used for educational and commissioning purposes. They would also help to define quality standards and contribute towards the BPS's strategy to improve the overall management of pain in the UK. The choice of membership for the BPS groups, coupled with the BPS's own ethical stance, satisfied the criteria put forward by Lenzer, et al, in their BMJ paper in 2013 (Table 2) [5].

The BPS decided to collaborate with the Map of Medicine, a highly experienced commercial provider of patient care pathways and they were determined that the pathways should be accessible by any healthcare professional, as well as by members of the public in England. They are now available via the British Pain Society's website for anybody viewing it from a UK-based internet connection. The maps are reviewed regularly and updated as new evidence is produced, or when valid comments are received from users of the maps.

Editorial methodology: The working party used secondary evidence from high quality sources including meta-analyses, systematic reviews and guidelines. They used the AGREE instrument to assess the quality of guidelines and they applied inclusion and exclusion criteria to systematic reviews and meta-analyses to ensure that only high quality information was selected. Where there was insufficient evidence, but a requirement to provide guidance was required, a panel agreement was reached and referenced accordingly in the document. The drafted care map was then developed and trialled by individuals of the group who had front line clinical experience (nominated by the BPS) with input from the editorial team at the Map of Medicine. The BPS's working party members included, amongst others, representatives from patient groups, primary care physicians, interventionist and non-interventionist pain medicine specialists, psychologists and physiotherapists. The working groups were supported by academics and others with experience in developing guidelines.

Map of Medicine pathways are constantly updated in response to new evidence and feedback is collected from users throughout the year. There is a quarterly publication cycle

TABLE 2 **Criteria from Lenzer**

Red flags that should raise substantial scepticism among guideline readers (and medical journals)

- Sponsor(s) is a professional society that receives substantial industry funding
- Sponsor is a proprietary company, or is undeclared or hidden
- Committee chair(s) have any financial conflict*
- Multiple panel members have any financial conflict*
- Any suggestion of committee stacking that would pre-ordain a recommendation regarding a controversial topic
- No, or limited, involvement of an expert in methodology in the evaluation of evidence
- No external review
- No inclusion of non-physician experts/patient representative/community stakeholders

*Includes a panelist with either or both a financial relationship with a proprietary healthcare company and/or whose clinical practice/specialty depends on tests or interventions covered by the guideline.

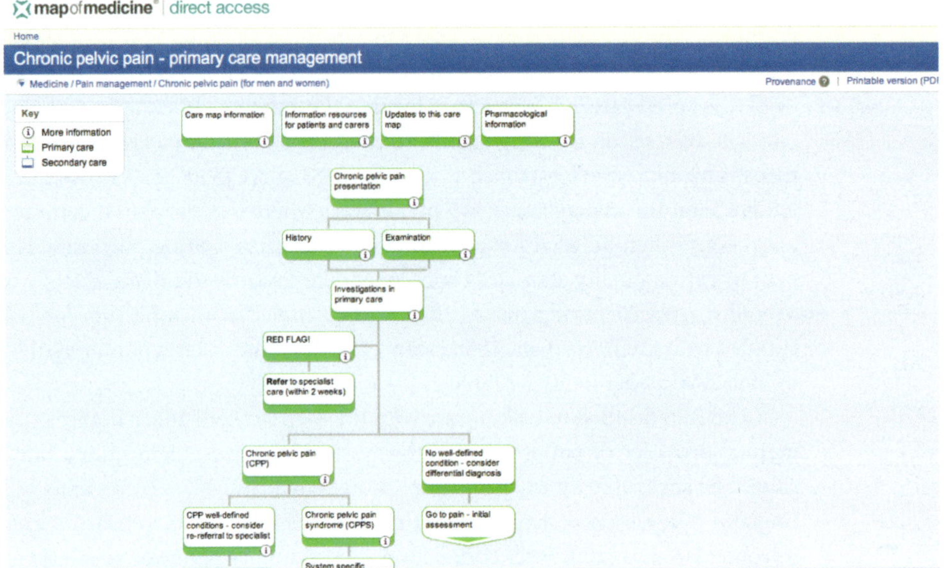

FIGURE 1 Map of Medicine Pelvic Pain Page for Primary Care.

for the maps and important changes are incorporated through this cycle. The Map of Medicine team have produced care maps for over 250 clinical topics and they have an active clinical editorial team, board of fellows and clinical stakeholders. The Map of Medicine can be adapted to local circumstances so that recommendations for further investigations or treatment can be directed to the appropriate local facility—they can even add telephone numbers, website addresses and other local details. The text can also be altered to reflect local resources and any local consensus agreements regarding the management of specific patient groups.

The map appears as a flow chart (see Fig. 1) and an information button is provided on many of the boxes. Clicking on the information button opens an information window which provides clear, yet concise information about the activity contained in the box. The information also contains references.

The whole map can be downloaded as a PDF document. In this form, the flow chart is contained on the first page of the document and the information boxes are reproduced on the subsequent pages. The primary care map translates into a 16 page PDF document and the secondary care (specialist care management) map translates into a 12 page document. The disadvantage of the downloaded documents is that they do not benefit from the updating process that is central to the Map of Medicine concept. However, the documents have proved popular in educational groups that the author has held both for primary care and secondary care colleagues. The primary care document is more detailed and prescriptive than the secondary care document and this has been found to be appropriate during teaching sessions using the map, with the non-specialist primary care audience appreciating the extra detail given.

PRACTICAL IMPLICATIONS

Approximately 1 million women in the UK have pelvic pain, with the prevalence of chronic pelvic pain in women being estimated at 38 per 1,000 [3], which is similar to the prevalence of asthma [1] or back pain. The prevalence in men has not been directly established, but referrals are common, with pain in the area of the prostate, testicles, penis and bladder. Clearly, it is not going to be possible for all of these patients to be treated in specialist clinics. Fortunately, if the care of these patients is properly coordinated, much, if not most, of their care can be delivered in primary care. The Map of Medicine pathways for patients with chronic pelvic pain make this possibility more of a reality, by giving clinicians the information that they need in a useable form that is evidence based and up to date.

The Map of Medicine pelvic pain pathway has been written by a multidisciplinary group and it can be used to break down the barriers between primary care and the different specialists that see and treat patients with chronic pelvic pain. Currently, the care a patient receives is often dependent more upon where they are seen, rather than the clinical condition from which they suffer. If it is used enthusiastically and adapted to local conditions, this BPS Map of Medicine pain pathway series will help all clinicians deliver the right care at the right time, making it more likely that patients will get greater benefit from their treatment. In the longer term this will reduce the wastage of healthcare resources and people's lives.

LOOKING AT THE FUTURE

The pathways will be kept up to date by the BPS team and the Map of Medicine editorial team. Most importantly, in addition to incorporating new scientific and clinical evidence, user feedback will help the teams to refine the pathways, to make them more user friendly. As a result, we can look forward to the organic development of these pathways, making them even more useful both as patient decision pathways and as teaching aids.

TAKE HOME MESSAGES

- Well written management pathways for patients with chronic pain, firmly based on current evidence, but written by active clinicians, are powerful additions to the clinician's armamentarium. The BPS's Map of Medicine pathways should enable clinicians at all levels to deliver evidence based care to patients with chronic pelvic pain, amongst other conditions. Patients receiving care from clinicians who use the pathways intelligently will receive timely, evidence based, integrated care that will give them the best chance of having the best outcome.
- The Map of Medicine pathways can be used as a tool to move much of the necessary care from secondary care to primary care facilities. Successful implementation requires commitment and engagement from all of the clinicians involved in caring for patients with chronic pelvic pain. When used in this way, primary care physicians will feel supported in their use of the pathway and a local network will have been established that will allow them to seek advice and further care for their patients appropriately.
- These pathways will reduce the use of unnecessary investigations and they will also reduce the wasteful use of treatments that are known either to be unnecessary or ineffective. The result of this will be a reduction in waste and an improvement in the timeliness of the use of the correct treatments for each patient.
- Readers should not underestimate the difficulties involved in introducing clinical pathways to a geographic or institutional locality. Many will feel threatened and

others will feel that their clinical autonomy is being undermined. However, if clinicians are allowed to take ownership of the pathway and modify it to suit the local conditions, the uptake of the pathway is much more likely to be successful. Furthermore, where clinicians realise that their local hospitals or CCGs are not offering the services required to follow the pathway, this in itself can be a spur to encourage the development of more appropriate local facilities.

- Any clinician who has the patient's interests at the centre of everything they do will quickly recognise the utility of these pathways in making it more likely that the patient will get the right treatment, delivered the right way, at the right time, thus giving them the chance of maximum benefit from their treatment.

FURTHER READING

There is no point producing guidelines and pathways if nobody actually uses them! Getting clinicians to use pathways requires the use of change management techniques. The National Institute for Health and Care Excellence (NICE) has a very good short guide to the techniques needed to implement change http://www.nice.org.uk/media/AF1/73/HowToGuideChangePractice.pdf (last accessed 26 May 2014).

The best book that I have read on changing practice in health care is edited by an Anglo-Dutch team—mirroring the Congress in Amsterdam. Its contents compare very favourably with the change management teaching on MBA degree courses and it is much more relevant to health care than more general "change management" books. Grol R, Wensing M, Eccles M, Davis D (Eds). Improving Patient Care: The Implementation of Change in Health Care (second edition). Chichester: Wiley-Blackwell BMJ Books, 2013

REFERENCES

1. Asthma UK. http://www.asthma.org.uk/asthma-facts-and-statistics (last accessed 30 April 2014).
2. British Pain Society/Map of Medicine: Chronic Pelvic Pain—Primary Care Management. Available via the internet: http://bps.mapofmedicine.com/evidence/bps/chronic_pelvic_pain_for_men_and_women_1.html (last accessed 30 April 2014).
3. Daniels JP, Khan KS. Chronic Pelvic Pain in Women. BMJ 2010; 341: c4834
4. Ferris JA, Pitts MK, Richters J, et al. National prevalence of urogenital pain and prostatitis-like symptoms in Australian men using the National Institutes of Health Chronic Prostatitis Symptoms Index. BJU International, 2010;105:373–379.
5. Lenzer J, Hoffman J, Furberg C, Ioannidis J. Ensuring the integrity of clinical practice guidelines: a tool for protecting patients. BMJ 2013;347:f5535.
6. Mathias SD, Kuppermann M, Liberman RF, et al. Chronic pelvic pain: prevalence, health-related quality of life, and economic correlates. Obstet Gynecol 1996;87(3);321–7
7. Right Care Commissioning for Value. www.rightcare.nhs.uk (last accessed 30 April 2014).
8. Secretary of State for Health (UK) https://www.gov.uk/government/publications/liberating-the-nhs-white-paper (last accessed 30 April 2014).

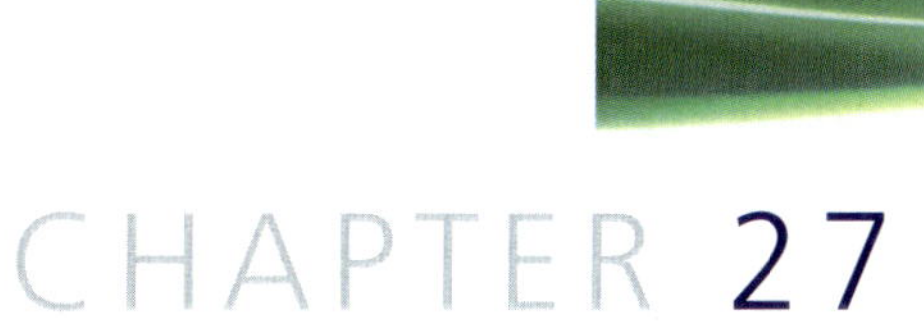

CHAPTER 27

Developing a Structure for Delivery of Care

Andrew Baranowski and Luke Mordecai

INTRODUCTION

This chapter looks at the difficulties and solutions around the provision of pain services for patients in England as an example of one national model of service delivery to bring seamless care for patients suffering and disabled with pain. The model presents care as being seamless from the patients' home up to specialized tertiary centers. Where as the model is England centric, the concepts about how change is being produced are applicable across the world. Developments of specialized services to meet the needs of those with abdominal and pelvic pain are a part of this model.

DESCRIBING THE SUBJECT

NHS England Focus as an Example of the Problem and Potential Solutions that May be Adapted

This chapter explores pain service delivery and in particular the provision of services for those suffering with pain perceived in the abdomen and pelvic regions. This area is a niche subspecialty, and pain perceived in these areas presents with unique diversity and polymorphism. Specific challenges exist within this demographic and failure to take onboard their needs can result in significant morbidity, often with iatrogenic overlay, and a disastrous effect on quality of life. Despite this the structural model of the service can evolve around a generic framework. The main thesis of this paper is that for specific subsets of patients, specialised and dedicated services need to be available but integrated within a seamless pathway of care.

The key management areas within seamless care are: early, clear diagnosis, avoidance of spurious terminology, the importance of re-assurance and education, empowerment for self-management, targeted, timely referral to those with the skills to manage pain as a condition in its own right and any co-morbidity. Co-morbidity is common in patients with abdominal and pelvic pain and needs input, support, diagnosis and management from dedicated multi-specialty teams.

This chapter focuses on England, the lead author holds a senior position within NHS England for delivery of Specialised Pain Services; however, the concepts hold generically true. Different but overlapping models of care exist but they should all have their origins in the key features detailed.

Burden of Pain and Issues Around Delivery of Care

Chief Medical Officers Report, 2008 [9]

In this report pain was featured as one of England's top five priorities. Additionally, concerns regarding the inequality of need and service provision were raised [10]. This was a generic report on pain and highlighted that:

- Chronic pain has a major impact on people's lives, causing sleeplessness and depression and interfering with normal physical and social functioning.
- All age groups are affected: a quarter of school-age children reported pain, as did most elderly nursing homes residents.
- Back pain alone costs the economy £12.3 billion per year. The report noted other significant causes, including pelvic pain in over a million women in the UK.
- Chronic pain and its consequences are not well controlled. Early intervention may stop pain becoming persistent.
- Specialist clinics are inundated with referrals, only 14% of people with pain have seen a pain specialist.
- Better coordination of services, designed around the patients' needs are essential.

High exposure reports like this have been key to placing pain on the agenda in England. The report went on to recommend a number of actions:

- Training in chronic pain should be included in the curricula of all healthcare professionals. This remains an issue and the general view still suggests that medical students spend less time learning about pain than vets.
- Consideration should be given to the inclusion of the assessment of pain in the Quality and Outcomes Framework (QOFs) for primary care. Managed by the National Institute for Health and Care Excellence (NICE) and based on Quality Standards, the QOF is a voluntary incentive scheme for GP practices in the UK, providing a financial reward for achieving clinical targets [14]. There are currently no NICE Quality Standards for pain and hence no possibility of a QOF. Pain specialists have lobbied for NICE Quality Standards and the following are suggestions as to what could be included (with thanks to those members of The British Pain Society, The Faculty of Pain Medicine Royal college of Anaesthetists and The Royal College of GP's amongst other agencies that formed the Shadow Quality Standards for Pain Committee):
  - Diagnosis and management in accordance with appropriate guidelines such as British Pain Society pain patient pathway maps.
  - Risk assessment of "problematic pain" using a structured questionnaire, including mental health, psychology, disability and work factors.
  - Production of a written and personalised action plan.
  - Access to appropriate care in primary, community, secondary and tertiary services. Where appropriate this should involve a MultiDisciplinary Team (MDT).
  - A minimum of an annual structured plan, which should include re-evaluation of biopsychosocial aspects and medications.
  - Provision of a self-management strategy for exacerbations with concomitant objective clinician reassessment.
  - People admitted to hospital with an exacerbation of pain should have a timely review by a member of a specialist inpatient pain team with formulation of an appropriate discharge plan, including review by their GP within 5 working days.
  - All acute facilities should have consultant-led pain services.

  - Pain management services must collect appropriate outcome data, such as Patient Reported Outcome Measures (PROM's) ideally using a national register. Services involved in delivering pain management must support and/or be involved in professional development.
- A pain score should be routinely monitored in all inpatients. There is no mandate for this to date.
- The feasibility of a national network of rapid-access pain clinics providing early assessment and treatment should be explored.
- A model pathway of care with clear standards should be developed by experts. The BPS has published guidelines [6]. These pathways of best care are based on evidence as well as consensus opinion to ensure equity of care and quality. They are now enshrined and mandated in the NHS England Service specification for Specialised Pain Services.
- All chronic pain services should supply comprehensive information to a National Pain Database.
- Agencies involved in the management of patients with chronic pain should form local networks to improve the quality of services.
- The Health Survey for England should routinely collect data on the impact of pain on quality of life.

The Health Survey for England, 2011 [7]

The Health and Social Care Centre provides national data to care organisations to improve standards. The National Health Survey for England published in 2011, included questions on the burden of pain. Their conclusions were:

- That chronic pain should be defined as "pain or discomfort that troubles a person, constantly or intermittently, for more than three months and also associates it with negative life outcomes and other organic pathology".
- Intersex variation in chronic pain, 31% of men and 37% of women meeting criteria, and an increasing prevalence with age.
- No significant variation in the prevalence of chronic pain across strategic health authorities.
- A strong socioeconomic correlation with 40% of men and 44% of women in the lowest income quintile of equivilised household income reporting chronic pain as compared to only 24% and 30% respectively in the highest.
- A Chronic Pain Grade was assigned based on the extent the pain interfered with usual activities and its intensity. Grades I and II indicate low interference pain at different intensities, while grades III and IV indicate pain with differing levels of restriction to usual activities. In the survey, the majority were assigned to Grade I or II (70% men and 68% women). The likelihood of obtaining a higher interference Grade III or IV increased with age and low socioeconomic status. These higher grade people also subjectively reported being in poorer health when compared to those with less limiting pain.
- The likelihood that those with chronic pain had attended a specialist pain service increased with the severity of Chronic Pain Grade. 61% of men and 54% of women classified as Grade IV reported attending, compared with 25% of men and 24% of women classified as Grade I.
- Those with chronic pain were more likely to suffer with anxiety or depression than those with no pain, and the prevalence of this increased with Chronic Pain Grade.

National Pain Audit, 2011–12 [8]

Whilst the Health Survey for England looked at the burden of pain, the British Pain Society in collaboration with Dr Foster Health™ undertook a survey to investigate NHS clinical pain management services and evaluate quality and level of provision.

The report identified that:

- Specialist pain services deliver care to a group of people who report a very poor quality of life.
- Regarding healthcare utilisation, 4,825 (20%) of respondents reported attending Accident and Emergency in the past six months all of whom had seen their GP. 3,469 (66%) had made more than three visits to healthcare providers.
- Access to MDT care, the essential requirement for specialist chronic pain services, was highly variable with only 81 out of 204 clinics (40%) meeting the minimum MDT standard with the presence of a psychologist, physiotherapist and physician.
- Services concentrate on spinal and musculoskeletal (MSK) pain despite a documented need for diversification into other subspecialties such as pelvic and non-MSK neuropathic pain.
- Positive outcome data was collected with 56.5% of clinics showing patients to have a mean improvement in quality of life after six months using the eq5d-3l. For disease specific change, measured by the Brief Pain Inventory (BPI), 70.6% of the clinics reported an overall reduction in pain severity by an average 0.22 adjusted health gain.
- Many patients report a good experience of their service, especially in terms of support and advice, yet this important activity has no recognised incentive for provision, nor is it captured via coding mechanisms. Simultaneously, 52% of patients reported difficulty in understanding chronic pain. Specialist and non-specialist services require greater integration to ensure delivery of a consistent message.

The report recommended:

- Identification of services.
  - A treatment specialty code (191) should be attached to all specialist pain services to identify them. Currently, Hospital Episode Statistics (HES) only apply to the acute setting. This should be extended to all settings, and ensure non-medical treatments delivered in the context of a documented specialist pain service are included.
- Access to services.
  - NHS Choices, and other recognised sources of information on services, should ensure that a minimum mandated standard of information on local pain services is available to patients.
  - The Royal College of Anaesthetists should adopt the International Association for the Study of Pain guidance on minimum waiting times in its Good Practice.
  - NICE should consider making access times that are "appropriate to need" a key standard for pain services.
- Staff skills mix
  - Given the high rate of anxiety and depression, the clear link between these and poor functioning, better access to physiotherapy and psychology is essential. Commissioners should ensure these skills are incorporated into local care pathways for pain.
  - Medical consultant doctors should underpin every specialist service.
  - Future audits should seek to understand the available skills mix and competencies in more detail.

  - Given the impact of pain on quality of life and in turn ability to work there needs to be more focus on helping those with pain return to employment.
- Staffing competencies
  - Specialty interest groups should provide guidance on which competencies and skills are required in order to meet patients' needs and to support commissioners in identifying what particular services are instituted.
- Multidisciplinary teams
  - Commissioners and providers should ensure a local health needs assessment is carried out to determine the degree to which specialist multidisciplinary care is required.
  - Clinical Commissioning Groups (CCG's) that commission local services should examine whether commissioned services match the Royal College of Anaesthetists' Faculty of Pain Medicine's recommended standards on staffing and structures.
  - CCG's should ensure procurement of an integrated multidisciplinary care model.
  - CCG's should ensure when a service cannot provide multidisciplinary care, it directs patients to accessible services which can.
- Assessing Quality of Care
  - NICE should draw upon the good practice demonstrated by specialist pain services in involving patients in decisions, this should be used as a standard for good practice. NICE should pursue the quality standard for pain with some degree of urgency to ensure services are able to meet need.

Stages to Correcting Inequalities

The burden of pain and inequalities within services are well documented. However, overhauling a national medical service is a significant undertaking. Several initiatives, following the CMO report, have occurred in parallel.

Pathways of Care

The CMO report correctly indicates that to improve care we need "Gold Standard" pathways to guide us.

- *British Pain Society (BPS) pathways of care.*

  There are 5 published and available pathways [6].

  The pathways clearly outline the early assessment, investigations and management that would be suitable in the primary care arena. Appropriate onward referral and secondary care management is also signposted. The inequality between need and provision clearly supports the role of early management close to the patient's home as is consistent for all "Long Term Conditions".

  Long-term conditions have been assigned their own domain because of the increasing burden on health expenditure they represent. 15.4 Million people suffer from long-term conditions, and the demographic accounts for 50% of all GP appointments and 70% of days spent in hospital beds. Pain is correctly allocated to this domain given it's often chronic, debilitating nature along with its association with other conditions.

  NHS England and CCG's have in partnership identified four action areas specific to this domain which are; helping patients take charge of their care, enabling good primary care, ensuring continuity of care and ensuring parity of esteem for mental health.

- *The BPS Chronic Pelvic Pain pathway (for men and women) [5]*
  This was written by representatives from multiple specialties and developed in collaboration with the Maps of Medicine editorial team, the BPS, and independent reviewers. It is based on best evidence and, when appropriate, consensus opinion, which was clearly identified. For the detailed editorial methodology, please see the pathway's provenance certificate [19]. Map of Medicine care pathways can be customised to reflect local commissioning needs and provide comprehensive, evidence based local guidance along with clinical decision support at the point of care.

  These pathways represent a seamless approach to this group of patients and represent the first step towards the essential integration of care.
- *European Association of Urology (EAU), Chronic Pelvic Pain (CPP) Guidelines*
  The EAU CPP guidelines were published in 2004. The latest version 2012 [16] clearly outlines the role of the different teams, and the evidence base to support this. The ten years of experience within this group supports a multispeciality and interdisciplinary approach to management [3].
- *International Association for the Study of Pain classification*
  Differences and spurious use of terminology have been known to result in inappropriate investigations and interventions [1] and even cause confusion regarding service provision. To combat this, the EAU and IASP SIG on Abdominal and Pelvic Pain (formally known as PUGO) commissioned working groups to look at classification, terminology and phenotyping. Following multiple publications by the EAU, their work was accepted by IASP in 2012 and will be published in the new IASP taxonomy [12].

  This work has been key in highlighting that in managing this group of patients it is essential to address functional issues (such as bowl and bladder disorders), emotional, cognitive, sexual and behavioural disorders as well as pain and teams need to be in place to support that approach.
- *England's Pain Summit*
  Whilst there are many differing models of health systems in the world, The Pain Summit [15] provided a forum for all interested parties and produced the following recommendations:
  - Clear standards and criteria must be agreed and implemented nationally for the identification, assessment, and initial management of problematic pain.
  - An awareness campaign should be run to explain the nature, extent, impact, prevention and treatment of chronic pain to the wider community.
  - Nationally agreed commissioning guidance must be developed and agreed, describing best value care in chronic pain to reduce unwarranted variation.
  - A data strategy for chronic pain should be agreed through creation of an epidemiology of chronic pain working group.
- *NHS England*
  The Health and Social Care Act, 2012, has precipitated the most extensive reorganisation of the NHS in its history. Specifically with regard to commissioning, the Primary Care Trusts (PCT's) and Strategic Health Authorities (SHA) that were previously responsible, have been replaced with Clinical Commissioning Groups (CCG's). CCG's are led by local clinicians, meaning they have direct influence over the commissioning of services for their specific patient population [13]. CCG's will negotiate over elective hospital care, rehabilitation, emergency care, and the majority of community and mental health services. As of March 2013, there were 211 CCG's [10] and they are held accountable by the also newly created NHS England.

Previously, commissioning of specialised services was performed by 10 separate Specialised Commissioning Groups (SCG's) with some services commissioned on a national basis. These SCG's were independent of each other leading to variation in services and inequality regarding access. The new system is focused on a single nationalised approach to specialised commissioning championing patient and public engagement in the process [11]. 74 Clinical Reference Groups (CRG's) develop recommendations regarding specialised service provision but are not decision-making bodies [11].

Specialised Pain Services

The primary, initial goal regarding Specialised Pain Services for England focused on what are the key standards and service delivery requirement to provide a specialised pain service. Those are defined in a national service specification. The model of care reflects services provided in a small number of tertiary level pain services, generally one tertiary specialised centre per region and several in London who serve a wider geographical catchment. Unlike secondary care centres the funding does not come from the many CCGs but direct from NHS England and as a consequence NHS England, through the CRG's, can set the standards of care. Clinical Reference Groups are the source of expert clinical advice and develop commissioning tools such as service specifications and quality dashboards that are clinically and patient led. Essentially, specialised pain service centres would represent the most comprehensive pain services, they may now and in the future work in a network model with smaller secondary care centres as well as community services to delivery pathways of care. Specialised pain providers are defined as such due to the multiple areas of specialisation such as an Abdominal and Pelvic Pain service (APPS) and a comprehensive Multi Disciplinary Team of at least two persons per discipline to support each service.

Policies. As well as defining the service, the CRG has been given the remit to produce policies for specific aspects of care for consideration and prioritisation by NHS England. For instance, the role of intrathecal drug delivery by implanted devices is being clearly described by the CRG, from indications through to standards of care expected. This policy is subjected to a number of stringent reviews and public consultation. It is envisaged that this evidence-based approach will also be used to define the role of Sacral Root Stimulation for pelvic pain in the not too distant future.

Quality Standards. As a part of defining specialised services and policies, national standards will be introduced and published with the aim of transparency. These National Standards will only apply to specialised tertiary services and not form mandates for primary, community and secondary care. Patients may only be referred to tertiary services if appropriate non-specialised management has already occurred. It is envisaged that over time each regional tertiary service may provide specialised Abdominal and Pelvic Pain Specialised services.

This model of seamless escalating levels of intervention and care will hopefully help to address standards of care within the health system of England. However, it will only work if greater resources are allocated to match the need and the provision of care.

- *Enhanced Pain Services for England.*

  This model aims to resolve the inequality around provision of care. Improving care around pain requires a significant financial investment to develop all tiers of care from primary to tertiary. The HSE and NPA have demonstrated the inequality but to make changes two key issues must be resolved by the CRG for specialized pain services. First, a Health Survey Analysis of costs needs to be undertaken which would involve a detailed assessment of the current expenditure, demand for specialised provision and current available capacity within existing specialised pain providers, the costs of enhancing the service and the savings that such an approach would realise. The second requires innovating a system that will be able to identify patients with pain through coding and facilitate the tracking of those patients and more importantly their response to interventions.

The Enhanced model of UGP care delivery in England. The BPS patient maps form the basis of a structured approach to the provision of care for those suffering with abdominal, pelvic and urogenital pain. They aim to clarify the process of early identification of problematic pain, as well as triage, support, education, and self-management. They emphasise the importance of multiple levels of care, combined with multispeciality and disciplinary input, along with a holistic approach.

PRACTICAL IMPLICATIONS

It is well recognised that patients suffering with abdominal, pelvic, and visceral pain have unique diversity requiring us to consider multiple tiers of seamless care depending upon the needs of the patient. A minimal number of specialist centres will not be capable of meeting the needs of this significant patient population and given their complexity a management regime involving solely primary and community care is not a feasible option. In recognition of this fact NHS England is investigating seamless care modeled on vertical integration with regional centres working closely, and communicating regularly, with secondary care centres, which in turn support community services. Equitable access depending on need must also remain a policy cornerstone.

Seamless care and integrated care are concepts that have been repeatedly used throughout this chapter and are topical regarding health policy. Current thinking regards them as a panacea for the inefficiency that almost inevitably accompanies any large corporation or institution. However, they are rather nebulous terms that neither identify the root cause of a problem nor offer a tangible solution? Currently primary, secondary and tertiary care all communicate with each other therefore is care not already integrated? Given the acknowledged power of leadership, teamwork, efficiency and knowledge sharing an integrated service indeed sounds like a panacea but how does one go about creating it functionally, and more interestingly why are we not employing these seemingly simple and obvious principles already?

The WHO defines integrated care as a concept bringing together inputs, delivery, management and organization services related to diagnosis, treatment, care rehabilitation and health promotion. Integration is a means to improve services in relation to access, quality, user satisfaction and efficiency. As an endpoint, this definition provides great clarity, however, the question remains as to how one might go about achieving it? To use a term first coined by Rittel and Webber creation of such a service is a proverbial "wicked" problem [18].

There are major obstacles aside from the lack of clinical resources. First is the issue of communication. The referral process still utilises the delivery of physical letters, and patient records are almost totally inaccessible between institutions, resulting in the slow and often neglected or erroneous passage of information. A universal network of electronic patient records is the first requirement for integration however recent costly failures in this area and the politically sensitive nature of accessible personal information has made this an unsavory concept in the NHS.

Another issue is around referral. Given the subjective nature of pain and the absence of reliable metrics, and despite the emergence of pathways to guide primary care, when is the correct juncture to refer patients? Additionally given the financial implication of sending patients to specialists, do primary care physicians delay referral in an attempt to avoid this cost when in fact it is merely delaying the inevitable at patient's expense? Does there need to be a paradigm shift whereby instead of primary care being in essence financially punished for referring patients, should they instead be rewarded for the timely referral of appropriate cases?

There is further complexity in payment. Broadly speaking primary care practices control their own budget, CCG's control the budgets for secondary care, and tertiary care is funded from a national pool. Payment and accounting is central to the efficient running and transparency of any institution, be it publically funded and not for profit or otherwise. Employing multiple and dynamic revenue streams depending on a patient's progression through the referral hierarchy is another systemic fault hindering the adoption of integration.

The Veterans Health Administration (VA) operating in the United States exemplifies real integration. It receives its budget from the federal government and from that employs its own physicians, runs it own hospitals and manages its own services. In the latter regard it is frequently compared with the NHS. It has not always run in this manner however and in the nineties it was plagued with bureaucracy and delivered mediocre care with different facets often working against each other and duplicating care [17]. A change of leadership precipitated creation of 21 independent networks each with responsibility for resources across all care settings, rigorous accountability, and universally agreed and widely disseminated performance and outcome measures. Huge investment in IT has also augmented data sharing and facilitated access to clinical guidelines and physician support tools [2]. Since adopting this vision for integrated care, the VA has reduced hospital bed days by 55% with no reported adverse consequences [2] and observed a 19% reduction in admissions along with high satisfaction scores [4].

The VA model proves that integrated care is more than a theoretical concept, however achieving it requires great leadership, significant investment and perhaps most importantly the ability to accept and embrace change.

LOOKING AT THE FUTURE

The burden of abdominal, pelvic, and visceral pain needs to be more widely accepted and acknowledged, as does the inequality in provision against need. Fragmented care will not provide the best services for patients and units with differing skills and expertise need to work together in an integrated fashion. This should not be considered a threat but rather an opportunity for the future.

TAKE HOME MESSAGES

- Specifically regarding pain services, there is significant inequality between the need and the provision of care.
- Due to the variable presentation of abdominal, pelvic and visceral pain, multiple disciplinary teams need to be involved, and tailored as appropriate to the needs of the patient.
- No single regional center can meet the need and smaller community centers will not be able to provide all aspects of care. Certain treatments should only be offered in specialised environments with appropriate competencies and transparent outcome measures.

- In light of this, seamless vertically integrated care needs to be developed with safeguards to ensure equitable access. Local surveys may need to be instigated to accomplish this and understand the unique diversity.
- This paper presents how engagement of patients, providers and fund holders may produce such a theoretical model based on sound evidence and pathways of care. Implementation is always more complex!
- Integrated care is a reality but requires investment, a willingness to embrace change and acceptance that trial and error will be required when reforming systems as cumbersome as health services.

FURTHER READING

Securing equity and excellence in commissioning specialised services http://www.england.nhs.uk/wp-content/uploads/2012/11/op-model.pdf

Everyone counts: planning for patients 2014/15 to 20018/19. http://www.england.nhs.uk/wp-content/uploads/2013/12/5yr-strat-plann-guid-wa.pdf

Specialised Pain Services for England. http://www.england.nhs.uk/ourwork/commissioning/spec-services/npc-crg/group-d/d08/

REFERENCES

1. Abrams P, Baranowski AP, Berger R, et al. A New Classification is needed for Pelvic Pain Syndromes: Existing Terminologies of Spurious Diagnostic authority are Bad for Patients? J Urology 2006, 175:1989–1990.
2. Ashton CM, Souchek J, Petersen NJ. Hospital use and survival among Veterans Affairs beneficiaries'. N Engl J Med 2003, 349:1637–46.
3. Engeler DS, Baranowski AP, Dinis-Oliveira P, et al. The 2013 EAU Guidelines on Chronic Pelvic Pain: Is Management of Chronic Pelvic Pain a Habit, a Philosophy, or a Science? 10 Years of Development. Eur Urol 2010;64(3):E43-e74.
4. Darkins A. Care Coordination/Home Telehealth: the systematic implementation of health informatics, home telehealth, and disease management to support the care of veteran patients with chronic conditions. Telemed J E-Health 2008;14:1118–26.
5. Chronic Pelvic Pain – Primary Care Management. *http://bps.mapofmedicine.com/evidence/bps/chronic_pelvic_pain_for_men_and_women_1.html Last Accessed July 2014*
6. Map of Medicine. *http://bps.mapofmedicine.com/evidence/bps/index.html Last Accessed July 2014*
7. Bridges S. Chronic Pain. *https://catalogue.ic.nhs.uk/publications/public-health/surveys/heal-surv-eng-2011/HSE2011-Ch9-Chronic-Pain.pdf*
8. National Pain Audit Final Report http://www.britishpainsociety.org/members_articles_npa_2012.pdf
9. http://www.avon.nhs.uk/kris/_Docs/CMO%20report.pdf
10. NHS England. *http://www.england.nhs.uk/about/*
11. *http://www.england.nhs.uk/npc-crg/*
12. http://www.iasp-pain.org/PublicationsNews/Content.aspx?ItemNumber=1673
13. Health and Social Care Act 2012 http://www.legislation.gov.uk/ukpga/2012/7/schedule/2
14. National Institute for Health and Care Excellence http://www.nice.org.uk/aboutnice/qof/qof.jsp?domedia=1&mid=A68618D5-19B9-E0B5-D43FB5A0D4317150
15. Pain Summit 2011. Summit Reports. http://www.painsummit.org.uk/node/7376
16. http://www.uroweb.org/gls/pdf/24_Chronic_Pelvic_Pain_LR%20II.pdf
17. Perlin JB, Kolodner RM, Roswell, RH. The Veterans Health Administration: quality, value, accountability, and information as transforming strategies for patient-centred care. Am J Managed Care 2004,10:828–36.
18. Rittel HW, Webber MM. Dilemmas in a general theory of planning. Policy Sciences 1973;4:155–169.
19. Map of Medicine. www.mapofmedicine.com

CHAPTER 28

Generating the Evidence Base for Chronic Pelvic Pain in the Future

Seema Tirlapur and Khalid Khan

INTRODUCTION

Chronic pelvic pain (CPP) is the most common cause for gynaecology outpatient referrals in the United Kingdom with an estimated prevalence similar to that of chronic back pain and asthma [1, 2]. The worldwide rates are variable with 59% due to dysmenorrhea, 13% dyspareunia and 10% non-cyclical pelvic pain [1]. CPP is often multi-factorial in nature with many pre-disposing factors such as pelvic pathology and psychological morbidity [3]. It is defined by the International Association of Pain as chronic or persistent pain perceived in structures related to the pelvis of either men or women. It is often associated with negative cognitive, behavioural, sexual and emotional consequences as well as with symptoms suggestive of lower urinary tract, sexual, bowel, pelvic floor or gynaecological dysfunction [5]. While surveys of specialist associations have identified areas in need of further research, it is important to engage clinicians and patients in order to discover new effective treatments and improve care quality [6]. Without engagement in research specialty development will be hindered.

DESCRIBING THE SUBJECT

Why Practitioners Should Engage in Research?

It is our duty as clinicians to strive to resolve the uncertainties about the effects of treatments [7]. This may be undertaken through research involving prevalence studies, diagnostic, prognostic or therapeutic trials. Participation in high quality gynaecology clinical trials has been increasing over the decades [8]. Large multi-centre clinical trials are needed to generate reliable, rapidly completed, generaliseable data. These trials generate robust data that influence clinical guidelines and change practice. Small studies are unreliable and often unfavourable. These studies risk falsely reporting that observations have no significance. The principal investigator is usually involved in the patients care and can convey the importance of participating in research, the clinical question being assessed, recruitment, consent and study details such as the length of participation and number of visits needed. It is useful to explain to patients how participation in research studies is hugely beneficial and the role they can play in influencing outcomes and future management.

Good Practice in Research Design

Randomised controlled trials (RCTs) are widely seen as the gold standard study design in clinical trials of treatment effectiveness. RCTs in gynaecology may assess medical or surgical management, and specialist or multidisciplinary care, involving a team of gynaecologists, pain specialists and clinical psychologists. This approach can provide very successful treatment as many women have a strong functional component to their pain, which may be best treated by non-surgical treatments [10]. These RCT's may involve phase 1 studies of treatment safety in a healthy population; phase 2 and 3 studies of efficacy and effectiveness in the affected target population and phase 4 studies of long-term safety and effectiveness. RCTs are not always suitable in surgical trials as it may not be possible for concealed allocations and blinding of clinicians or patients in these studies. Large trials are needed to show small differences in effect size in benign gynaecological conditions, such as pelvic pain, which are common. Small studies may show non-significant results. A power of 80% is often used, ie. there is an 80% chance of finding a genuine effect. When calculating the sample size it is based on the anticipated difference between the outcome of the comparison and intervention groups. The standardised difference is calculated; a standard deviation of 0.2 is a small effect size; 0.5 is medium and 0.8 is large [11]. Table 1 shows the number of patients needed in test accuracy and effectiveness of treatment studies at varying prevalence and power levels. Larger sample sizes are needed for robust studies, as small studies may not be reliable as the statistical difference may not be clinically relevant.

Clinicians should strive to minimise bias with adequate randomisation, concealment and allocation methods to minimise selection bias, double blinding to avoid performance bias, blinding the outcome measurer (triple blinding where possible) to minimise measurement bias and performing intention to treat analysis with completeness of follow up data to avoid attrition bias. Compliance with allocation and treatment, along with withdrawals is difficult to predict but can be overcome by carefully selected patients during screening for eligibility, commencing treatment soon after randomisation and educating patients about what is to be expected. Recruiting patients from multiple centres allows for generaliseable data with external validity, free from local peculiarities. When choosing outcomes, it is important to remember that the end-point may be an improvement or change in symptoms as complete

TABLE 1 **Sample Sizes for Different Research Questions**

a. Treatment effectiveness studies (11)

	Standardised effect size		
Power	0.5	0.33	0.20
80%	128	292	788
90%	172	388	1054

b. Test accuracy studies
Sample size at 80% Power

Sensitivity	Sensitivity to exclude	No. of patients	Total number of patients		
			30% prevalence	40% prevalence	50% prevalence
60%	45%	82	273	205	164
70%	55%	76	253	190	152
80%	65%	69	230	173	132

disease resolution is difficult in chronic conditions [11]. Outcome measures should be clearly defined as primary or secondary with methods of testing stated. The CROWN (core outcomes in women's health) initiative is aiming to identify and prioritise core reporting outcomes for common conditions in obstetrics and gynaecology in order to minimise inconsistencies in the reporting of outcomes and avoid reporting bias [12]. Follow up data can be hard to collect but keeping questionnaires short, providing pre-paid envelopes, and financial incentives may help.

MEDAL: An Exemplar of a Multi-Centre Study

Surveys of the British Society of Gynaecological Endoscopy (BSGE) identified pelvic pain as an area in need of further research [6]. The MEDAL study (Magnetic resonance imaging [MRI] to establish a diagnosis against laparoscopy in unexplained chronic pelvic pain) is a diagnostic accuracy study that was developed to assess if a pelvic MRI scan is as effective as a diagnostic laparoscopy at triaging patients and to evaluate the cost-effectiveness [13]. This national institute for health research (NIHR) portfolio trial has recently completed recruitment to target sample size in 26 centres. Figure 1 shows the centres spread across the United Kingdom that participated in the study. The trial aims to identify if MRI can replace diagnostic laparoscopy in all or a sub-group of patients with chronic pelvic pain.

PRACTICAL IMPLICATIONS

We need to encourage clinicians and patients to participate in research studies in order to identify what is best practice. In order to participate in large multi-centred trials, practitioners need to take on the role of principal investigator (PI). This responsibility involves the local recruiting of patients. The PI needs basic mandatory research training, for example good clinical practice (GCP) training and an understanding of local funding methods. Their efforts are

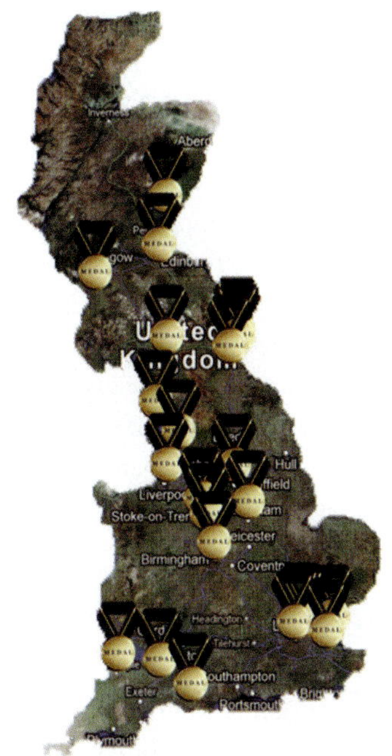

FIGURE 1 Map of the United Kingdom showing centres participating in the MEDAL study.

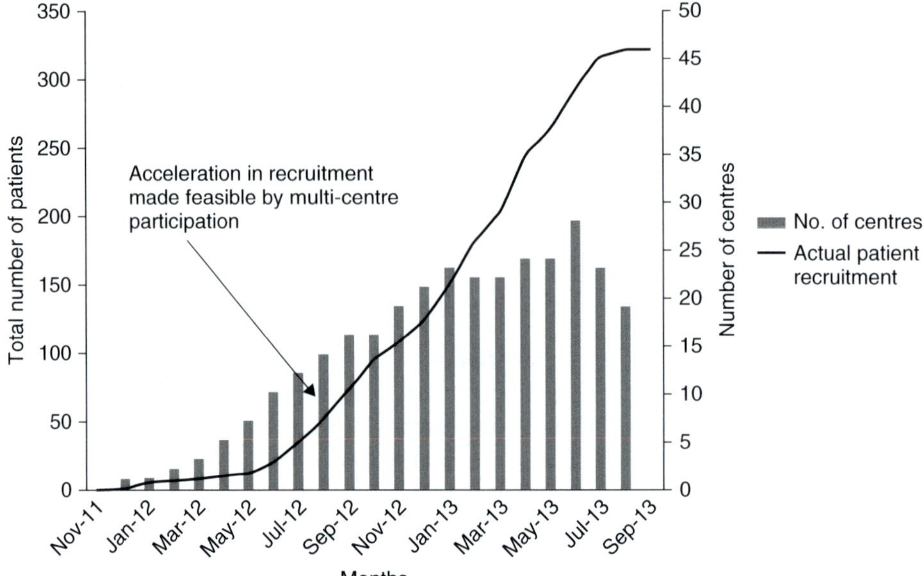

FIGURE 2 MEDAL study recruitment graph.

recognised as part of appraisals, revalidation, and publication [9]. Patient involvement can be increased by engaging with support groups through their websites and social media, and using local media sources that may be able to help generate interest in research projects. Figure 2 shows the recruitment graph for the MEDAL study, which demonstrates how trial recruitment often starts slowly and with the introduction of additional centres, recruitment accelerates.

LOOKING AT THE FUTURE

How can we translate what is learned from clinical trials into everyday practice? The first step is to keep updated on the latest research and evidence-based practice emerging around the world. National and international guidelines draw from the available literature from studies and should be adhered to where possible to provide standardised, good quality care for patients. Clinicians could also learn from the results of new studies and incorporate them into daily practice where feasible [14]. Some barriers to implement changes are skepticism, fear of loss of autonomy, poor motivation and resistance to change [15].

The development of care pathways to guide primary care givers how to triage patients with pelvic pain and commence initial management has been welcomed in the United Kingdom and are being created with key stakeholders. As chronic pelvic pain is multifactorial and may have more than one cause or pathological process, a multi-disciplinary approach to therapy with involvement of several specialties would be beneficial. The prevalence and financial burden of chronic pelvic pain warrants the undertaking of further studies to improve the management of this condition.

TAKE HOME MESSAGES

- Many evidence-based interventions remain under-utilised.
- Research improves patient outcomes in future practice.

- Participants in research fair better than non-participants in terms of outcomes.
- Both clinicians and patient should be actively encouraged to participate in research.
- Large multi-centre studies produce robust evidence for guiding practice.
- Participation in research is a key means to improve care quality.
- A day without participation in research is a day without progress.

FURTHER READING

Initial management of chronic pelvic pain – Green Top guideline no. 41, May 2012, Royal College of obstetricians and Gynaecologists

ACKNOWLEDGEMENTS

The MEDAL study, MRI to establish a diagnosis in chronic pelvic pain, a project funded by the National Institute for Health Research Health Technology Assessment (NIHR HTA) (ref: 09/22/50) (http://www.ukctg.nihr.ac.uk/trialdetails/ISRCTN13028601). The views and opinions expressed are those of the authors and do not necessarily reflect those of the HTA programme, NIHR, NHS or Department of Health.
Conflict of interest: Both authors are members of the MEDAL study management group.

REFERENCES

1. Latthe P, Latthe M, Say L, et al. WHO systematic review of prevalence of chronic pelvic pain: a neglected reproductive health morbidity. BMC Public Health. 2006;6:177.
2. Zondervan KT, Yudkin PL, Vessey MP, et al. Prevalence and incidence of chronic pelvic pain in primary care: evidence from a national general practice database. Br J Obstet Gynaecol. 1999;106(11):1149–55.
3. Latthe P, Mignini L, Gray R, et al. Factors predisposing women to chronic pelvic pain: systematic review. BMJ. 2006;332(7544):749–55.
4. Royal College of Obstetricians and Gynaecologists. Initial management of chronic pelvic pain. 2012.
5. Baranowski A, Abrahms P, Berger R, et al. Classification of Chronic Pain. 2 ed. International Association for the Study of Pain. 2011.
6. Tirlapur SA, Leung E, Ball E, et al. Future research in gynaecological surgery. Best Pract Res Clin Obstet Gynaecol. 2013;27(3):471–8.
7. Good Medical Practice. General Medical Council. 2012.
8. Raza A, Chien PF, Khan KS. Multicentre randomised controlled trials in obstetrics and gynaecology: an analysis of trends over three decades. BJOG. 2009;116(8):1130–4.
9. Thangaratinam S, Khan KS. Participation in research as a means of improving care quality: Role of a Principal Investigator in Multicentre Clinical Trials (In press).
10. Cheong Y, Stones R. Management of chronic pelvic pain: evidence from randomised controlled trials. Obstet Gynaecol 2006; (8):32–8.
11. Khan KS. Gynaecology randomized control trials. In: Gad SC (ed). Clinical trials handbook. 2009:523–33.
12. Kirkham JJ, Gargon E, Clarke M, Williamson PR. Can a core outcome set improve the quality of systematic reviews?—a survey of the Co-ordinating Editors of Cochrane Review Groups. Trials 2013;14:21.
13. UK Clinical Research Network: Portfolio Database. http://public.ukcrn.org.uk (Accessed 24th Oct 2013).
14. Kulier R, Gee H, Khan KS. Five steps from evidence to effect: exercising clinical freedom to implement research findings. BJOG. 2008;115(10):1197–202.
15. Deshpande N, Publicover M, Gee H, Khan KS. Incorporating the views of obstetric clinicians in implementing evidence-supported labour and delivery suite ward rounds: a case study. Health Info Libr J. 2003;20(2):86–94.

CHAPTER 29

The Future of Abdominal and Pelvic Pain Management

Maria Adele Giamberardino, Claudio Tana, Giannapia Affaitati, Francesca Massimini, and Raffaele Costantini

INTRODUCTION

Pain in the abdomen or pelvis is a very common experience. Community surveys demonstrate, for example, that 25% of people have intermittent abdominal pain and 24% of women have pelvic pain [29,56]. The symptom can originate from different structures of the abdominal and pelvic area. Especially in the chronic form, however, it most often results from multiple conditions with the global experience of pain being not merely the sum of symptoms from all conditions but rather the result of a complex interaction among them [30]. Pain at abdominal and pelvic level can also be the local expression of a generalized pain condition such as fibromyalgia [37]. Management of the symptom remains difficult at the moment and still represents a challenge for the medical community. Treatment interventions have traditionally targeted specific biomedical conditions with variable success [33]. Future management of this pain needs to take into account the complexity with a personalized, integrated multidisciplinary and multimodal strategy. This chapter will focus on the fundamental principles of the therapeutic approach to patients complaining of chronic abdominal and pelvic pain, based on the most recent available data from the literature on the diagnostic process and pathophysiology of the symptom.

BASIC ASPECTS

As underlined in the introduction, abdominal and pelvic pain can occur in a high number of algogenic diseases affecting the numerous structures of the abdominal and pelvic area but can also manifest in the context of diffuse pain conditions involving central sensitization [6] (Table 1). The correct identification is not always easy in current medical practice but is, on the other hand, an indispensable step towards establishing an effective therapy. A proper diagnosis involves the detection of the main sources of the pain and all their possible interactions, as detailed in the following section.

TABLE 1 Origin of Abdomino-Pelvic pain

A. Abdomino-pelvic
- Musculoskeletal
- Neuropathic
- Visceral (digestive and genito-urinary organs)

B. Extra abdomino-pelvic
In the context of generalized pain conditions, e.g., fibromyalgia

DESCRIBING THE SUBJECT

Pain of Abdominal and Pelvic Origin

Musculoskeletal Origin

A number of abdominal and pelvic pain conditions derive primarily from the musculoskeletal system, particularly myofascial pain syndromes (MPS) from active trigger points (TrPs) in various muscle structures such as rectus abdominis, lateral abdominalis, iliocostalis lumborum, obliquus externus, iliopsoas, multifidi, quadratus lumborum, levator ani, glutei or piriformis. As for any other body location, TrPs are formed mainly as a consequence of micro-traumatic events to muscle structures, due to several factors such as poor posture, mechanical overload or habits and activities involving repetitive movements of the same muscle groups. Identification of "taut bands" at muscle level, and reproduction of the spontaneous pain complaint by stimulation of the TrP within the band is key to the diagnostic process [20,48].

Neuropathic Origin

Several abdominal and pelvic pains are neuropathic in nature, as in the case of the pudendal or sciatic nerve entrapment syndromes, where the nerves are entrapped or compressed, due to pregnancy, accidents, scarring from surgery or repetitive activities such as heavy and prolonged bicycling. A burning-lancinating quality of the pain, together with a location radiating along the typical nerve distribution are among the most indicative elements suggestive of the diagnosis of neuropathic pain [38].

Visceral Origin

Internal organs are by far the most frequent [24, 37] source of abdominal and pelvic pain conditions: irritable bowel syndrome (IBS), dysmenorrhea - primary or secondary, endometriosis, or Bladder Pain Syndrome/ interstitial cystitis (BPS/IC) are just a few examples [2,8,12,35]. Particular emphasis will thus be placed here on visceral pain phenomena through which the symptom can manifest: (1) referred somatic pain and hyperalgesia, (2) visceral hyperalgesia, (3) viscero-visceral hyperalgesia (VVH) [24,44].

- Referred somatic pain and hyperalgesia. Pain from internal organs typically project to somatic areas including the neuromeric fields of the affected viscus, where tissue hypersensitivity (secondary hyperalgesia) most often develops. This hyperalgesia has been characterized in a number of clinical studies with various abdominal and pelvic pain conditions including: IBS, primary dysmenorrhea, pelvic pain from endometriosis and urinary colics from calculosis. Evaluating pain thresholds to various stimuli (e.g. mechanical, electrical) in the relative areas of referral or projection, has shown that thresholds are decreased in the three tissues of the abdominal and pelvic body wall (skin, subcutis and muscle), particularly in the muscle. Muscle pain threshold decrease is a function of the number of previous visceral pain episodes, i.e., the higher this number, the greater the threshold decrease and thus the hyperalgesia. Muscle hyperalgesia is a long-lasting phenomenon, persisting in the pain-free interval and often, though to a lesser extent, after elimination of the primary visceral trigger, e.g., elimination of the stone in urinary calculosis or laser ablation of endometriotic lesions [5,10,21,23,26,54,55]. Referred muscle hyperalgesia is frequently accompanied by trophic changes in the referred area, including thickening of the subcutaneous tissue and decreased thickness/section area of the muscle. Thickness is the height of muscle tissue from skin to inferior fascia of the muscle. Section area is the area of a transverse section of the muscle (i.e., perpendicular to the major axis of muscle fibers) both are measured with ultrasound evaluation.

These phenomena have been documented in patients by measuring tissue thickness/section area using ultrasound [21,54]. Interestingly, they are not modulated by the visceral algogenic input, since they do not decrease or increase with decreasing or increasing numbers of visceral pain episodes. They seem a rather on-off phenomenon, that is, once they have taken place they tend to persist for a long time rather independently of further visceral algogenic activity. Mechanisms beyond sensory referred changes are probably both central, i.e., sensitization of viscero-somatic convergent neurons, and peripheral [11]. In the latter case, activation of reflex arcs has been claimed to be involved, where the afferent branches of the arcs are represented by sensory fibers from the affected viscera and the efferent branches by sympathetic efferents towards the skin and subcutis. The somatic efferents transport signals towards the muscle where a sustained contraction would be induced, with local secondary sensitization of nociceptors, which further contributes to the hyperalgesia. Mechanisms of referred trophic changes, however, must involve reflex mechanisms, since these are objective changes that cannot be explained on the basis of central mechanisms only [24]. Independently of mechanisms, trophic changes are of crucial importance clinically in that they profoundly modify tissue structure in the referred pain area. In particular, they involve a dystrophic or atrophic reaction in the muscle which is likely to impair tissue function for a long time, predisposing the abdominal and pelvic pain patient to further complications at the musculoskeletal level [4,21].

- Visceral hyperalgesia. Hypersensitivity of an internal organ (visceral hyperalgesia), is a typical feature of most forms of abdominal and pelvic pain. Examples are: vaginal hyperalgesia in endometriosis or dysmenorrhea (expressed clinically as dyspareunia), intestinal hyperalgesia in IBS (manifesting as abdominal and pelvic pain during the normal intestinal transit or dyschezia), and bladder pain upon bladder distension during urinary bladder inflammation [6,47]. Visceral hyperalgesia has been clearly attributed to phenomena of peripheral sensitization first, with threshold lowering of "high threshold" receptors and activation of previously unresponsive receptors (recruitment of silent nociceptors) and subsequent central sensitization due to the massive afferent barrage from the periphery [7,11].

- Viscero-visceral hyperalgesia. Most visceral pain syndromes of the abdominal and pelvic area tend to co-exist in the same patients, particularly women. It has been shown that over 50% of women with IBS also have dysmenorrhea and about 50% of women with dysmenorrhea also have IBS symptoms. Forty-six per cent of patients with IBS also exhibit urinary symptoms, some of which are consistent with a diagnosis of BPS/IC, and up to 52% of patients with BPS/IC also have symptoms compatible with IBS diagnosis [2,8,12,18]. The co-occurrence of several visceral algogenic diseases in the same patient can give rise to phenomena of viscero-visceral hyperalgesia when the affected organs share at least part of their central sensory projection. Viscero-visceral hyperalgesia consists of an enhancement of both direct and referred symptoms from all involved districts, producing intricate clinical pictures [25,27]. VVH takes place when IBS co-exists with dysmenorrhea: patients with both conditions present more painful menstrual cycles and referred muscle hyperalgesia from the uterus than patients with dysmenorrhea only and more numerous and intense IBS pain episodes and referred muscle hyperalgesia from the intestine than patients with IBS only (common sensory projection between colon and uterus: T10-L1). Similarly, patients with dysmenorrhea, primary or secondary to endometriosis, plus urinary calculosis present more numerous and intense urinary colics and more pronounced referred muscle hyperalgesia at lumbar level (site of referred pain from the urinary tract) than patients with calculosis only and more painful menstrual cycles and referred muscle hyperalgesia from the uterus than patients with dysmenorrhea only (common projection between uterus and upper urinary tract: T10-L1). The pathophysiology of VVH is still under investigation, but probable contributing mechanisms involve sensitization of neurons receiving convergent input from multiple visceral structures, as well as from the somatic areas of referral from the involved viscera (viscero-viscero-somatic convergence) [9,39,40,43,51].

Though the initial origin of abdominal and pelvic pain can be specifically from the musculoskeletal, neural or visceral compartments of the abdominal or pelvic areas, in time the symptom is most often the result of a combination of all these origins [30]. As reported above, visceral pain projects to musculoskeletal structures, provoking secondary hyperalgesia which may persist beyond the primary visceral insult, frequently through formation and activity of secondary trigger points in the referred area [24], while a neuropathic pain component often develops in conjunction with both a musculoskeletal and a visceral pain disease of long duration [25,38]. The diagnostic process must therefore carefully consider not only the actual characteristics of the symptom but also the modalities of its development in time since its onset [20].

Pain of Extra- Abdominal and Extra-Pelvic Origin

Abdominal and pelvic pain may also occur in the context of pain conditions involving a generalized increase in pain sensitivity (decreased pain thresholds in both painful and non-painful areas), such as fibromyalgia or headache with a high frequency of crises [1,34–36,41,42,45,50]. In these cases, the symptom is likely to be rather the local manifestation of a generalized process than a regional entity; indeed, it most frequently improves with treatment of the main pain condition [17].

PRACTICAL IMPLICATIONS

The first step for the clinician in the approach to the patient complaining of abdominal and pelvic pain is to identify all specific conditions and diseases, not only in the abdominal and pelvic area but also at extra-abdominal and extra-pelvic level, that might provoke and/or influence the symptom presentation. With this respect it is important to detect not only current but also previous pain conditions, whose long-lasting traces may have repercussions on the current symptomatology. The second step assesses all possible disease and structure interactions among the identified conditions and affected structures (Table 2). This is key to establishing the correct management plan.

Management

With the above-described premises, the initial management plan must involve treatment of the specific pain conditions that are identified and treatment of their possible interactions. Treatment of the pain as such also follows if these measures are not sufficient for satisfactory relief [46](Table 2).

Treatment of Pain Diseases

Management of an identified disease is ideally handled at a specialist level, e.g., gynecological for diseases of the female reproductive organs, urological for those from the urinary tract, or gastroenterological for conditions of the digestive system. Many other competences may, however, be needed, such as psychiatric and psychological intervention to handle affective disorder co-morbidity, frequent in all forms of chronic pain, or physical therapy to address rehabilitation needs. If specialist consultations are important in order to set up targeted therapies for each specific condition, a unifying medical figure is also essential to collect and evaluate comparatively all information thus obtained, identify possible conflicts and interactions among the prescribed therapies and act as the point of reference for the patient. Although there are several differences in the organization of medical assistance in

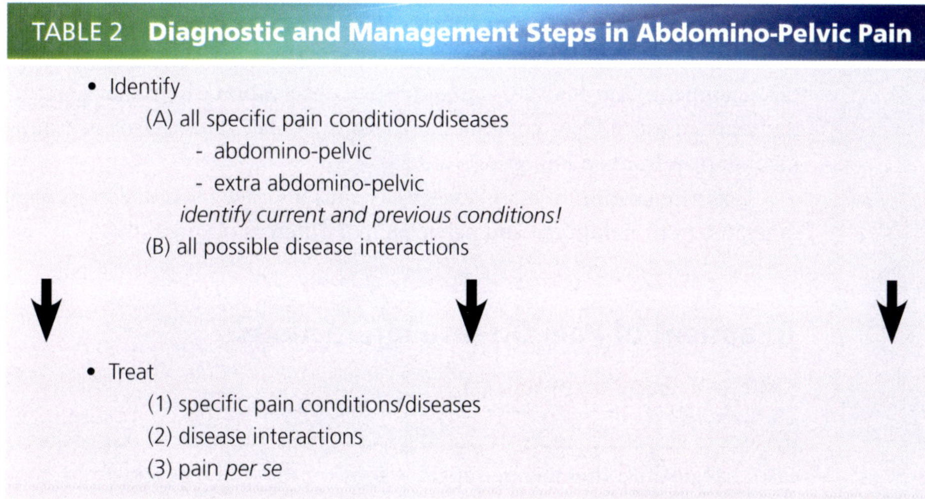
TABLE 2 **Diagnostic and Management Steps in Abdomino-Pelvic Pain**

- Identify
  - (A) all specific pain conditions/diseases
    - abdomino-pelvic
    - extra abdomino-pelvic

    identify current and previous conditions!
  - (B) all possible disease interactions

↓ ↓ ↓

- Treat
  - (1) specific pain conditions/diseases
  - (2) disease interactions
  - (3) pain *per se*

different countries, even in the same geographic area (e.g., within Europe) it is, in fact, often observed in clinical practice that communication among different professional figures is lacking, and the patient is left alone to handle the data from the different specialists [30]. It is the personal view of the authors that the specialty of the coordinating physician is of only relative importance. Whether it is pain therapy, anesthesiology, internal medicine or any other field, what really counts is the ability and willingness of this figure to combine all the specialist information coherently and implement these with careful evaluation of the interactions, to optimize the final therapy for the patient.

Specialist treatment of each identified condition comprises multiple approaches, e.g., pharmacological, surgical, behavioral, physical therapy, and interventional pain management measures. It is not the aim of this paper to describe a protocol for each condition, which is referred to in specific chapters of this book. However, it must be underlined that in each specialty field a multimodal management regimen has been shown to provide better results than a single modality intervention and should always be preferred [30,33].

In the case of multiple identified diseases as the basis of abdominal and pelvic pain, an important element in the therapeutic approach to the patient is to try to identify common treatments, i.e., useful for more than one condition, as happens when targeting common pathophysiological mechanisms. One example is provided by the overactivity of mast cells that is an established concept in pain of neuropathic origin [14,31] but has also been documented in several visceral diseases manifesting with pain at abdominal and pelvic level. In patients with IBS, for instance, rectal hypersensitivity is associated with the presence and activation of mast cells in the mucosa [52]. In BPS/IC a high number of intravesical mast cells has been found [35], while the presence of increased activated and degranulating mast cells has also been shown in deep infiltrating endometriosis [3,49]. These observations provide the rationale for the use of compounds that down-regulate mast cell activity, such as the endogenous cannabimimetic and anandamide analogue N-palmitoyl-ethanolamine (PEA), in various abdominal and pelvic pain conditions. PEA has indeed been shown to significantly attenuate the effects of experimentally induced visceral hyperalgesia in rats, i.e., NGF/turpentine-induced bladder hyperalgesia: bladder hyper-reflexia, referred thermal somatic hyperalgesia and c-fos expression in the spinal cord [15,16]. In recent preliminary research studies in an animal model of viscero-visceral hyperalgesia from experimental endometriosis plus ureteral calculosis in female rats, prolonged administration of PEA has also proven to reduce mast cells overexpression at the level of the endometrial lesions, in parallel with a reduction of the behavioral indices of abdominal and pelvic pain and referred hyperalgesia [22, Giamberardino et al, 2014, unpublished observation]. In humans, promising results of the adjuvant use of PEA (combined with transpolydatin) have also been shown in the treatment of pain from endometriosis [13,28].

Down-regulation of mast cell activity thus appears a useful complementary approach to treatment of abdominal and pelvic pain of different origins.

Treatment of Pain Disease Interactions

Viscero-Visceral Interactions

In cases of suspected viscero-visceral hyperalgesia, treatment of one of the two visceral diseases has positive therapeutic repercussions on the other, as shown by clinical controlled studies [25]. Dietary treatment of IBS also relieves spontaneous and referred symptoms from dysmenorrhea and hormonal treatment of dysmenorrhea also relieves direct and referred intestinal pain/hyperalgesia in patients with IBS-dysmenorrhea co-morbidity. Similarly, stone expulsion promoted by extracorporeal shock-wave lithotripsy relieves dysmenorrhea symptoms and hormonal treatment of primary dysmenorrhea or laser treatment of endometriosis lesions in secondary dysmenorrhea also relieves urinary direct and referred pain symptoms in patients with dysmenorrhea and urinary calculosis comorbidity [25,27].

It is interesting to note that VVH also takes place when one of the two visceral diseases is latent with respect to spontaneous pain, e.g., women with silent endometriosis (i.e., endometriosis not giving rise to pelvic pain, discovered by chance at laparoscopy performed for infertility reasons) plus urinary calculosis present more urinary pain episodes and enhanced referred lumbar muscle hyperalgesia than women with calculosis only. In this case it has been shown that laser treatment of endometriosis produces a reduction of the urinary pain [25].

Viscero-Muscular Interactions

The relationship between myofascial trigger points and visceral pain is complex. On one hand a number of primary TrPs in abdominal and pelvic muscles, formed because of microtraumatic events, can give rise to pain mimicking visceral pain syndromes. It is the case of TrPs at various levels in the rectus abdominis, which can mimic the pain of dysmenorrhea or of appendicitis, or that of pain in the lateral abdominals, mimicking urinary pain [20,48].

On the other hand, visceral pain from various diseases of internal organs can produce the formation of secondary trigger points in the referred pain area, which can persist in time and be responsible for the persistence of the visceral-like pain even after the visceral focus has been eliminated. It has been shown, for instance, that 22% of patients with urinary calculosis who have spontaneously eliminated the stone still present colic-like symptoms and 88% of them still have residual lumbar muscle hyperalgesia 3 years after stone elimination. Physical examination of the referred area in these cases reveals the presence of trigger points, developed as a consequence of the visceral process, whose stimulation reproduces the typical visceral pain attack and whose extinction with local treatment reverts the visceral pain symptomatology. It has also been shown that 39% of patients with painful endometriosis who have been subjected to laser removal of lesions continue to experience spontaneous pain and 96% of them still present residual abdominal muscle hyperalgesia 1 year afterwards. Physical examination of the referred area in these cases reveals the presence of secondary trigger points whose stimulation reproduces the typical spontaneous pain and whose extinction with local treatment attenuates the visceral pain symptomatology [32,53].

Recent clinical studies have shown the implications for therapy of these visceromuscular interactions in the case of multiple, though not contemporary, visceral pain syndromes in the same patient. The impact of previous urinary calculosis on pain from endometriosis has been investigated. It has been shown that women with endometriosis who had previously suffered from urinary colics from calculosis but had spontaneously eliminated the stone a long time prior to examination showed viscero-visceral hyperalgesia by presenting more painful menstrual cycles and referred muscle hyperalgesia from the uterus than women with dysmenorrhea from endometriosis without previous urinary calculosis. Physical examination in these women showed the presence of active TrPs in the lumbar region whose stimulation reproduced a colic-like pain. Local therapy of these TrPs was able to reduce the dysmenorrhea pain and also the referred hyperalgesia from the uterus in a prospective 6-month study. Other studies in women with urinary calculosis and previous endometriosis showed similar results. Women with recurrent urinary colics from calculosis who had previously suffered from endometriosis, subsequently cured by laser ablation of lesions, presented more numerous and intense urinary colics and more marked referred lumbar muscle hyperalgesia than women with calculosis only (i.e., without previous endometriosis). Physical examination of the rectus abdominis in the lower abdominal quadrants in co-morbid women showed the presence of active myofascial trigger points whose stimulation reproduced the typical uterine pain perceived at the time of active endometriosis. Local extinction of these TrPs with anesthetic injection produced a significant reduction of the urinary pain and of referred lumbar muscle hyperalgesia in a prospective 6-month study [Giamberardino et al, 2014, unpublished observation].

The presence of myofascial trigger points in a referred pain area from an internal organ can thus modify pain perception not only from that organ but also from other neuromerically connected organs [20].

Abdominal and Pelvic and Extra-Abdominal and Extra-Pelvic Interactions

Abdominal and pelvic pain occurring in the context of fibromyalgia [FS] or headache at a high frequency of crises (H) may significantly improve with effective specific pharmacologic prophylaxis of these conditions [17]. Vice-versa, treatment of a determined abdominal and pelvic visceral pain disease, which is co-morbid with FS or H, can also have an impact on the extra-abdominal and extra-pelvic symptoms (diffuse musculoskeletal pain and tenderness, headache crises). In patients with IBS or dysmenorrhea associated with FS, dietary treatment of IBS or hormonal treatment of dysmenorrhea for 6 months (vs no treatment) also produces a reduction of the intensity of FS pain and of the diffuse somatic tissue hyperalgesia (in both painful and non-painful areas). Similar visceral pain treatment in patients with concurrent IBS or dysmenorrhea and headache also decreases the number and intensity of headache crises as well as of the generalized diffuse somatic hyperalgesia in a prospective study of 6 months [Giamberardino et al, 2014, unpublished observation].

An integrated therapy of the abdominal and pelvic and extra-abdominal and extra-pelvic conditions must thus be carefully designed in co-morbid patients.

Treatment of The Pain

Pain symptoms need to be treated *per se* when disease-based interventions fail or are not sufficient. It is not our aim here to describe all possible measures to achieve this goal: from pharmacologic to non-pharmacologic, from systemic to local, these are numerous and discussed in detail and specifically in other chapters of this book. However, some general considerations can be made with this respect. Pure symptomatic pain treatment should not be performed too early, at least not before the probable origin/s of the pain have been identified with reasonable approximation. Pain, in its various characteristics of site, spatial discrimination or accompanying signs is, in fact, a precious source of information to identify the underlying diseases; cancelling it immediately may impair the diagnostic process, thus delaying or compromising the possibility of a mechanism-based therapy. At the same time, once the sources of the pain have been detected, the pain should be treated as early as possible, even if it is not of high intensity, to avoid long-term consequences of the persisting algogenic input, such as the hyperalgesia and the hypotrophy reaction in muscles [18]. Paradoxically this appears exactly the opposite of the current attitude in many medical environments, where prompt pain relief is provided to patients as soon as the pain occurs, while further treatment is discouraged when the diagnosis is clear and the symptoms are no longer of particular intensity.

In summary, the phenomena described in this chapter show that the experience of abdominal and pelvic pain is intricate and unique for each patient; as a consequence the management plan needs to be personalized and involve an integrated multidisciplinary, multimodal and multilevel approach.

LOOKING AT THE FUTURE

Achieving the goal of full control of abdominal and pelvic pain in the future is necessarily based on a better understanding of the mechanisms beyond single disease entities and their interactions as well as of individual factors that influence symptom presentation. Future research areas in the field must thus involve more clinical and experimental studies on the: disease pathophysiology, to enhance the possibility of mechanism-based therapies; genetic and gender–related factors (increasingly being shown as crucial in modulating the individual pain occurrence/maintenance), to help personalize therapies; and co-morbidity (Table 3). The latter is of particular importance, since the co-occurrence of multiple medical pain and non-pain conditions is becoming more the rule than the exception in the clinical setting. The set-up of experimental models of co-morbid diseases will hopefully allow a better understanding of disease interactions and consequently help the clinician to combine and/or integrate therapies in the suffering patient [1,18,19,42].

TAKE HOME MESSAGES

- Abdominal and pelvic pain is most often the result of a complex interaction among algogenic conditions from different structures, both at abdominal and pelvic and extra-abdominal and extra-pelvic level.
- Each patient with abdominal and pelvic pain presents a unique combination of diseases and disease interactions.
- Ideal management of abdominal and pelvic pain requires a personalized, multidisciplinary and multimodal approach.
- Improvement of abdominal and pelvic pain management will hopefully be achieved through future pathophysiological, genetic, gender-related and co-morbidity studies.

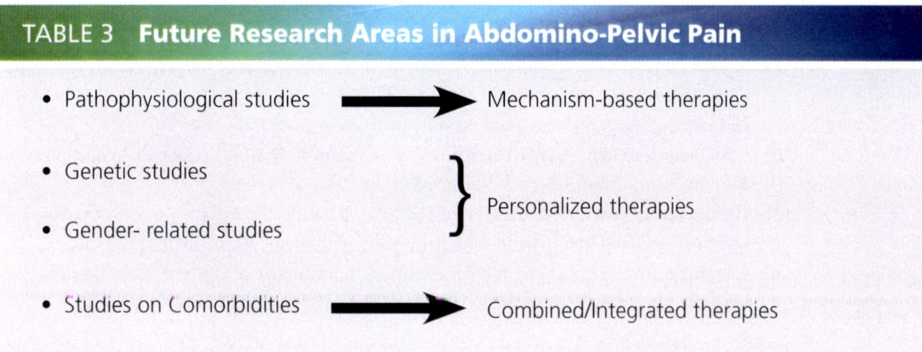

TABLE 3 **Future Research Areas in Abdomino-Pelvic Pain**

• Pathophysiological studies	→	Mechanism-based therapies
• Genetic studies	}	Personalized therapies
• Gender- related studies	}	Personalized therapies
• Studies on Comorbidities	→	Combined/Integrated therapies

FURTHER READING

Cervero F. Understanding Pain. Cambridge: The MIT Press, 2012:192.

Chaitow L, Lovegrove Jones R (eds). Chronic Pelvic Pain and Dysfunction. Philadelphia: Churchill Livingstone, Elsevier, 2012:429.

Giamberardino MA, Jensen TS (eds). Pain Comorbidities: understanding and treating the complex patient. Seattle: IASP Press, 2012:507.

REFERENCES

1. Ablin JN, Cohen H, Buskila D. Mechanisms of Disease: genetics of fibromyalgia. Nat Clin Pract Rheumatol 2006;2:671–8.
2. Altman G, Cain KC, Motzer S, et al. Increased symptoms in female IBS patients with dysmenorrhea and PMS. Gastroenterol Nurs 2006;29:4–11.
3. Anaf V, Chapron C, El Nakadi I, et al. Pain, mast cells, and nerves in peritoneal, ovarian, and deep infiltrating endometriosis. Fertil Steril 2006;86:1336–43.
4. Arendt-Nielsen L, Schipper KP, Dimcevski G, et al. Viscero-somatic reflexes in referred pain areas evoked by capsaicin stimulation of the human gut. Eur J Pain 2008;12:544–51.
5. Bajaj P, Bajaj P, Madsen H, Arendt-Nielsen L. Endometriosis is associated with central sensitization: a psychophysical controlled study. J Pain 2003;4:372–80.
6. Berkley KJ. A life of pelvic pain. Physiol Behav 2005;86:272–80.
7. Bradesi S, Herman J, Mayer EA. Visceral analgesics: drugs with a great potential in functional disorders? Curr Opin Pharmacol 2008;8:697–703.
8. Brinkert W, Dimcevski G, Arendt-Nielsen L, et al. Dysmenorrhoea is associated with hypersensitivity in the sigmoid colon and rectum. Pain 2007;132:46–51.
9. Brumovsky PR, Gebhart GF. Visceral organ cross-sensitization – an integrated perspective. Auton Neurosci Basic Clin 2010;153(1–2):106–15.
10. Caldarella MP, Giamberardino MA, Sacco F, et al. Sensitivity disturbances in patients with irritable bowel syndrome and fibromyalgia. Am J Gastroenterol 2006;101:2782–89.
11. Cervero F. Visceral pain-central sensitization. Gut 2000;47:56–7.
12. Choung RS, Herrick LM, Locke GR 3rd, et al. Irritable bowel syndrome and chronic pelvic pain: a population-based study. J Clin Gastroenterol 2010;44:696–701.
13. Cobellis L, Castaldi MA, Giordano V, et al. Effectiveness of the association micronized N-Palmitoylethanolamine (PEA)-transpolydatin in the treatment of chronic pelvic pain related to endometriosis after laparoscopic assessment: a pilot study. Eur J Obstet Gynecol Reprod Biol 2011;158:82–6.
14. Di Cesare Mannelli L, D'Agostino G, Pacini A, et al. Palmitoylethanolamide is a disease-modifying agent in peripheral neuropathy: pain relief and neuroprotection share a PPAR-alpha-mediated mechanism. Mediators Inflamm 2013;2013:328797. doi:10.1155/2013/328797.
15. Farquhar-Smith WP, Jaggar SI, Rice AS. Attenuation of nerve growth factor-induced visceral hyperalgesia via cannabinoid CB(1) and CB(2)-like receptors. Pain 2002;97:11–21.
16. Farquhar-Smith WP, Rice AS. Administration of endocannabinoids prevents a referred hyperalgesia associated with inflammation of the urinary bladder. Anesthesiology 2001;94:507–13.
17. Gerwin RD. Chronic Pain Perspectives: diagnosing fibromyalgia and myofascial pain syndrome: a guide. J Fam Pract 2013; 62:S19–25.
18. Giamberardino MA. Women and visceral pain: are the reproductive organs the main protagonists? Mini-review at the occasion of the "European Week Against Pain in Women 2007". Eur J Pain 2008;12:257–60.
19. Giamberardino MA, Affaitati G, Costantini R. Concurrent visceral pain syndromes: the concept of viscerovisceral hytperalgesia. In: MA Giamberardino, TS Jensen (Eds). Pain Comorbidities: understanding and treating the complex patient. Seattle: IASP Press, 2012: 309–30.
20. Giamberardino MA, Affaitati G, Fabrizio A, Costantini R. Myofascial pain syndromes and their evaluation. Best Pract Res Clin Rheumatol 2011;25:185–98.
21. Giamberardino MA, Affaitati G, Lerza R, et al. Relationship between pain symptoms and referred sensory and trophic changes in patients with gallbladder pathology. Pain 2005;114:239–49.
22. Giamberardino MA, Berkley KJ, Affaitati G, et al. Influence of endometriosis on pain behaviors and muscle hyperalgesia induced by a ureteral calculosis in female rats. Pain 2002; 95:247–57.

23. Giamberardino MA, Berkley KJ, Iezzi S, et al. Pain threshold variations in somatic wall tissues as a function of menstrual cycle, segmental site and tissue depth in non-dysmenorrheic women, dysmenorrheic women and men. Pain 1997;71:187–97.
24. Giamberardino MA, Cervero F. The neural basis of referred visceral pain. In: Parischa PJ, Willis WD, Gebhart GF (eds). Chronic abdominal and visceral pain: theory and practice. New York, London: Informa Healthcare, 2007:177–92.
25. Giamberardino MA, Costantini R, Affaitati G, et al. Viscero-visceral hyperalgesia: characterization in different clinical models. Pain 2010;151:307–22.
26. Giamberardino MA, de Bigontina P, Martegiani C, Vecchiet L. Effects of extracorporeal shock-wave lithotripsy on referred hyperalgesia from renal/ ureteral calculosis. Pain 1994;56:77–83.
27. Giamberardino MA, De Laurentis S, Affaitati G, et al. Modulation of pain and hyperalgesia from the urinary tract by algogenic conditions of the reproductive organs in women. Neurosci Lett 2001;304:61–4.
28. Gugliano E, Cagnazzo E, Soave I, et al. The adjuvant use of N-palmitoylethanolamine and transpolydatin in the treatment of endometriotic pain. Eur J Obstet Gynecol Reprod Biol 2013;168:209–13.
29. Halder SLS, Locke GR III. Epidemiology and social impact of visceral pain. In: Giamberardino MA, editor. Visceral pain: clinical, pathophysiological and therapeutic aspects. Oxford: Oxford University Press, 2009:1–8.
30. Herbert B. Chronic pelvic pain. Altern Ther Health Med 2010;16:28–33.
31. Hesselink JM, Hekker TA. Therapeutic utility of palitoylethanolamide in the treatment of neuropathic pain associated with various pathological conditions: a case series. J Pain Res 2012; 5.437–42.
32. Jarrell J, Giamberardino MA, Robert M, Nasr-Esfahani M. Bedside testing for chronic pelvic pain: discriminating visceral from somatic pain. Pain Res Treat 2011;2011:692102. doi: 10.1155/2011/692102.
33. Jarrell JF, Vilos GA, Allaire C, et al. Chronic Pelvic Pain Working Group; SOGC. Consensus guidelines for the management of chronic pelvic pain. J Obstet Gynaecol Can 2005;27:781–826.
34. Karp BI, Sinaii N, Nieman LK, et al. Migraine in women with chronic pelvic pain with and without endometriosis. Fertil Steril 2011; 95:895–9.
35. Kelada E, Jones A. Interstitial cystitis. Arch Gynecol Obstet 2007; 275:223–9.
36. Kurland JE, Coyle WJ, Winkler A, Zable E. Prevalence of irritable bowel syndrome and depression in fibromyalgia. Dig Dis Sci 2006; 51:454–60.
37. Labat JJ, Riant T, Delavierre D, et al. Global approach to chronic pelvic and perineal pain: from the concept of organ pain to that of dysfunction of visceral pain regulation systems. Prog Urol 2010;20:1027–34.
38. Labat JJ, Robert R, Delavierre D, et al. Symptomatic approach to chronic neuropathic somatic pelvic and perineal pain. Prog Urol 2010;20:973–81.
39. Malykhina AP. Neural mechanisms of pelvic organ cross-sensitization. Neurosci 2007;149:660–72.
40. Malykhina AP, Qin C, Greenwood-van Meerveld B, et al. Hyperexcitability of convergent colon and bladder dorsal root ganglion neurons after colonic inflammation: mechanism for pelvic organ cross-talk. Neurogastroenterol Motil 2006;18:936–48.
41. Mulak A, Paradowski L. Migraine and irritable bowel syndrome. Neurol Neurochir Pol 2005;39:S55–60.
42. Nyholt DR, Gillespie NG, Merikangas KR, et al. Common genetic influences underlie comorbidity of migraine and endometriosis. Gener Epidemiol 2009; 33:105–13.
43. Pezzone MA, Liang R, Fraser MO. A model of neural cross-talk and irritation in the pelvis: implications for the overlap of chronic pelvic pain disorders. Gastroenterology 2005;128:1953–64.
44. Sengupta JN. Visceral pain: the neurophysiological mechanism. Handb Exp Pharmacol 2009;194:31–74.
45. Shaver JL, Wilbur J, Robinson FP, et al. Women's health issues with fibromyalgia syndrome. J Womens Health (Larchmt). 2006;15:1035–45.
46. Shin JH, Howard FM. Management of chronic pelvic pain. Curr Pain Headache Rep 2011;15:377–85.
47. Sikandar S, Dickenson AH. Visceral pain: the ins and outs, the ups and downs. Curr Opin Support Palliat Care 2012;6:17–26.
48. Simons DG, Travell JG, Simons LS. Upper half of body. In: Travell & Simons' myofascial pain and dysfunction. The trigger point manual. 2nd edition, Volume 1. Baltimore: Williams & Wilkins, 1999: 1038.
49. Sugamata M, Ihara T, Uchiide I. Increase of activated mast cells in human endometriosis. Am J Reprod Immunol 2005;53:120–5.
50. Tietjen GE, Bushnell CD, Herial NA, et al. Endometriosis is associated with prevalence of comorbid conditions in migraine. Headache 2007;47:1069–78.
51. Ustinova EE, Fraser MO, Pezzone MA. Cross-talk and sensitization of bladder afferent nerves. Neurourol Urodyn 2010;29:77–81.

52. van Hoboken EA, Thijssen AY, Verhaaren R, et al. Symptoms in patients with ulcerative colitis in remission are associated with visceral hypersensitivity and mast cell activity. Scand J Gastroenterol 2011;46:981–7.
53. Vecchiet L, Giamberardino MA, de Bigontina P. Referred pain from viscera: when the symptom persists despite the extinction of the visceral focus. Adv Pain Res Ther 1992;20:101–10.
54. Vecchiet L, Giamberardino MA, Dragani L. Referred muscular hyperalgesia from viscera: clinical approach. Adv Pain Res Ther 1990;13:175–82.
55. Vecchiet L, Giamberardino MA, Dragani L, Albe-Fessard D. Pain from renal/ ureteral calculosis: evaluation of sensory thresholds in the lumbar area. Pain 1989;36:289–95.
56. Zondervan KT, Yudkin PL, Vessey MP, et al. The community prevalence of chronic pelvic pain in women and associated illness behaviour. Br J Gen Pract 2001;51:541–7.

CHAPTER 30

The Role of Patient Organizations

Judy Birch, Françoise Watel, Jane Meijlink, Lisa Kruse, Sally Crowe, and Jennifer Birch

INTRODUCTION

While persistent abdominal and pelvic pain is potentially disabling and difficult to live with, it is an "invisible" condition that has received little recognition. This may indeed be the reason why sufferers are particularly motivated to obtain a diagnosis, find out about treatment options and about what they can do to help themselves. They want to learn more about pelvic pain, as well as seek peer support online and liaise with "expert patients". These "expert patients" have developed a unique expertise in their own field of disease that they can share with other patients. Their knowledge is not only theoretical, but is also experiential as they live with the condition on a daily basis. This capacity can be enhanced by specific education (university courses, for example in France). They can play a valuable and significant role when supported by a patients' association. In today's world, medical knowledge is no longer solely in the hands of health professionals.

DESCRIBING THE SUBJECT

The International Pelvic Pain Partnership (IPPP) was initiated in March 2012 with a meeting in London of patient representatives interested in collaborating on development of research and services for chronic pelvic pain. While these groups already showed a high degree of communication and interaction, the IPPP endeavoured to put this work on a more formal and recognizable footing and to agree on priorities for shared activity.

Key aspirations of the IPPP include:

- Better awareness, education, understanding, and experience of physicians to take chronic pelvic pain seriously and to diagnose and treat it effectively;
- Better access to (integrative and interdisciplinary) pain management;
- Improving quality of life and comfort, with more respect for the condition;
- Empowering more men and women to ask for better treatment, care, and to encourage self management;
- Less confusion regarding terminology and definitions;
- Better research to underpin all of the above.

To this end, the IPPP developed a statement of intent and the 1st World Congress on Abdominal & Pelvic Pain in Amsterdam was the first arena at which the IPPP introduced itself:

> "The IPPP is committed to substantially improving education, early and accurate diagnosis, effective treatment, management, and realistic prognosis for neuropathic chronic and visceral pelvic and perineal pain. We intend to increase the participation of people in research and services development, so that these objectives are achieved in the next decade".

At the congress, the IPPP aimed to convey a clear message about the role of patient organizations, to work with a small, specifically interested group of professionals on research priorities and ensure that personal experiences of chronic abdominal and pelvic pain be presented to congress delegates. The IPPP delivered a congress presentation entitled "The Role of Patient Organizations from Local to Worldwide". We discussed what has changed and what is currently changing in relation to patients, clinicians and collaboration between the two parties. A new kind of patient is emerging: patients who want to be equal partners in their healthcare. The amount of time patients spend with health professionals is very small compared to the time they spend managing their health condition(s). In today's world, many patients are seeking support and information online. IPPP also organised a successful and thought-provoking workshop during the congress for patient representatives, clinicians and researchers entitled "What are the research gaps and priorities in abdominal and pelvic pain diagnosis, treatment and management?"

Some Important Ways in Which Patient Organizations Can Support Patients

Communication and Collaboration

The role of patient support groups has evolved over the years, enabling them to network both locally and globally (Figs. 1 and 2).

Patient organizations help patients to communicate more clearly with health professionals and to provide key information about their situation. They may encourage patients to use questionnaires, diaries and also to ask the questions to which they are seeking answers, even if answers do not yet exist.

This is increasingly happening through the use of technology, message boards, forums, social media, networks and blogs. Video clips of patient to patient interviews highlighted the value to patients of being able to discuss their pain with other patients. One patient said about an online forum:

> "it helped me a lot to identify if I had the same kind of level of disease as other patients because it's so hard to define it. When somebody asks you about your pain, it's really so personal, so reading forums helped me to identify that it was quite serious"

Patient organizations have a responsibility to direct patients to accredited and certified information, such as that of the National Institute for Health and Care Excellence (NICE) evidence and The Information Standard for patient information (www.theinformationstandard.org) in the United Kingdom. These sources of information are extremely useful as

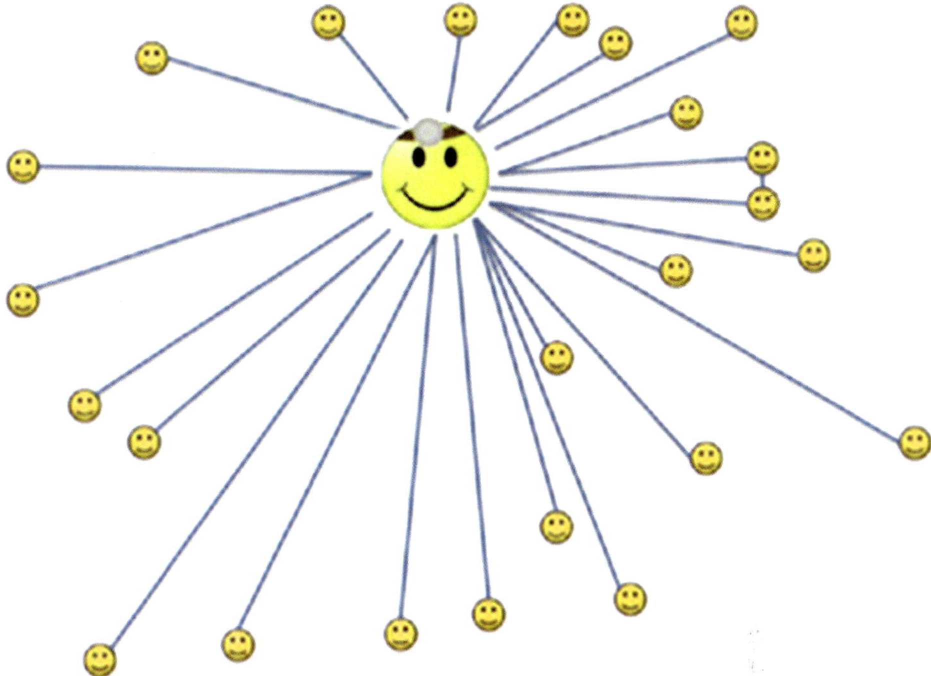

FIGURE 1 Centralized Medical Knowledge.

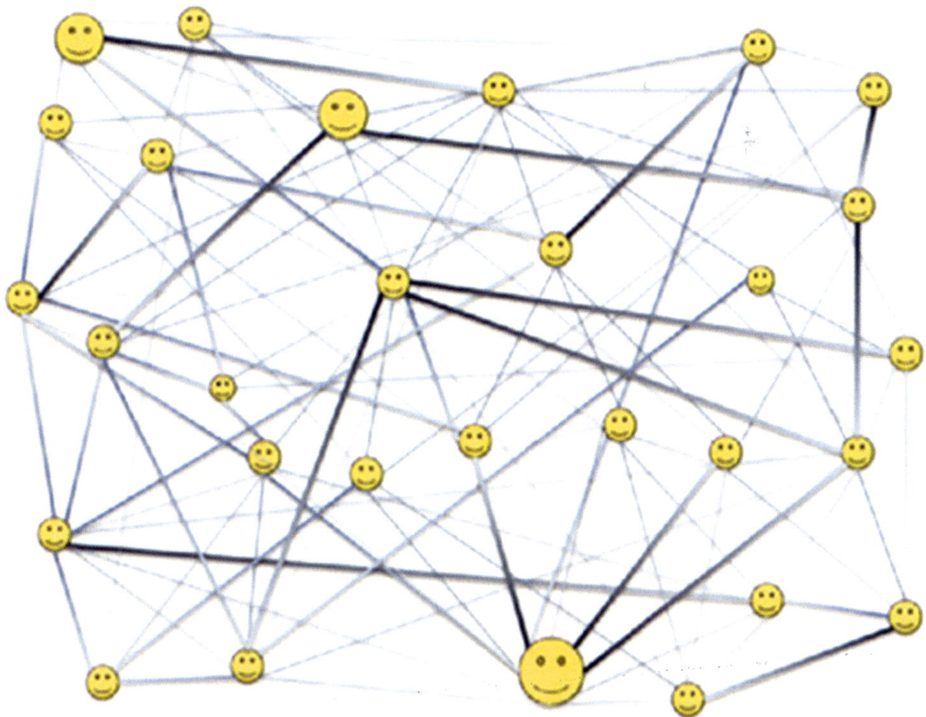

FIGURE 2 Peer-to-Peer Shared Medical Knowledge.

they are evidence-based and frequently the only information in patient accessible language. Guidelines and patient pathways such as the Map of Medicine chronic pelvic pain (in men and women) pathway may also be helpful.

Patient organizations in the partnership already provide very informative newsletters and updates, organize speakers, seminars, information booths at medical conferences, workshops, and meetings.

In the field of abdominal and pelvic pain, there are many organizations and initiatives with which the organizations in the IPPP work closely, some specifically relating to chronic pain such as Pain Alliance Europe (PAE), the Societal Impact of Pain (SIP), Active Citizenship Network (ACN), and Patients Rights' activities relating to pain and the International Alliance of Patients Organizations (IAPO). The latter is currently developing a focus on chronic pain with various organizations and countries working together.

Representatives of patient organizations contribute to Cochrane reviews and updates, disease specific international, national and local guidelines, standardization projects, scientific journal articles as well as contributing chapters to medical books. They may also contribute to World Health Organization (WHO) work on International Classification of Diseases (ICD) coding and classification. Furthermore, IPPP members work at EU policy level, contributing to initiatives such as the European Patients' Academy on Therapeutic Innovation (EUPATI).

The importance of the role of patient organizations is increasingly recognized by political and social authorities at national levels and in the European Union. Laws to emphasize this have been in existence in England and France for several years and have been strengthened during the last decade.

At a wider level, patient organizations themselves need to collaborate or are already collaborating to:

- exchange information
- exchange good practice
- associate to raise awareness
- advocate patient-centred management

at national, European and international levels.

They can do this informally (exchange of information through regular meetings, such as the IPPP) or formally by setting up national networks, such as the Réseau Douleurs Chroniques Pelvi-périnéales (RDCP) in France, a federation of national patients associations working in the field of pelvic pain, or setting up European umbrella associations for specific diseases, such as MICA for interstitial cystitis/bladder pain syndrome in Europe.

Input to the Medical Curriculum

In 1988, A. Kleinmann called for new ways of teaching and training programmes with patient narrative central to the education process. In 2010, the Frenck independent commission called for major reform in health professional education. A recent survey of the undergraduate curriculum in the UK indicates that pain content is woefully inadequate. [2]

Recently, a General Practitioner who is a patient with persistent pelvic pain, wrote: "during the undergraduate course, I do not recall any input regarding management of

Chronic Pelvic Pain as a general condition ... I don't recall any undergraduate teaching regarding the basic science, assessment, management, biopsychosocial aspects, self-management of chronic pain"

Following a number of recent publications, work has started to try to improve this situation (see list). However, there is little evidence of any patient or patient organization input into this as yet.

- Chief Medical Officer (CMO) Public Health Report 2008 "Pain: breaking through the barrier" [3]
- UK pain curricula survey and Centre for the Advancement of Interprofessional Education [2,1]
- International Association for the Study of Pain (IASP): Interprofessional, Uniprofessional [7]
- European Federation of IASP Chapters (EFIC) - Societal Impact of Pain, Education taskforce
- North America [6]
- UK Royal College of Obstetricians and Gynaecologists (RCOG) national undergraduate curriculum

The British Medical Association (BMA) has stated that "patients should be actively involved in the development, review and implementation of undergraduate and post graduate medical curricula" and that "patients should be actively involved in teaching during undergraduate and post graduate training". In a literature review on this subject, Wykurz and Kelly concluded that involving patients as teachers has important educational benefits for learners [8]. Patients offer unique qualities that can enhance the acquisition of skills and change attitudes towards patients. In addition, patients themselves enjoy such involvement. Howe and Anderson suggested involving patients in education as an approach to overcoming some of the difficulties of opportunistic learning in clinical settings [5]. In 2006, the Picker Institute stated that greater use should be made of patients as teachers [4]. Both real and simulated patients have a potentially useful part to play in medical education and there is considerable scope for extending and developing their role. It was also noted that there are currently few examples of good practice. The social sciences have much to contribute to the education of doctors in this field. There is an extensive body of published research evidence on patients' attitudes and expectations, their experiences of being ill and receiving treatment, and their values and preferences.

Research has shown advantages of involving patient teachers in a variety of educational activities (including physical examination skills, diagnostic skills and communication skills training), with the role of the patient teacher typically involving presentations, facilitating seminars, demonstrating to small groups, and giving feedback on individual doctors' performance. Videos of patients talking about the experience of being ill and receiving treatment can also prove helpful for training purposes. [4]

> "Well, in the UK you cannot get an appointment with a specialist before you see a GP, so you go on for years like this because your GP says no, there's nothing wrong or it's just epression or it's just your tummy and we'll do everything for your tummy and then you realize, no, it wasn't this and then you see a specialist."

Current Situation: Undergraduate

While there are several examples of patient involvement in the delivery of the undergraduate curriculum, these are usually in other disease areas. However, Leeds University is expanding its patient input delivered by the UK's Pelvic Pain Support Network in the field of pelvic pain as part of the chronic pain module for nurses due to its success and positive evaluation by students.

Another initiative is at the Royal College of Surgeons in Dublin where there is ongoing patient input in the training of surgeons in gynaecology by patient input from the Endometriosis Association of Ireland. This has not yet been extended to postgraduate medical education or continuing medical education in anything other than a sporadic manner, with patient organization representatives occasionally speaking at local and national meetings for health professionals usually on more general topics.

Health Services and Research

Patient organizations can and do make a significant contribution to the development of health services and research.
Many patients and careers know about:

- living with a chronic disease or condition and living with multiple conditions
- the impact of side-effects
- issues such as costs, availability of services
- what could make an intervention *more* acceptable or *less* acceptable
- what questions they want addressed for their benefit

There are many examples of good practice and collaboration in this field including:

- INVOLVE National Institute Health Research (NIHR) funded advisory group that supports greater public involvement in NHS, public health and social care research in the UK;
- UK Health Technology Assessment study: e.g. multi-centre MEDAL;
- James Lind Alliance UK NIHR Evaluation, Trials and Studies Coordinating Centre (NETSCC) Research Priority Setting Partnerships
- National Health Service (NHS) Quality, Innovation, Productivity and Prevention programme.

Ideally patient input is integral throughout the study, from suggesting topics for research to developing the proposal and disseminating the results.

As part of the 1st World Congress on Abdominal & Pelvic Pain, members of the International Pelvic Pain Partnership (patient organisations with a common aim) worked with clinicians and researchers to discuss and explore uncertainties in the diagnosis, treatment and management of chronic abdominal and pelvic pain. The title of the workshop was "What are the research gaps and priorities in abdominal and pelvic pain diagnosis, treatment and management? Patient and Professional Perspectives". Following some input on research methods relevant to persistent abdominal and pelvic pain, small discussion groups used the Map of Medicine Pathway (UK) to help structure dialogue and maintain focus. The atmosphere in the workshop was collaborative and respectful, with participants debating the relative merit of research ideas to address issues such as:

- the initial presentation/primary care, especially how to ensure that this first contact with services is useful for both health professional and patient;

- diagnosis, in particular how to improve communication between patient and clinician;
- how to reduce duplicated or unnecessary investigations;
- personalising treatments, phenotyping;
- dealing with side-effects, managing expectations when treatments don't work;
- improving multidisciplinary team effectiveness so that patients are not part of a 'pinball' experience of services.

A health professional, also patient representative wrote:

> "I had hoped to have had the privilege of being with you and speaking to you in person today. Unfortunately, international travel is now impossible for me as I cannot sit nor stand for very long without being in a great deal of pain. Until two years ago, I was a woman with a full and active life. I enjoyed a 30-year career as an OB/GYN nurse and was working in a position that I loved. So I reach out to you today as both a professional and a patient. When I developed severe urethral pain unlike anything I had experienced before, I thought a quick round of antibiotics would do the trick and I would be fine. I prided myself on being a woman who was never sick. I then began a nightmare that lasted all day every day. The pain became something I can only describe as inhumane and yet still, I could not get an accurate diagnosis. I was seen in the ER and was misdiagnosed as having kidney stones. I underwent an unnecessary 6-hour laparoscopic hysterectomy. I saw more physicians and had more tests in 3 months than I had in 57 years and still, no diagnosis. The pain persisted and intensified. One night, in desperation, after having searched on the Internet hundreds of times for pelvic pain, I searched for pelvic nerve. And there it was: A textbook case of pudendal neuralgia. In 30 years, I had never heard of it nor had any of my colleagues. Only then was I able to be fiercely proactive in my quest for appropriate treatment. I should never have had to endure the unrelenting intractable pain of this horrible affliction for as long as I did. Pelvic pain has steadily unravelled every thread that was the fabric of my life. As a health care professional, I did not have the vaguest notion of the staggering impact of neuropathic pain. I most certainly had never heard of CNS sensitization. You are the stewards of information that can prevent patients from enduring what I did. Please educate your colleagues and primary care providers. And know that the work you do, is powerfully transformative" (Figs. 3–6).

LOOKING AT THE FUTURE

Patient organizations have a key role in the future diagnosis, treatment and management of abdominal and pelvic pain by writing, producing and editing information in collaboration with health professionals based on the existing evidence base (combined with patient preferences and values).

Promoting partnerships with patients is on the policy agenda. It is emphasised in professional guidance and codes and it is beginning to appear explicitly in medical curricula. It now needs to be taken to the next stage, i.e. developing practical methods for teaching and assessing the necessary skills and providing an effective challenge to inappropriate role models.

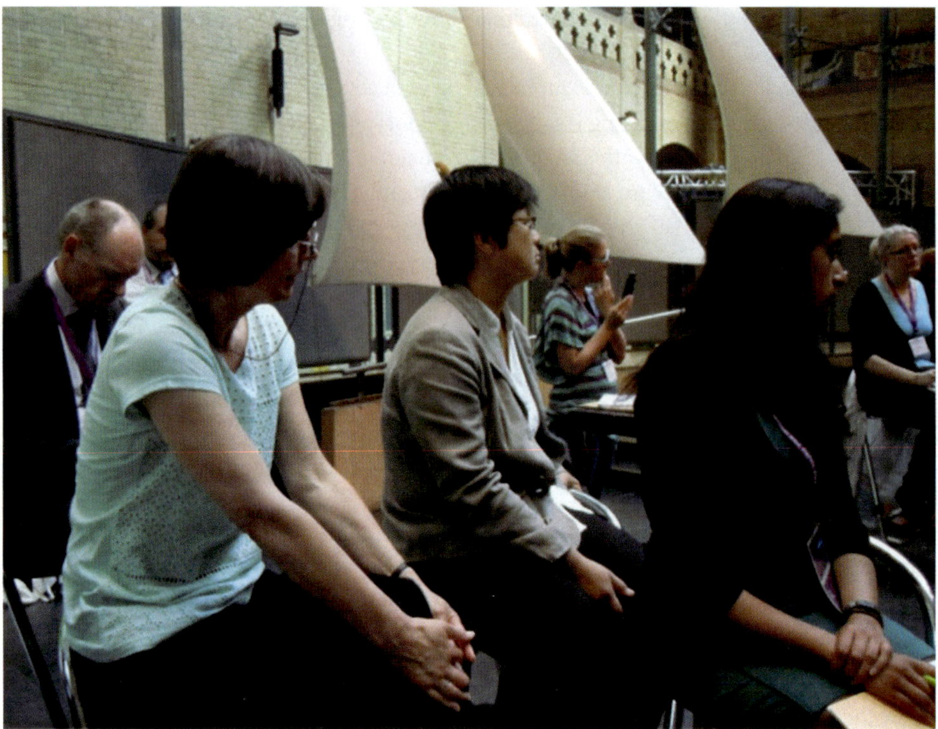

FIGURE 3 Start of the patient organisations day during the 1st World Congress on Abdominal and Pelvic Pain.

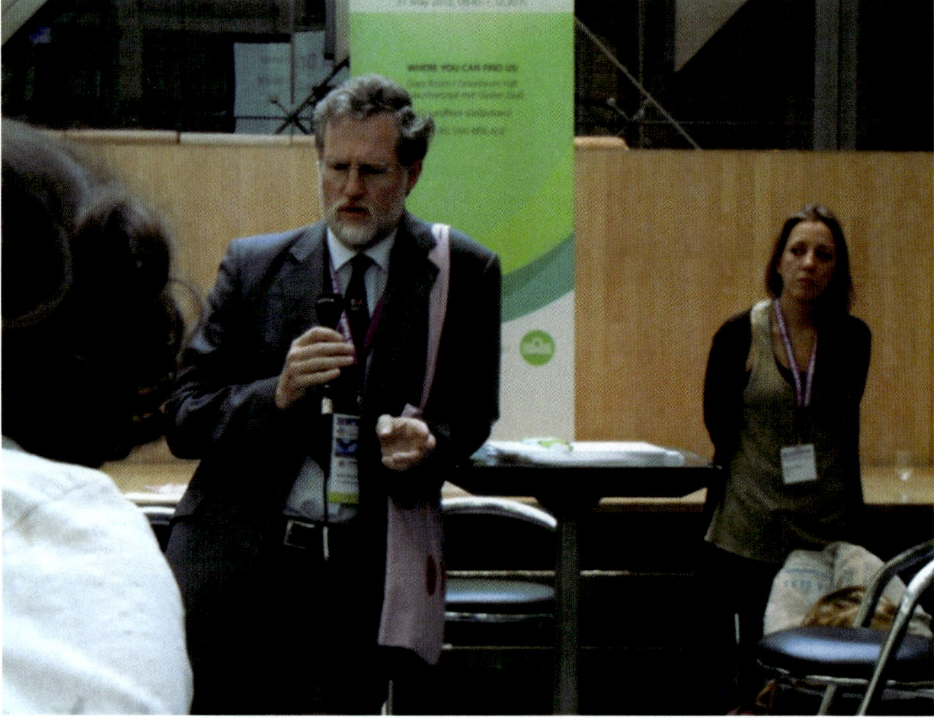

FIGURE 4 Patients and doctors working together during the 1st World Congress on Abdominal and Pelvic Pain.

Crowe Associates Ltd
PERSONALISING TREATMENT
what are treatment challenges when 'different' conditions overlap?
HOW DO WE IMPROVE LISTENING? FOR BETTER TREATMENT
PHENOTYPING MAY REDUCE TRIAL + ERROR IN TREATMENT
LOOKING FOR 'SYMPTOMS' RATHER THAN
TREATING WOMEN WHO WANT TO GET PREGNANT?

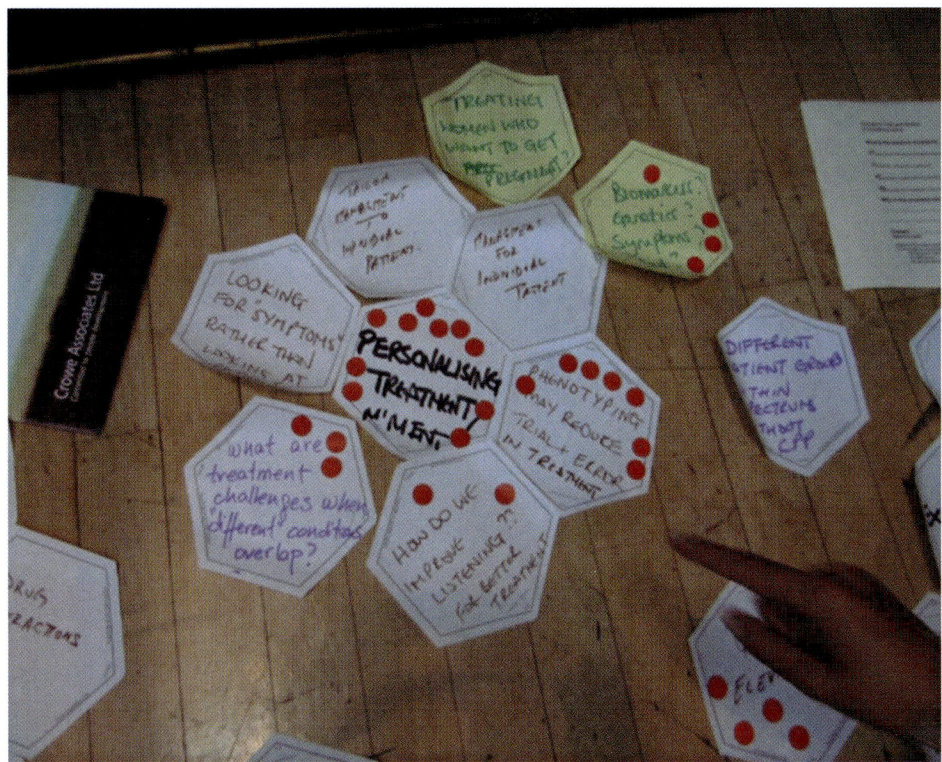

FIGURE 5 Working in groups at the patient organisations day during the 1st World Congress on Abdominal and Pelvic Pain.

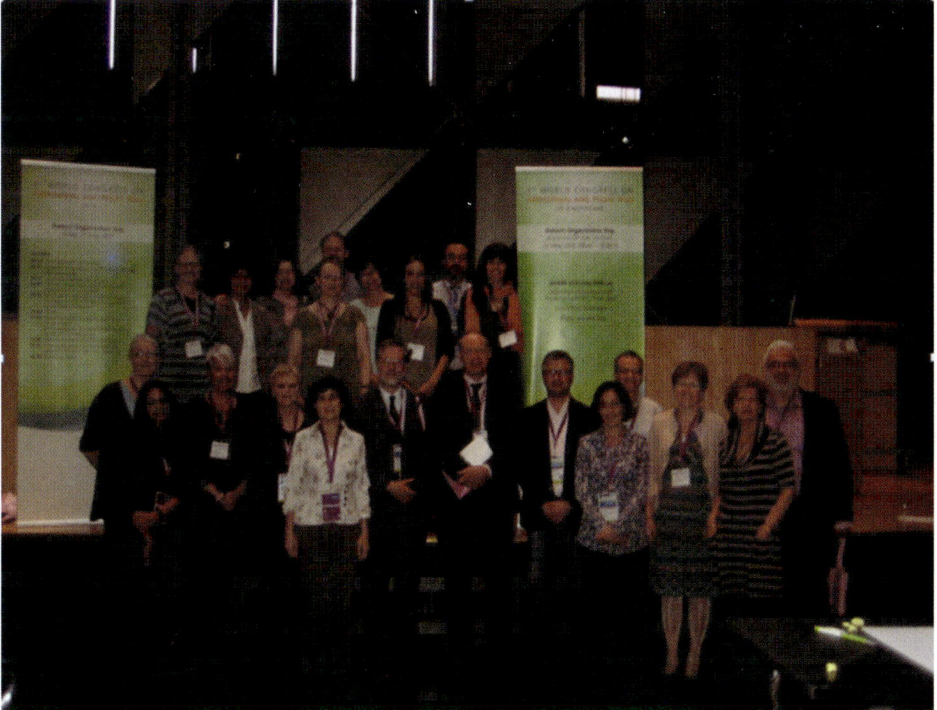

FIGURE 6 All participants of the patient organisations day during the 1st World Congress on Abdominal and Pelvic Pain.

Patient organizations have the ability to reach large numbers of patients and are a useful asset and resource for input to clinical trials as well as qualitative studies. They can act as a link between health professionals to encourage multi-disciplinary management and treatment in a patient-centred approach. This multi-disciplinary approach can and must include not only health professionals in the widest sense but also expert patients.

TAKE HOME MESSAGES

- The role of patient organizations, patients and health professionals continues to evolve.
- Patient organizations are collaborating and linking up in the field of persistent pelvic pain and working more closely with health professionals.
- We need patients to be involved at whatever level they are able and willing to contribute, whether locally, nationally or internationally, and for health professionals to support and work with us to help us meet our objectives.
- Patient organization is defined here as "not-for-profit". In the case of the IPPP, member organisations are volunteer-led and neutral with regard to industry funding.
- A patient recently wrote: "That's the problem with the pelvis isn't it, there are so many different specialists involved . . . from my point of view as a pelvic nerve pain sufferer, I would like to see the recognition of all pelvic pain problems being understood by the separate medical modalities. . . . chronic pain is so common and the psychosocial aspects need to be addressed and more patient support services need to be made available".

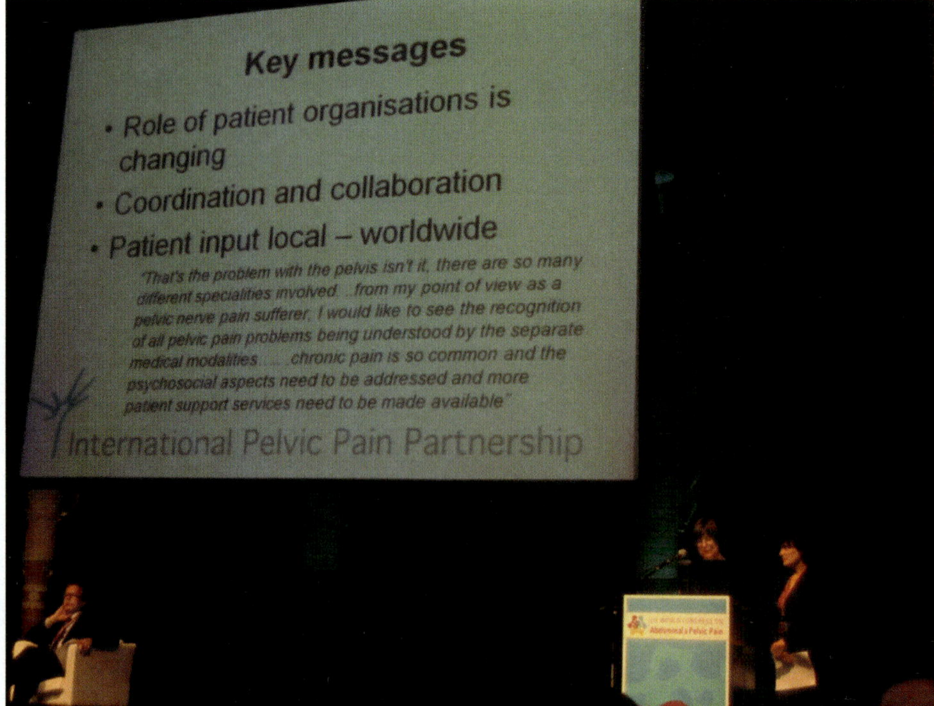

FIGURE 7 The key messages from the patient organisations day presented at the plenary session of the Congress.

REFERENCES

1. Barr H, Low H. Interprofessional Education in Pre-registration courses: guide for Commissioners and Regulators of Education CAIPE 2012 Jan (Centre for the Advancement of Interprofessional Education UK) www.caipe.org.uk
2. Briggs EV, Carr C, Whittaker. Survey of undergraduate pain curricula for healthcare professionals in the United Kingdom. Eur J Pain. 2011;15(8):789–95.
3. Donaldson L. Pain: breaking through the barrier. CMO's 150 years Public Health Report, 2008 http://webarchive.nationalarchives.gov.uk/20130107105354/http://www.dh.gov.uk/en/Publicationsandstatistics/Publications/AnnualReports/DH_096206
4. Hasman A, Coulter A, Askham J "Education for partnership-developments for medical education" 2006 May Picker Institute Europe www.pickereurope.org
5. Howe A, Anderson J. "Involving patients in medical education" BMJ 2003;327 (7410):326–8.
6. Mezei L, Murinson BB. Pain education in North American medical schools; Johns Hopkins Pain Curriculum Development Team. J Pain. 2011;12(12):1199–208.
7. Watt-Watson J, Hunter J, Pennefather P, et al. An integrated undergraduate pain curriculum, based on IASP curricula, for six health science faculties. Pain. 2004;110(1–2):140–8.
8. Wykurz G, Kelly D. Developing the role of patients as teachers: literature review. BMJ 2002; 325 (7368):818–21.

INDEX

NOTE: Page numbers followed by "*f*" and "*t*" denote figures and tables, respectively.

A

Abdominal pain, 251–252
  chronic, 224–225
  epidemiology of, 221–222
  future of, 9–10
  gender, role of, 49–55
  incidence and prevalence of, 4–5
  management, future of, 301–305
  neuromodulation of, 247–253
  origin of, 298*t*
  physical therapy treatment for, 73–74
  practical implications of, 9
  primary care management of, 221–226
    future of, 225
    practical implications for, 225
    SOEP methodology, 222–224
  problem definition, 3–4
  social impact of, 3–10
  soft tissue phenomena and, 69–74
ABRUPT neurons, 39
Acceptance and Commitment Therapy (ACT), 242
Active Citizenship Network (ACN), 312
Active MTrPs, 69–70, 72
Adhesions, 161
Adrenocorticotrophic hormone (ACTH), 52
Alpha-blockers, for prostate pain syndrome, 153
American Committee of Obstetrics and Gynaecology, 21
American Urological Association, 21, 62, 136
Analgesia, sex differences in, 51
Anesthetics injections
  for generalized unprovoked vulvodynia, 194
  for provoked vestibulodynia, 194
Angiotensin converting enzyme inhibitors, and functional gastro-intestinal disorders, 205
Angiotensin II type receptor (AT2), 263
Anorectal dysfunction
  and chronic pain, 212–217
  future of, 216
  pathophysiology of, 213–216
  practical implications of, 216
Anorectal function, normal
  continence, 210–211
  defecation, 210–211
  horizontal links, 211
  vertical links, 211–212
Anorectal pain disorders, 164*t*
Anorectum, anatomy of, 209–210
Antibiotics, and functional gastro-intestinal disorders, 205
Antimicrobial therapy, for prostate pain syndrome, 153
Anti-progestogens, for endometriosis associated pain, 175
Anus, 209–210
Anxiety, and abdominal/pelvic pain, 54
Aromatase inhibitors (AIs), for endometriosis associated pain, 176, 177
Arousal, influence on sensory perception, 125*t*
Austrialian New Zealand Clinical Trial Registry, 263

B

Bacterial vaginosis (BV), 188*f*
Beta-blockers, and functional gastro-intestinal disorders, 205
Bladder pain syndrome (BPS), 6, 50, 270, 271*f*
Bladder pain syndrome/interstitial cystitis (BPS/IC), 87, 88, 111, 135–143, 260, 302
  animal models for, 140–141
  biomarkers to identify, 140
  catastrophizing in, 91–92, 94–95
  clinical phenotypes of, 91
  comorbid conditions, 141–142
  defined, 96, 136
  epidemiology of, 137
  etiology of, 135, 139
  in female patient 137, 142
  future of, 143
  in male patient, 135, 142
  pathophysiological mechanisms, 139–141
  practical implications for, 142–143
  relations in, 95
  social relations in, 92–93, 92*f*
  urogenital floor, 137–139, 138*f*
Body–mind–brain, in pelvic pain, 59–65
  biopsychosocial perspective, 60
    biomedical versus, 61–62
  central sensitization, 60
  future of, 65
  persistent pain mechanisms, 59
  practical implications, 62–65
BOTOX, 127

Bradykinin, 171
Brain derived neurotropic factor (BDNF), 171, 174
Brief Pain Inventory (bpi), 284
British Medical Association (BMA), 313
British Pain Society (BPS), 21, 237
  basic aspects, 276
  future of, 279–280
  Map of Medicine, 10
  patient pathways, 275–276
  practical implications, 278–279
  subject, 276–278
British Society for the Study of Vulval Disease (BSSVD), 21
British Society of Gynaecological Endoscopy (BSGE), 293

C

Capsaicin
  for generalized unprovoked vulvodynia, 194
  for provoked vestibulodynia, 194
Carbamazepine, and functional gastro-intestinal disorders, 205
Central pain mechanisms, 59, 60, 61
Central sensitization
  definition, 60
  importance of, 35–45
    dorsal horn components of sensation, 35–39, 37*f*, 38*f*, 39*f*
    future of, 45
    models of disease, 42–44, 44*f*
    practical implications, 44–45
    visceral pain, features of, 40–41
    visceroceptive neurons, using nocigenic inhibition, 39–40, 41*f*, 42*f*
Chief Medical Officers Report, 282–283
Chronic abdominal pain, 224–225
Chronic abdominal pelvic pain (CAPP), 227
  pain management physiotherapy for
    desensitisation, 232
    exercise, 233–234
    pain education, 231–232
    stretches, 232–233
Chronic anorectal pain, 270, 272*f*
Chronic low back pain, 61
  biopsychosocial model of, 60
Chronic pain
  defined, 283
  intersex variation in, 283
Chronic Pain Grade, 283
Chronic pelvic pain (CPP), 4
  causes of, 160*t*
  clinical history and examination for, 164–165
  defined, 4, 18, 157
  evidence base for, 291–295
  future of, 165–166, 294
  gynaecological aspects of, 157–166, 158*t*
  management of, 165
  MEDAL study, 293
  patient needs, understanding, 165
  practical implications for, 293–294
  practitioners in research, 291
  psychosexual components of. *See* Chronic pelvic pain, psychosexual components of in research design, 292–293
  sexual dysfunction related to, 99–106
    in men, 103–105
    in women, 99–103
  in women, aetiology of, 159–164
Chronic Pelvic Pain Guidelines, 286
Chronic pelvic pain, psychosexual components of, 111–117
  anxiety in medical and physical therapy treatment of, 114
    addressing anxiety, trauma and abuse, 115
    history taking, 114–115
    mindfulness based insertion therapy, 116–117
    patient anxiety and fear aversion, 115–116
  biopsychosocial components to integrative approach, 113–114
  bio-psycho-social paradigm, 112–113
  female sexual pain disorders, 112
  future of, 117
Chronic pelvic pain syndrome (CPPS), 18, 61, 79, 87, 157, 250–251
  catastrophizing in, 89–90, 90*f*, 93
  definitions, 18, 96
  prevalence rates, 88
  relations in, 94
  social relations in, 90–91
  symptoms of, 89
Chronic prostatitis (CP), 87
  catastrophizing in, 89–90, 90*f*, 93
  definitions, 96
  prevalence rates of, 88
  relations in, 94
  social relations in, 90–91
  symptoms of, 89
Chronic visceral pain, as disease, 136
Clinical Commissioning Groups (CCGs), 276, 285
Clinical Reference Groups (CRG), 287
Clinician-patient-relatives model, 268
Cognitive behavioral therapy (CBT), 128, 227–228, 241, 242
  for generalized unprovoked vulvodynia, 194
  for provoked vestibulodynia, 194
Cogwheeling, 60
Combined oral contraceptive pills (COCPs), 128–129
Co-morbidities, and functional gastro-intestinal disorders, 204
Complex Regional Pain Syndrome (CRPS), 61, 232
Concentric mechanical stressors, 70
Conditioned Pain Modulation (CPM), 42–43

Connective tissue manipulation (CTM), 73
Connective tissue restrictions, 72–73
 active MTrPs, 72
 defined, 72
 neurotrophic reflexes, 72
 peripheral nerve inflammation, 72–73
 viscerosomatic reflex, 72
Construct validity, 23, 26–28
Contact dermatitis (CD), 189
Continence, 210–211
Corticotrophin releasing factor (CRF), 25
CPCI (Chronic Pain Coping Inventory), 87
CROWN (core outcomes in women's health), 293
Cyclical bleeding within lesions, 170
Cyclical or recurrent pain, 18
Cyclophosphamide-induced cystitis, 141

D

Danazol
 for endometriosis associated pain, 175, 176
 for pelvic congestion/varicosity syndrome, 162
Defecation, 210–211
 impaired, and anorectal pain, 215
Delivery of care, 281–290
 burden of pain and issues around, 282–285
 correcting inequalities in, 285–288
 future of, 289
 pathways of care, 285–287
 practical implications, 288–289
 problem and potential solutions, 281
 Specialised Pain Services, 287–288
Depression, and abdominal/pelvic pain, 54
Desensitisation, for chronic abdominal pelvic pain, 232
Desipramine, 127
Desquamative inflammatory vaginitis (DIV), 187, 188*f*, 189*f*
Diagnostic and Statistical Manual of Mental Disorders, 99, 100
Dienogest, for endometriosis associated pain, 175
Dopamine, 53
Dorsal horn neuronal sensitization, mechanisms of, 36*t*
Dry needling, 71
Dual Uptake Inhibitors, 64
Dynamometry, 83
Dysmenorrhoea, 50, 250
Dysorgasmia, 128
Dyspareunia, 99, 102, 103, 106, 112
 associations of, 123*t*
 defined, 122, 130

E

Eccentric mechanical stressors, 70
Ejaculation, 104
Elastometry, 83
EMA-401, 263
Endometriosis associated pain, 5, 160, 161*f*, 169–178, 303
 cyclical bleeding within lesions, 170
 future of, 177
 immune and inflammatory factors associated with, 170–171
 neuroangiogenesis, 173–174
 neuropathic pain, 172–173
 pelvic nerves, irritation and invasion of, 171–172
 practical implications for, 177
 treatment for, 175–176
 visceral nociceptors and, 172
England's Pain Summit, 286
Enhanced Pain Services for England, 287–288
Epidermal growth factors, 171
Epididymectomy, for scrotal pain syndrome, 151
Equity and Excellence: Liberating the NHS, 276
Etiopathogenesis
 induced models of
  noxious environmental stimuli, 25
  noxious local stimuli, 24
  noxious systemic stimuli, 24–25
 naturally occurring models of, 25–26
Etonogestrel subdermal implants (Implanon)
 for endometriosis associated pain, 175
European Association of Urology (EAU), 4, 17, 17*t*, 21, 147, 237, 267–269
 assessment, 269
 Chronic Pelvic Pain Guidelines, 17, 286
 future, 273
 management plan, 269–270
 pelvic pain, taxonomy for, 20*f*
 practical implications, 270–273
European Patients' Academy on Therapeutic Innovation (EUPATI), 312
Exercise, for chronic abdominal pelvic pain, 233–234
"Explain Pain" model, 115
Extra-abdominal and extra-pelvic interactions, 304

F

Face validity, 23–24
Fear Aversion Model (FAM), 115
Female genital pain, 185–196
 differential diagnosis of, 185–190
 examination for, 193–194
 future of, 195
 generalized unprovoked vulvodynia, 190
 generalized vulvar pain syndrome, 190
 history taking, 192
 patient assessment for, 192
 provoked vestibulodynia, 190, 191–192
 provoked vulvar pain syndrome, 190, 191–192
 treatment for, 194–195
Female orgasmic pain, 128–129
Female pelvic pain, incidence and prevalence of, 5–6
Female sexual pain disorders, 112
Fibromyalgia, 77

5-Fluorouracil, for endometriosis associated pain, 176, 177
Food and Drug Administration (FDA), 257
Fulranumab, 261
Functional abdominal pain syndrome (FAPS), 5
Functional gastro-intestinal disorders (FGID), 199–206
  co-morbidities and, 204
  consultation for, 204
  diagnosis of, 203
  drugs and, 205
  epidemiology of, 202–203
  future of, 205
  mechanisms of, 200–202
  practical implications for, 205
  pre clinic work up for, 203–204
  relationship with participating events, 204–205
  Rome III criteria for, 200, 201*t*
  somatization and, 204
  taxonomy of, 200
  terminology, 199
Functional magnetic resonance imaging (fMRI), 248

G

Gabapentin, 127, 258, 264
  for endometriosis associated pain, 176
  for generalized unprovoked vulvodynia, 194
  for provoked vestibulodynia, 194
Gastrointestinal problems, and chronic pelvic pain, 162
Gender, role in abdominal and pelvic pain, 49–55
  anxiety and depression, 54
  epidemiology, 50–51
  future of, 54–55
  gender bias in pain treatment, 53
  gender roles, 53
  history, 49
  hormonal influences on pain, 52
  pain modulation, effect of sex hormones on, 52–53
  practical implications, 54
  sex differences
    with non-pharmacological treatments, 51
    in pain and analgesia, 51
  sex hormones, 53–54
  stress, coping and catastrophising, 53
Generalized unprovoked vulvodynia (GVD), 190
  treatment for, 194–195
Generalized vulvar pain syndrome (GVPS), 190
Genital pain, 249–250
Genito-pelvic pain/penetration disorder, 99–100
  characteristics of, 100
  prevalence of, 101
  subtypes of, 100
Gestrinone (ethylnorgestrienone, R2323)
  for endometriosis associated pain, 176
Glial cell–derived neurotrophic factor (GDNF), 174
GnRH agonists, for endometriosis associated pain, 175, 176, 177
Gray (neuronal) matter, 249

H

Headaches
  attributed to spontaneous low CSF pressure, 129
Health and Social Care Centre, 283
Health Related Quality of Life (HRQOL), 8
Hebbian axiom, 248
Histamine, 171, 173
Hormonal contraceptives, for endometriosis associated pain, 175
Hormone
  effects of sex, on pain modulation, 52–53
  influences on pain, 52
Hospital Episode Statistics (HES), 284
Hunner's ulcers, 136
Hyperalgesia, 173, 298–299
Hysterectomy, for endometriosis associated pain, 175

I

Immune cells, role in endometriosis associated pain, 170–171
Implanon. *See* Etonogestrel subdermal implants
Inferior hypogastric plexus, 137
Inflammatory Bowel disease, 4–5, 221
Inflammatory factors, role in endometriosis associated pain, 170–171
Information Standard for patient information, The, 312
Inguinal hernia repair, for scrotal pain syndrome, 153
Inherited erythromelalgia (IEM), 262
Inhibition susceptible (IS) neurons, 38, 43
  MNN neurons versus, 40
  schematic description of, 38*f*
Initiative on Methods, Measurement, and Pain Assessment in Clinical Trials (IMMPACT), 240
Integrated care, 288
Interleukin 1 (IL-1), 171
Interleukin 6 (IL-6), 170
Intermittent footshock sessions, effects of stress by, 42*f*
International Alliance of Patients Organizations (IAPO), 312
International Association for the Study of Pain (IASP), 16, 21, 23, 27, 136, 147, 157, 159, 190, 257, 286
  pelvic pain, taxonomy for, 19*t*
  Taxonomy Taskforce, 17
  Taxonomy Working Group, members of, 17*t*
International Classification of Headache Disorders, 129
International Consultation on Incontinence, 21
International Continence Society, 159
International Pelvic Pain Partnership (IPPP), 309–310, 314
International Prostate Symptom Score (I-PSS), 149
International Society for the Study of Bladder Pain Syndrome (ESSIC), 17*t*, 136

International Society for the Study of Vulvovaginal Disease (ISSVD), 99, 185, 187, 190
Interstitial cystitis (IC), 6. *See also* Bladder pain syndrome/interstitial cystitis
Irritable bowel syndrome (IBS), 5, 199, 251–252, 264
  Rome criteria for, 203*f*
Irritable bowel syndrome with constipation (IBS-C), 212

L

Lamotrigine, 127
Laparoscopic uterosacral nerve ablation (LUNA), for endometriosis associated pain, 175
Laparotomy, for endometriosis associated pain, 175
Leeds University, 314
Leukotrienes, 171
Levator ani syndrome, and anorectal pain, 214–215
Levonorgestrel-releasing intrauterine system (Lng-IUS), for endometriosis associated pain, 175
Lichen planus (LP), 190
Lichen sclerosus (LS), 189
Lipase inhibitors, and functional gastro-intestinal disorders, 205
Lithium, and functional gastro-intestinal disorders, 205

M

Male ejaculatory/post-orgasmic pain, 128
Male genital pain, 147–154
  diagnosis of, 148
  future of, 153
  general, 147–148
  penile pain, 149–150, 153
  post-inguinal hernia repair and, 152
  post vasectomy pain syndrome, 151–152
  practical implications for, 152–153
  prostate pain syndrome, 148–149, 153
  scrotal pain syndrome, 150–151, 153
  terminology, 147
  treatment for, 148
  urethral pain syndrome, 150, 153
Male pelvic pain, incidence and prevalence of, 6
Mannosebinding lectin (MBL), 191
Map of Medicine pathways, 275, 277–279, 278*f*, 314–315
Matrix metalloproteinases (MMP), for endometriosis associated pain, 175, 176
MEDAL study, 293, 294
Medically unexplained symptoms, 239
Mefipristone. *See* RU486
Melanocortin-1 receptor (MC1R) gene, 191
Melatonin, for endometriosis associated pain, 176, 177
Men, sexual dysfunction related to CPP in, 103–105
  etiology, 104–105
    pain perception, 105
    pelvic floor overactivity, 105
    psychological mechanisms, 104
    relational mechanisms, 105
    sexual abuse, 104
  prevalence, 104
  terminology and assessment, 103–104
Men with chronic pelvic pain, 112
Menstrual pain, 250
Messendiak Cognitive Somatic Therapy, 115
Mindfulness based insertion therapy, 116–117
Monocyte chemoattractant protein 1 (MCP-1), 170
Multidimensional Sexuality Questionnaire, 240
Multisynaptic Nociceptive Network (MNN) neurons, 37, 38, 43
  IS neuron versus, 40
  schematic description of, 39*f*
Muscle hyperalgesia, 299
Muscle pain threshold, 299
Myofascial pain, 77, 162
Myofascial pain syndromes (MPS), 298
Myofascial trigger points (MTrPs), 69–70
  evaluating, 70
  injections, 71
  interpreting response to, 71

N

National Health Survey for England, 283, 286–287
National Institute for Health and Care Excellence (NICE), 282–283, 312
National institute for health research (NIHR), 293
National Institute of Health (NIH), 17*t*, 87, 142–143
National Institutes of Health Chronic Prostatitis Symptom Index (NIH-CPSI), 149
National Pain Audit, 3, 284–285
  access to services, 284
  identification of services, 284
  multidisciplinary teams, 285
  Quality of Care, 285
  staffing competencies, 285
  staff skills mix, 284–285
Nav1.7 sodium channel, 262
Neonatal bladder inflammation, 141
Nerve growth factor (NGF), 171, 174, 258–263
Neuroangiogenesis, 173–174
Neuromatrix, 35
Neuromodulation, of abdominal and pelvic pain, 247–253
  abdominal pain, 251–252
  basic aspects, 248–249
  future of, 253
  genital pain, 249–250
  menstrual pain, 250
  practical implications, 252–253
  urological pelvic pain, 250–251
Neuropathic pain, endometriosis associated, 172–173
Neuropathic pain, pharmacotherapy in, 257–265
  compounds in clinical development for, 258
    angiotensin II type receptor, 263
    nerve growth factor, 258–263
    n-type calcium channels, 263
    for visceral pain, 263–264

Neuropathic pain *(continued)*
current treatments for, 257–258
future of, 265
practical implications, 264–265
NGF/turpentine-induced bladder hyperalgesia, 302
NMDA receptor antagonists, for endometriosis associated pain, 176
Nocigenic inhibition (NI), 37, 38, 43
visceroceptive neurons and, 39–40, 41*f*, 42*f*
Non-organic signs of pain, 60
Non-pharmacological treatments, sex differences with, 51
Non-steroidal anti-inflammatory drugs, for pelvic congestion/varicosity syndrome, 162
Norepinephrine reuptake inhibitor (SNRI), 259
N-type calcium channels, 263

O

Oestrogen, 51, 52, 53
Oral contraceptives (OCs), for endometriosis associated pain, 175
Orchiectomy, for scrotal pain syndrome, 151
Organ-based stressors, 70
Orgasmic headache, 129
Orgasm, influence on sensory perception, 125*t*
Orgasm pain, in women, 103
Ovarian remnant syndrome, 161
Overactive bladder (OAB), 111

P

Pain
abdominal. *See* Abdominal pain
from biomedical to biopsychosocial approach, 63–64
chronic pelvic, 157–166
defined, 15, 62–63, 87–88
education, 63
endometriosis associated, 169–178
female genital, 185–196
hormonal influences on, 52
male genital, 147–154
management, algorithm for, 272*f*
mechanisms, in vulval pain, 124*f*
modulation, sex hormones effects on, 52–53
non-organic signs of, 60
pelvic. *See* Pelvic pain
pharmacological intervention for, 64
psychological components of, 87–96
sex differences in, 51
of sex-specific organs, 50–51
treatment, 304–305
gender bias in, 53
Pain Alliance Europe (PAE), 312
Pain Catastrophization Scale, 64, 65, 90*f*, 93
Pain education, for chronic abdominal pelvic pain, 231–232
Painful bladder syndrome, 136
Pain management physiotherapy
assessment of, 228, 229–230*t*
for chronic abdominal pelvic pain
desensitisation, 232
exercise, 233–234
pain education, 231–232
stretches, 232–233
evidence-based, 227–228
future perspective of, 234
one-to-one, 228, 231
Pain management programmes (PMPs), 229, 231
Pain of Urogenital Origin (PUGO), 4, 16, 17*t*
Special Interest Group on Abdominal and Pelvic Pain, 16
N-Palmitoyl-ethanolamine (PEA), 302
Pancoast's syndrome, 172
Pancreatitis, chronic, 5
Patient controlled analgesia (PCA), 51
Patient organizations, role of, 309–318
communication and collaboration, 310–312, 311*f*
future of, 315, 318
health services and research, 314–315, 316–317*f*
input to medical curriculum, 312–313
International Pelvic Pain Partnership (IPPP), 309–310
undergraduate curriculum, 314
Patient Reported Outcome Measures (PROM's), 283
Pelvic congestion/varicosity syndrome, 162
Pelvic floor dysfunction, 113
sexual abuse and, 115
Pelvic floor muscle (PFM)
evaluation and investigations, 82–83
future of, 84
objective assessment signs, 80–82
overactivity of, 78, 102–103, 105, 106
pain, 77–84
practical implications, 83
pressure-pain thresholds, 83
primary pain generator, confirmation of, 79
subjective assessment symptoms, 79–80
tension, 77–78, 82, 83
terminology, 77–79, 78*f*
Pelvic floor relaxation, 103
Pelvic girdle pain, 6
Pelvic Inflammatory Disease (PID), 5
acute, 161
chronic, 161
Pelvic nerves, irritation and invasion of, 171–172
Pelvic organ, quantification of, 269
Pelvic pain, 87
body, mind and brain in, 59–65
female, 5–6
gender, role of, 49–55
IASP taxonomy for, 19*t*
male, 6
management, future of, 301–305

neuromodulation of, 247–253
origin of, 298*t*
physical therapy treatment for, 73–74
practical implications of, 9
primary care management of, 221–226
future of, 225
practical implications for, 225
SOEP methodology, 222–224
problem definition, 3–4
social impact of, 3–10, 6–9
soft tissue phenomena and, 69–74
Pelvic pain syndrome, 270
Penile pain, 149–150, 153
Pentosan polysulphate, for prostate pain syndrome, 153
Pentoxifylline, for endometriosis associated pain, 176, 177
Perineal pain syndrome, 161–162, 163*t*
causes of, 163–164*t*
Persistent pelvic pain, 59
barriers for biopshycosocial approach to, 61–62
PF physiotherapy
for generalized unprovoked vulvodynia, 194
for provoked vestibulodynia, 194
Phenotyping, 267
Placebo-controlled randomized trials (PCRT), 194
Platelet-derived growth factor (PDGF), 171
PLISSIT model, 114–115
Post-gynaecology oncology surgery pain, 162, 164
Post-inguinal hernia repair, 152
Post-urogynaecology surgery pain, 162, 164
Post vasectomy pain syndrome, 151–152
Predictive validity
defined, 23
induced models of treatment, 28–29
naturally occurring models of treatment, 29–30
Pregabalin
for endometriosis associated pain, 176
for neuropathic pain, 258, 264
and prostate pain syndrome, 153
Preganglionic efferents, 137
Preorgasmic headaches, 129
Presacral neurectomy, for endometriosis associated pain, 175
Pressure manometry, 83
Proctalgia, 214–215
Progestogens, for endometriosis associated pain, 175
Prostaglandins (PGs), 171
Prostate pain, 50–51
Prostate Pain Syndrome (PPS), 87, 148–149, 153, 250–251, 270, 271*f*
catastrophizing in, 89–90, 90*f*, 93
definitions, 96
prevalence rates, 88
relations in, 94
social relations in, 90–91
symptoms of, 89
Proton pump inhibitors (PPIs), and functional gastro-intestinal disorders, 205
Provoked vestibulodynia (PVD), 190
treatment for, 194–195
Provoked vulvar pain syndrome (PVPS), 190
causes of, 191–192
Provoked vulvodynia (PVD), 99
Psychology, in pain assessment and management, 237–243
Pudendal nerve, 139
Pudendal nerve entrapment syndromes, 298

Q

Q-tip test, 193, 193*f*
Quality and Outcomes Framework (QOF), 282
Quality of Life (QoL), 87, 88
Quinolones, for prostate pain syndrome, 153

R

Randomised controlled trials (RCTs), 292
Real-time ultrasound, 83
Rectal intraganglionic laminar endings (rIGLEs), 210
Rectum, 210
Relief of pain, 269
Réseau Douleurs Chroniques Pelvi-périnéales (RDCP), 312
Residual ovarian syndrome, 161
Rosenbaum Protocol, 115–116
Royal College of Obstetrics and Gynaecology, 21
Royal College of Surgeons, 314
RU486 (mefipristone), for endometriosis associated pain, 176, 177

S

Sacral nerve, 139
Schwann cell proliferation, 171
Sciatic nerve entrapment syndromes, 298
Scrotal pain, 147
Scrotal pain syndrome, 150–151, 153
Second-order neurons, 35, 37
Selective estrogen receptor modulators (SERMs)
for endometriosis associated pain, 176, 177
Selective progesterone receptor modulators (SPRMs)
for endometriosis associated pain, 176, 177
Sensitization, 213–214
Serotonin, 53, 171, 259
Serotonin and norepinephrine reuptake inhibitors, for endometriosis associated pain, 176
Sex hormones, role of, 51–52
Sex-related pain, 121–130
assessment of, 126
associations, 123, 123*t*
causes of, 127*t*
defined, 121
epidemiology, 122–123

Sex-related pain *(continued)*
  future of, 130
  mechanisms of, 124–125, 124*f*
  phenotyping, 123–124
  practical implications for, 129–130
  research into, 122–128
  special cases, 128–129
    female orgasmic pain, 128–129
    male ejaculatory/post-orgasmic pain, 128
    sexual headache, 129
  treatment of, 125–126, 127*t*, 128
Sexual abuse, 238, 240
Sexual dysfunction, 99–107
  future of, 106
  male genital pain and, 147–148
  practical implications, 105–106
  related to CPP in men, 103
    etiology, 104–105
    prevalence, 104
    terminology and assessment, 103–104
  related to CPP in women, 99–103
    etiology, 101–103
    prevalence, 101
    terminology and assessment, 99–101
Sexual headache disorders, 129
Sexual pain disorders (SPD), 112, 113
Short-Form 36 Health Questionnaire (SF-36), 7, 9
Sleep deprivation, 270
Societal Impact of Pain (SIP), 312
SOEP (Subjective, Objective, Evaluation, Plan) methodology, 222–224
Soft tissue phenomena, 69–74
  connective tissue manipulation, 73
  connective tissue restrictions, 72
    active MTrPs, 72
    definition, 72
    neurotrophic reflexes, 72
    peripheral nerve inflammation, 72–73
    viscerosomatic reflex, 72
  future of, 74
  myofascial trigger points, 69–70
    dry needling, 71
    injections, 71
    interpreting response to, 71
    manual therapy, 70
  physical therapy treatment for APP, 73–74
  practical implications, 73–74
Somatic efferents, 299
Somatic pain, 298–299
Somatisation, 238
  and functional gastro-intestinal disorders, 204
Specialised Pain Services, 287–288
Spinifex Pharmaceuticals, 263
Spousal responses, categories of, 90–91
Steroids
  for generalized unprovoked vulvodynia, 194
  for provoked vestibulodynia, 194
Stretches, for chronic abdominal pelvic pain, 232–233
Subarachnoid haemorrhage (SAH), 129
Subcutaneous panniculosis. *See* Connective tissue restriction
Surface EMG, 83
SUSTAINED neurons, 39, 40

T

Tampa Scale of Kinesiophobia, 64, 65
Tanezumab, 260–261
Terminology, development of, 16–17
Testosterone, 51–52
Tetracyclines, for prostate pain syndrome, 153
TGF-beta, 171
Topical lidocaine, 127
Transforming growth factors (TGFs), 170
Treatment emergent adverse events (TEAEs), 261
Trichomoniasis, 188*f*
Tricyclic antidepressants (TCA), 258
  for endometriosis associated pain, 176
  for neuropathic pain, 148
Trigger points, 77, 298
  myofascial, 69–70, 71
Tropomyosin-related kinase A (TrkA), 258
Tumor necrosis factor (TNF), 170, 171
Tumor necrosis factor- alpha (TNF-alpha), 171

U

UPOINT classification system for pelvic pain, 253
Urethral pain disorders, 163*t*
Urethral pain syndrome, 150, 153
Urethral syndrome (US), 6
Urinary nerve growth factor (NGF), 140
Uroflowmetry, 148
Urogenital floor, 137–139, 138*f*
Urological chronic pelvic pain syndromes (UCPPS), 83, 87, 88, 95
  biopsychosocial model for, 88*f*
  characteristics of, 88
  definitions, 96
  future of, 95
Urological pelvic pain, 250–251

V

Vaginal pressure algometer, 83
Vaginismus, 100, 103, 113, 126, 130
Vascular endothelial growth factor (VEGF), 171, 174
Veterans Health Administration (VA), 289
Visceral hyperalgesia, 299
Visceral nociceptors, and endometriosis associated pain, 172

Visceral pain, 35, 247
  features of, 40–41
  models of, 42
  neuropathic pain treatments in clinical development for, 263–264
  sensitization mechanisms with, *37f*
Visceroceptive neurons, 36
  using nocigenic inhibition-related criteria, 39–40
Viscero-muscular convergence in anorectal pain, relevance of, 215–216
Viscero-muscular interactions, 303–304
Viscero-visceral hyperalgesia, 24, 300
Viscero-visceral interactions, 302–303
Voltage-gated calcium channels (VGCCs), 263
Vulval pain
  disorders, 163*t*
  pain mechanisms in, 124*f*
Vulval tissue, 83
Vulvar pain syndrome (VPS), 99, 101, 106, 185, 186*t*, 249–250
Vulvar Vestibulitis Syndrome (VVS), 62
Vulvodynia, 185, 249–250
Vulvovaginal atrophy, 187, 188*f*, 189*f*
Vulvovaginal pain, 100
Vulvo-vaginal pain disorders, 163*t*

W

White (axonal) matter, 249
Women
  chronic pelvic pain in, 112
    aetiology of, 159–164
  pelvic organ, quantification of, 269
  with recurrent urinary colics, 303–304
  sexual dysfunction related to CPP in, 99–103
    etiology, 101–103
    prevalence, 101
    terminology and assessment, 99–101
World Health Organisation (WHO)
  World Mental Health Survey, 3

X

XEN402, 262

Y

Yeast Infection, and vulvovaginitis, 187, 188*f*

Z

Z160, 263
Zalicus Pharmaceuticals, 263
Zymosan, acute inflammation produced by, 41*f*, 44*f*